T0264038

Update in Endocrinology

Editors

ELIZABETH H. HOLT
SILVIO E. INZUCCHI

MEDICAL CLINICS OF NORTH AMERICA

www.medical.theclinics.com

Consulting Editor
JACK ENDE

November 2021 • Volume 105 • Number 6

ELSEVIER

1600 John F. Kennedy Boulevard • Suite 1800 • Philadelphia, Pennsylvania, 19103-2899

http://www.theclinics.com

MEDICAL CLINICS OF NORTH AMERICA Volume 105, Number 6
November 2021 ISSN 0025-7125, ISBN-13: 978-0-323-81052-4

Editor: Katerina Heidhausen
Developmental Editor: Arlene Campos

© **2021 Elsevier Inc. All rights reserved.**

This periodical and the individual contributions contained in it are protected under copyright by Elsevier, and the following terms and conditions apply to their use:

Photocopying
Single photocopies of single articles may be made for personal use as allowed by national copyright laws. Permission of the Publisher and payment of a fee is required for all other photocopying, including multiple or systematic copying, copying for advertising or promotional purposes, resale, and all forms of document delivery. Special rates are available for educational institutions that wish to make photocopies for non-profit educational classroom use. For information on how to seek permission visit www.elsevier.com/permissions or call: (+44) 1865 843830 (UK)/(+1) 215 239 3804 (USA).

Derivative Works
Subscribers may reproduce tables of contents or prepare lists of articles including abstracts for internal circulation within their institutions. Permission of the Publisher is required for resale or distribution outside the institution. Permission of the Publisher is required for all other derivative works, including compilations and translations (please consult www.elsevier.com/permissions).

Electronic Storage or Usage
Permission of the Publisher is required to store or use electronically any material contained in this periodical, including any article or part of an article (please consult www.elsevier.com/permissions). Except as outlined above, no part of this publication may be reproduced, stored in a retrieval system or transmitted in any form or by any means, electronic, mechanical, photocopying, recording or otherwise, without prior written permission of the Publisher.

Notice
No responsibility is assumed by the Publisher for any injury and/or damage to persons or property as a matter of products liability, negligence or otherwise, or from any use or operation of any methods, products, instructions or ideas contained in the material herein. Because of rapid advances in the medical sciences, in particular, independent verification of diagnoses and drug dosages should be made.

Although all advertising material is expected to conform to ethical (medical) standards, inclusion in this publication does not constitute a guarantee or endorsement of the quality or value of such product or of the claims made of it by its manufacturer.

Medical Clinics of North America (ISSN 0025-7125) is published bimonthly by Elsevier Inc., 360 Park Avenue South, New York, NY 10010-1710. Months of publication are January, March, May, July, September, and November. Business and editorial offices: 1600 John F. Kennedy Boulevard, Suite 1800, Philadelphia, PA 19103-2899. Periodicals postage paid at New York, NY, and additional mailing offices. Subscription prices are USD $304.00 per year (US individuals), $910.00 per year (US institutions), $100.00 per year (US Students), $381.00 per year (Canadian individuals), $965.00 per year (Canadian institutions), $200.00 per year (foreign students), $100.00 per year for (Canadian students), $422.00 per year (foreign individuals), and $965.00 per year (foreign institutions). To receive student/resident rate, orders must be accompanied by name of affiliated institution, date of term, and the signature of program/residency coordinator on institution letterhead. Orders will be billed at individual rate until proof of status is received. Foreign air speed delivery is included in all Clinics' subscription prices. All prices are subject to change without notice. **POSTMASTER:** Send address changes to *Medical Clinics of North America*, Elsevier Health Sciences Division, Subscription Customer Service, 3251 Riverport Lane, Maryland Heights, MO 63043. **Customer Service: Telephone: 1-800-654-2452** (U.S. and Canada); **1-314-447-8871** (outside U.S. and Canada). **Fax: 314-447-8029. E-mail: journalscustomerserviceusa@ elsevier.com** (for print support); **journalsonlinesupport-usa@elsevier.com** (for online support).

Reprints. For copies of 100 or more of articles in this publication, please contact the Commercial Reprints Department, Elsevier Inc., 360 Park Avenue South, New York, NY 10010-1710. Tel.: 212-633-3874; Fax: 212-633-3820; E-mail: reprints@elsevier.com.

Medical Clinics of North America is also published in Spanish by McGraw-Hill Interamericana Editores S. A., P.O. Box 5-237, 06500 Mexico, D.F., Mexico.

Medical Clinics of North America is covered in *MEDLINE/PubMed (Index Medicus), Current Contents, ASCA, Excerpta Medica, Science Citation Index,* and *ISI/BIOMED.*

PROGRAM OBJECTIVE
The goal of the *Medical Clinics of North America* is to keep practicing physicians up to date with current clinical practice by providing timely articles reviewing the state of the art in patient care.

TARGET AUDIENCE
All practicing physicians and other healthcare professionals.

LEARNING OBJECTIVES
Upon completion of this activity, participants will be able to:
1. Review the evaluation and management of thyroid nodules, subclinical thyroid disease, and elevated parathyroid hormone levels.
2. Explain current pharmaceutical treatment and technological approaches to diabetes management.
3. Discuss the assessment, diagnosis, and management of adrenal and pituitary gland disorders.

ACCREDITATION
The Elsevier Office of Continuing Medical Education (EOCME) is accredited by the Accreditation Council for Continuing Medical Education (ACCME) to provide continuing medical education for physicians.

The EOCME designates this journal-based CME activity for a maximum of 11 *AMA PRA Category 1 Credit*(s)™. Physicians should claim only the credit commensurate with the extent of their participation in the activity.

All other healthcare professionals requesting continuing education credit for this enduring material will be issued a certificate of participation.

DISCLOSURE OF CONFLICTS OF INTEREST
The EOCME assesses conflict of interest with its instructors, faculty, planners, and other individuals who are in a position to control the content of CME activities. All relevant conflicts of interest that are identified are thoroughly vetted by EOCME for fair balance, scientific objectivity, and patient care recommendations. EOCME is committed to providing its learners with CME activities that promote improvements or quality in healthcare and not a specific proprietary business or a commercial interest.

The planning committee, staff, authors, and editors listed below have identified no financial relationships or relationships to products or devices they or their spouse/life partner have with commercial interest related to the content of this CME activity:
Layla A Abushamat, MD, MPH; Anika K. Anam, MD; Baha M. Arafah, MD, FACP; Richard J. Auchus, MD, PhD; Regina Chavous-Gibson, MSN, RN; Nadine El-Asmar, MD; Joshua M. Evron, MD; Maria Fleseriu, MD; Samuel Gnanakumar; Mona Gossmann, MD; Xin He, MD, MBA; Elizabeth H. Holt, MD, PhD; Karl Insogna, MD; Fabienne Langlois, MD; Grace S. Lee, MD; Beatrice C. Lupsa, MD; Merlin Packiam; Maria Papaleontiou, MD; Patricia R. Peter, MD; Aman Rajpal, MD; Jane EB Reusch, MD; Anu Sharma, MBBS; Corrine K. Welt, MD

The planning committee, staff, authors and editors listed below have identified financial relationships or relationships to products or devices they or their spouse/life partner have with commercial interest related to the content of this CME activity:
W. Scott Butsch, MD: Consultant/advisor: Novo Nordisk, Rhythm Pharmaceuticals

Natalie E. Cusano, MD, MS: Consultant/advisor: Shire, Radius Pharmaceuticals; Research support: Shire

Silvio E. Inzucchi, MD: Speaker: Boehringer Ingelheim, AstraZenca; Consultant/advisor: Abbott, AstraZeneca, Boehringer Ingelheim, Esperion, Merck, Novo Nordisk, Pfizer, VTV Therapeutics

Ania M. Jastreboff, MD, PhD: Consultant/advisor: Boehringer Ingelheim, Lilly, Novo Nordisk; Research support: Lilly, Novo Nordisk

UNAPPROVED/OFF-LABEL USE DISCLOSURE
The EOCME requires CME faculty to disclose to the participants;
1. When products or procedures being discussed are off-label, unlabelled, experimental, and/or investigational (not US Food and Drug Administration [FDA] approved); and
2. Any limitations on the information presented, such as data that are preliminary or that represent ongoing research, interim analyses, and/or unsupported opinions. Faculty may discuss information about pharmaceutical agents that is outside of FDA-approved labelling. This information is intended solely for CME

and is not intended to promote off-label use of these medications. If you have any questions, contact the medical affairs department of the manufacturer for the most recent prescribing information.

TO ENROLL
To enroll in the *Medical Clinics of North America* Continuing Medical Education program, call customer service at 1-800-654-2452 or sign up online at http; //www.theclinics.com/home/cme. The CME program is available to subscribers for an additional annual fee of USD 324.00.

METHOD OF PARTICIPATION
In order to claim credit, participants must complete the following;
1. Complete enrolment as indicated above.
2. Read the activity.
3. Complete the CME Test and Evaluation. Participants must achieve a score of 70% on the test. All CME Tests and Evaluations must be completed online.

CME INQUIRIES/SPECIAL NEEDS
For all CME inquiries or special needs, please contact elsevierCME@elsevier.com.

MEDICAL CLINICS OF NORTH AMERICA

FORTHCOMING ISSUES

January 2022
Substance Use Disorder
Melissa B. Weimer, *Editor*

March 2022
Update in Preventive Cardiology
Douglas S. Jacoby, *Editor*

May 2022
Disease-Based Physical Examination
Paul Aronowitz, *Editor*

RECENT ISSUES

September 2021
An Update in ENT for Internists
Erica Thaler, Jason Brant, and Karthik
Rajasekaran, *Editors*

July 2021
Dermatology
Jeffrey P. Callen, *Editor*

May 2021
Ophthalmology
Paul J. Bryar and Nicholas J. Volpe, *Editors*

SERIES OF RELATED INTEREST

Primary Care: Clinics in Office Practice
Endocrinology & Metabolism Clinics

VASCULAR PLANTS OF NORTH AMERICA

Contributors

CONSULTING EDITOR

JACK ENDE, MD, MACP
The Schaeffer Professor of Medicine, Perelman School of Medicine, University of Pennsylvania, Philadelphia, Pennsylvania, USA

EDITORS

ELIZABETH H. HOLT, MD, PhD
Professor of Medicine, Section of Endocrinology, Diabetes, and Metabolism, Yale School of Medicine, New Haven, Connecticut

SILVIO E. INZUCCHI, MD
Professor of Medicine, Section of Endocrinology, Diabetes, and Metabolism, Yale School of Medicine, New Haven, Connecticut

AUTHORS

LAYLA A. ABUSHAMAT, MD, MPH
Clinical Fellow/Instructor, Division of Endocrinology, Metabolism, and Diabetes, University of Colorado School of Medicine, Aurora, Colorado, USA

ANIKA K. ANAM, MD
Department of Internal Medicine, Section of Endocrinology, Yale Bone Center, Yale School of Medicine, New Haven, Connecticut, USA

BAHA M. ARAFAH, MD
Division of Clinical and Molecular Endocrinology, Assistant Professor of Medicine, University Hospitals Cleveland Medical Center, Case Western Reserve University, Cleveland, Ohio, USA

RICHARD J. AUCHUS, MD, PhD
The James A. Shayman and Andrea S. Kevrick Professor of Translational Medicine, Professor of Internal Medicine and Pharmacology, Division of Metabolism, Endocrinology, and Diabetes, Department of Internal Medicine, Department of Pharmacology, University of Michigan, Ann Arbor Veterans Affairs Medical Center, Ann Arbor, Michigan, USA

W. SCOTT BUTSCH, MD
Departments of Surgery, and Internal Medicine and Geriatrics, Bariatric and Metabolic Institute, Cleveland Clinic, Cleveland, Ohio, USA

NATALIE E. CUSANO, MD, MS
Associate Professor of Medicine, Donald and Barbara Zucker School of Medicine at Hofstra/Northwell, Division of Endocrinology, Department of Medicine, Lenox Hill Hospital, New York, New York, USA

NADINE EL-ASMAR, MD
Assistant Professor of Medicine, Division of Clinical and Molecular Endocrinology, University Hospitals Cleveland Medical Center, Case Western Reserve University, Cleveland, Ohio, USA

JOSH M. EVRON, MD
Assistant Professor, Division of Endocrinology and Metabolism, Department of Internal Medicine, The University of North Carolina at Chapel Hill, Chapel Hill, North Carolina, USA

MARIA FLESERIU, MD
Professor, Departments of Medicine (Division of Endocrinology, Diabetes and Clinical Nutrition) and Neurological Surgery, Pituitary Center, Oregon Health & Science University, Portland, Oregon, USA

MONA GOSSMANN, MD
Clinical Endocrinology Fellow, Department of Internal Medicine (Endocrinology and Metabolism), Yale School of Medicine, New Haven, Connecticut, USA

XIN HE, MD, MBA
Clinical Instructor, Division of Metabolism, Endocrinology, and Diabetes, Department of Internal Medicine, University of Michigan, Ann Arbor, Michigan, USA

ELIZABETH H. HOLT, MD, PhD
Associate Professor, Department of Internal Medicine, Section of Endocrinology, Diabetes and Metabolism, Yale School of Medicine, New Haven, Connecticut, USA

KARL INSOGNA, MD
Department of Internal Medicine, Section of Endocrinology, Yale Bone Center, Yale School of Medicine, New Haven, Connecticut, USA

ANIA M. JASTREBOFF, MD, PhD
Associate Professor, Department of Internal Medicine (Endocrinology and Metabolism), Associate Professor, Department of Pediatrics (Pediatric Endocrinology), Yale School of Medicine, New Haven, Connecticut, USA

FABIENNE LANGLOIS, MD
Associate Professor, Division of Endocrinology, Department of Medicine, Centre intégré universitaire de santé et de services sociaux de l'Estrie - Centre Hospitalier Universitaire de Sherbrooke, Sherbrooke, Quebec, Canada

GRACE S. LEE, MD
Assistant Professor, Section of Endocrinology, Department of Internal Medicine, Yale School of Medicine, VA Connecticut Healthcare System, West Haven, Connecticut, USA

BEATRICE C. LUPSA, MD
Assistant Professor, Section of Endocrinology, Department of Internal Medicine, Yale School of Medicine, Yale-New Haven Hospital, New Haven, Connecticut, USA

MARIA PAPALEONTIOU, MD
Assistant Professor, Division of Metabolism, Endocrinology and Diabetes, Department of Internal Medicine, University of Michigan, Ann Arbor, Michigan, USA

PATRICIA R. PETER, MD
Assistant Professor in Medicine (Endocrinology), Section of Endocrinology, Department of Internal Medicine, Yale School of Medicine, New Haven, Connecticut, USA

AMAN RAJPAL, MD
Case Western Reserve University, Assistant Professor of Medicine, Louis Stokes VA Medical Center, Cleveland, Ohio, USA

JANE E.B. REUSCH, MD
Professor of Medicine, Bioengineering and Physiology, Division of Endocrinology, Metabolism, and Diabetes, University of Colorado School of Medicine, Ludeman Family Center for Women's Health Research, Rocky Mountain Regional Veteran Affairs Medical Center, Aurora, Colorado, USA

ANU SHARMA, MD
Assistant Professor of Medicine, Division of Endocrinology, Metabolism and Diabetes, University of Utah, Salt Lake City, Utah, USA

CORRINE K. WELT, MD
Professor of Medicine, Division of Endocrinology, Metabolism and Diabetes, University of Utah, Salt Lake City, Utah, USA

Contents

Foreword: From One Benchmark to Another   xv

Jack Ende

Preface: Update in Endocrinology   xvii

Elizabeth H. Holt and Silvio E. Inzucchi

Evolving Concepts of Type 2 Diabetes Management   955

Layla A. Abushamat and Jane E.B. Reusch

> With the concept of patient-centered care in mind, this article outlines the current diabetes medications available for glucose lowering and the characteristics of each of these medications that need to be considered in shared decision-making for durable and effective therapy. Important patient characteristics such as weight, risk for hypoglycemia, cost, social determinants of health, and medical literacy need to be considered. The evidence-base informing the use of antihyperglycemic agents has changed dramatically due to 2008 FDA guidance for cardiovascular safety and cardiorenal protection with antihyperglycemic agents. New evidence supports an approach to diabetes management that addresses pre-existing cardiorenal disease.

Continuous Glucose Monitoring for the Internist   967

Grace S. Lee and Beatrice C. Lupsa

> Continuous glucose monitoring system is a convenient wearable device that provides glucose readings from the interstitial fluid every few minutes. Continuous glucose monitoring has revolutionized diabetes care. Patients with type 1 diabetes mellitus and type 2 diabetes mellitus, regardless of the type of treatment regimen, can benefit from continuous glucose monitoring. Continuous glucose monitoring systems provide patients with diabetes and their providers with an ambulatory glucose report that summarizes and also gives graphical representations of the glucose data. This wealth of information helps to better understand patients' glycemic patterns, and thereby reduces hemoglobin A_{1c} and hypoglycemia.

Treating the Chronic Disease of Obesity   983

Mona Gossmann, W. Scott Butsch, and Ania M. Jastreboff

> Obesity is a treatable chronic disease. Primary care providers play an essential role in diagnosis, treatment, and comprehensive care of patients with obesity. In recent years, treatment approaches have continued to rapidly evolved, increasing effective and safe therapies. In this review, we provide practical information on the care of patients with obesity with a focus on antiobesity pharmacotherapy within the context of currently available therapeutic modalities including intensive lifestyle interventions and bariatric surgery.

Current Evaluation of Thyroid Nodules   1017

Elizabeth H. Holt

Thyroid nodules may be discovered in a variety of settings. Familiarity with their management is important for medical specialists. Workup should start with history and physical examination, proceed to laboratory studies, and then to imaging. Nodules are selected for fine needle aspiration (FNA) biopsy based on imaging criteria. Most nodules can be accurately diagnosed on cytopathology, but some may require additional molecular testing to evaluate risk of malignancy. Patients with malignant lesions require additional investigation before referral to an experienced thyroid surgeon. Those who have benign lesions may require monitoring by periodic ultrasound to identify nodules requiring reevaluation.

Decision Making in Subclinical Thyroid Disease   1033

Josh M. Evron and Maria Papaleontiou

Subclinical thyroid disease is frequently encountered in clinic practice. Although overt thyroid dysfunction has been associated with adverse clinical outcomes, uncertainty remains about the implications of subclinical thyroid disease. Available data suggest that subclinical hypothyroidism may be associated with increased risk of cardiovascular disease and death. Despite this finding, treatment with thyroid hormone has not been consistently demonstrated to reduce cardiovascular risk. Subclinical hyperthyroidism has been associated with increased risk of atrial fibrillation and osteoporosis, but the association with cardiovascular disease and death is uncertain. The decision to treat depends on the degree of thyroid-stimulating hormone suppression and underlying comorbidities.

Approach to the Patient with an Incidental Adrenal Mass   1047

Xin He, Patricia R. Peter, and Richard J. Auchus

Adrenal masses are frequently incidentally identified from cross-sectional imaging studies, which are performed for other reasons. The intensity of the approach to the patient with such a mass is tailored to the clinical situation, ranging from a quick evaluation to a detailed work-up. In all cases, the three components of the evaluation are clinical assessment, review of the images, and biochemical testing with the goal of ruling out malignancy and identifying hormonally active lesions. This article incorporates recent information to produce a logical, systematic assessment of these patients with risk stratification and proportionate follow-up.

Primary Hyperaldosteronism: Approach to Diagnosis and Management   1065

Nadine El-Asmar, Aman Rajpal, and Baha M. Arafah

Hyperaldosteronism is a relatively more common disorder than previously recognized. Patients with hyperaldosteronism are at high risk for cardiovascular events. Patients suspected of having hyperaldosteronism should undergo initial screening and subsequent confirmatory testing to establish a biochemical diagnosis. Although adrenal computed tomography/magnetic resonance imaging scans often define a disease's subtype, adrenal vein sampling, in order to determine lateralization, may be necessary in some patients who are surgical candidates. Medical therapy using optimal doses of mineralocorticoid receptor antagonists can control symptoms and normalize plasma renin activity. The long-term outcome of patients treated with either surgical or optimal medical therapy appears similar.

What to Do with Incidentally Discovered Pituitary Abnormalities?   1081

Fabienne Langlois and Maria Fleseriu

Pituitary incidentalomas are discovered in approximately 10% to 40% of brain images. A complete patient history, physical examination, and dedicated pituitary function testing are needed, and subsequent results should lead to appropriate patient management. However, most lesions are asymptomatic pituitary adenomas or Rathke cleft cysts with a benign course. Many lesions can be clinically significant, including prolactinomas or other pituitary adenomas that warrant specific pituitary disease treatment. In other cases, mass effect causing visual compromise or refractory headache indicates a need for surgery. Here, various facets of a complex evaluation and treatment algorithm for pituitary incidentalomas are reviewed.

Practical Approach to Hyperandrogenism in Women   1099

Anu Sharma and Corrine K. Welt

The approach to hyperandrogenism in women varies depending on the woman's age and severity of symptoms. Once tumorous hyperandrogenism is excluded, the most common cause is PCOS. Hirsutism is the most common presenting symptom. The woman's concern about her symptoms plays an important role in the management of disease. Although measurement of testosterone is useful in identifying an underlying cause, care must be taken when interpreting the less accurate assays that are available commercially. Surgical resection is curative in tumorous etiologies, whereas medical management is the mainstay for non-tumorous causes.

Update on Osteoporosis Screening and Management   1117

Anika K. Anam and Karl Insogna

Osteoporosis is a metabolic bone disease characterized by low bone mass and microarchitectural deterioration of bone tissue leading to an increased risk of fragility fractures. Central dual-energy X-ray absorptiometry measurements are the gold standard for determining bone mineral density. A well-balanced diet containing adequate amounts of calcium and vitamin D, exercise, smoking cessation, and limited alcohol intake are important to maintain bone health. Pharmacologic agents should be recommended in postmenopausal women who are at high risk for fractures. Newer anabolic therapies including teriparatide, abaloparatide, and romosozumab have emerged for use in severe osteoporosis.

Evaluation and Management of Elevated Parathyroid Hormone Levels in Normocalcemic Patients   **1135**

Natalie E. Cusano

Primary hyperparathyroidism is a common endocrine disorder. It used to present as a highly symptomatic disease before the advent of the multichannel autoanalyzer, now usually presenting as mild asymptomatic hypercalcemia. A newer presentation has been increasingly identified in the past two decades, normocalcemic primary hyperparathyroidism, presenting with elevated parathyroid hormone concentrations and consistently normal serum calcium. These patients are usually symptomatic, with parathyroid hormone levels measured in the evaluation for kidney stones or osteoporosis. It is important to exclude causes of secondary hyperparathyroidism. This review will focus on the evaluation and management of elevated parathyroid hormone levels in normocalcemic patients.

Foreword

From One Benchmark to Another

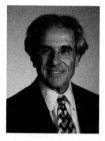

Jack Ende, MD, MACP
Consulting Editor

Ever wonder how far we have come in our understanding of our patients' clinical problems? I have. I suggest we look back to where we were when internal medicine first found its voice and was established as a discipline. I know of no better benchmark than the first textbook of internal medicine. I refer, of course, to *The Principles and Practice of Medicine* by arguably the father of internal medicine and indisputably the most prominent physician of his age, Sir William Osler. What did Osler have to say about endocrinology in his landmark, single-authored text, published in its first edition in 1892, nearly 130 years ago?

In fact, very little. Osler provided brief chapters on diabetes mellitus and diabetes insipidus, included in the section on Constitutional Diseases, and even briefer chapters on Addison disease and diseases of the thyroid, included in the section, Diseases of the Blood and Ductless Glands. Endocrinology was late in developing its identity as a field. Indeed, today's Endocrine Society was called, until 1952, the Association for the Study of Internal Secretions.

Despite the late start, the field of endocrinology certainly has caught up and come a long way. If advances in the management of type 2 diabetes mellitus is an example, the progress made in the past few years is, in fact, as far reaching as it is game changing. Similar advances have been made in our approach to diseases of the thyroid, adrenal, and pituitary glands, along with our understanding of diseases of bone-mineral metabolism—all covered in this issue. "Update in Endocrinology" provides an important, modern-day benchmark for the field. If the first edition of Osler's textbook serves as a benchmark for what endocrinology did or did not entail in the late nineteenth century, then this issue of *Medical Clinics of North America* serves as a benchmark for the knowledge base comprising the field today. Guest Editors, Silvio E. Inzucchi and Elizabeth H. Holt, have done a splendid job selecting the topics of greatest importance for practicing clinicians. Their authors have focused on what is impactful, evidence based, and new, and what practitioners need to know to diagnose and manage the

Med Clin N Am 105 (2021) xv–xvi
https://doi.org/10.1016/j.mcna.2021.09.004
0025-7125/21/© 2021 Published by Elsevier Inc.

endocrinologic problems they will encounter in their offices. It is a fine benchmark indeed.

Jack Ende, MD, MACP
The Schaeffer Professor of Medicine
Perelman School of Medicine
University of Pennsylvania
5033 West Gates Pavilion
3400 Spruce Street
Philadelphia, PA 19104, USA

E-mail address:
jack.ende@pennmedicine.upenn.edu

Preface

Update in Endocrinology

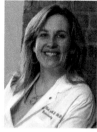 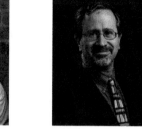

Elizabeth H. Holt, MD, PhD Silvio E. Inzucchi, MD
Editors

Essentially, every biological process in the human body is regulated, at least in part, by hormones produced by the endocrine glands. The field of endocrinology is unique among the medical subspecialties because it encompasses multiple glandular organs, each with its own function, regulation, and physiology. The signals produced by these glands include peptides, steroids, neurotransmitters, and other small molecules. The endocrine system responds to external cues, such as light-dark cycles and environmental stress, as well as internal signals ranging from nutritional cues to volume status to pregnancy. An understanding of the normal function of the key parts of the endocrine system, and the care of their associated disease states, is therefore valuable for any clinician, particularly those in primary care, where endocrine disorders first manifest. Producing a collection of updates on important parts of the endocrine system by a group of recognized authorities was our goal in editing this issue of *Medical Clinics of North America:* Update in Endocrinology.

The topics chosen for this issue were based on the major endocrine diseases facing internists in the United States today, as well as the pattern of referrals we receive in our clinical practices. Given the growing epidemic of diabetes and obesity today, we elected to devote three articles to diabetes and obesity. These address the increasingly complex world of type 2 diabetes treatment, the incorporation of continuous glucose monitoring into diabetes management, and the rapidly evolving strategies of treating the disease of obesity. Thyroid disorders are a common problem, and one that many nonspecialists find vexing. The articles on management of thyroid nodules and the evaluation of and approach to mild thyroid function abnormalities elucidate the latest research findings and management guidelines for these conditions. In today's world of readily available imaging studies, incidental lesions of the endocrine glands are common and require evaluation. Individual articles reviewing the evaluations of incidental adrenal and pituitary masses are also covered herein. Hyperaldosteronism is now recognized as the most common cause of secondary hypertension, and a

Med Clin N Am 105 (2021) xvii–xviii
https://doi.org/10.1016/j.mcna.2021.09.003
0025-7125/21/© 2021 Published by Elsevier Inc.

state-of-the-art evaluation of this condition and its pitfalls is delineated here. Hyperandrogenism in women is another frequent presentation to primary care clinicians, and a practical approach to its evaluations is included in this issue. With the aging of our population, osteoporosis is another major health concern. Its treatment options have become varied in recent years, so a review of screening and management of osteoporosis was essential and is included here. Finally, patients with elevated PTH but normal calcium concentrations are a growing portion of the referrals we see, and the article here will help clarify a confusing area of calcium metabolism.

We would like to extend our thanks to the esteemed article authors, without whose expertise and clarity this issue would not have been possible. In addition, we would like to recognize the hard work and expertise of the team at Elsevier, particularly Arlene B. Campos and Katerina Heidhausen, whose hard work made this issue possible.

Elizabeth H. Holt, MD, PhD
Section of Endocrinology, Diabetes
and Metabolism
Yale School of Medicine
PO Box 208020
New Haven, CT 06520-8020, USA

Silvio E. Inzucchi, MD
Section of Endocrinology, Diabetes
and Metabolism
Yale School of Medicine
PO Box 208020
New Haven, CT 06520-8020, USA

E-mail addresses:
elizabeth.holt@yale.edu (E.H. Holt)
silvio.inzucchi@yale.edu (S.E. Inzucchi)

Evolving Concepts of Type 2 Diabetes Management

Layla A. Abushamat, MD, MPH[a],*, Jane E.B. Reusch, MD[a,b,c]

KEYWORDS

- Type 2 diabetes • Atherosclerotic cardiovascular disease • Heart failure
- Microvascular complications • Obesity • Cost • Patient-centered care

KEY POINTS

- Patient-centered goal-directed glucose management is a successful strategy for durable glucose control that is possible but not routinely achieved in practice.
- Metformin is inexpensive and highly effective and should be used first-line in all people without contraindication or pre-existing cardiovascular or significantly progressed renal disease.
- Combination therapy of metformin with other glucose-lowering agents needs to factor in patient characteristics including cardiorenal disease, cost, comorbidities, hypoglycemia, and complexity.
- The evidence base generated in more than 190,000 patients under the auspices of the cardiovascular outcomes trials has changed the landscape of diabetes medication use.
- The best therapy for an individual with diabetes is one that can be executed by the patient in a durable fashion for sustained efficacy.

INTRODUCTION

The prevalence of type 2 diabetes (T2D) in the United States has been steadily increasing over the last two decades, reaching 34.2 million.[1] A diagnosis of diabetes mellitus (DM) is burdensome for individuals with the disease and the health care system. In 2017, DM was the seventh leading cause of death in the United States. However, the attributable risk of death in diabetes is 11.5% to 11.9%, thus making it the third leading cause of death.[2] One in four 2017 health care dollars is dedicated to diabetes with total direct and indirect cost of $327 billion.[1]

People with T2D often have multiple comorbidities that enhance the risk for diabetes-related complications, including obesity and cardiovascular disease (CVD)

[a] Division of Endocrinology, Metabolism, and Diabetes, University of Colorado School of Medicine, MS 8106, 12801 East 17th Avenue, Room 7103, Aurora, CO 80045, USA; [b] Ludeman Family Center for Women's Health Research, 12348 East Montview Boulevard, Mail Stop C-263, Aurora, CO 80045 USA; [c] Rocky Mountain Regional Veteran Affairs Medical Center, 1700 North Wheeling Street, Aurora, CO 80045, USA
* Corresponding author.
E-mail address: layla.abushamat@cuanschutz.edu

Med Clin N Am 105 (2021) 955–966
https://doi.org/10.1016/j.mcna.2021.06.003
0025-7125/21/© 2021 Elsevier Inc. All rights reserved.

risk factors such as hypertension, hyperlipidemia, and physical inactivity, thereby contributing to additional morbidity and mortality from the disease.[1] In particular, people with T2D have a 2- to 6-fold increase in morbidity and premature mortality from clinical CVD.[3,4] Excess risk for premature CVD needs to be addressed in the comprehensive management of T2D.

In the 21st century, there has been a significant advancement in glucose-lowering medications and a major increase in prospective randomized studies to direct therapeutic decision-making. In addition, in response to a 2008 Food and Drug Administration (FDA) guidance, a robust evidence base supports cardiorenal benefits of newer agents including sodium-glucose cotransporter 2 inhibitors (SGLT2i) and glucagon-like peptide-1 receptor agonists (GLP-1 RAs), allowing for a more patient-tailored approach to therapy given the breadth of options. The data from the cardiovascular outcomes trials mandate an expansion of the treatment paradigm beyond glycemic control to include primary and secondary prevention of outcomes associated with atherosclerotic CVD (ASCVD), chronic kidney disease (CKD), and heart failure (HF). At the same time, real-world data reveal that the use of these agents when indicated for secondary prevention of ASCVD was instituted in only 6.9% of patients with diabetes, indicative of poor uptake by providers and patients.[5] The reasons underlying poor uptake include both patient and provider factors and remain incompletely understood. This article will review the evolution of T2D management with the availability of new pharmacologic therapy, identify the barriers to instituting optimal therapy, and discuss how the approach to the care of T2D in the clinic is affected.

Background and History

The options for oral and injectable antihyperglycemic therapy have expanded in the 21st century. Before this time, oral diabetes medications included sulfonylureas (SUs, est. 1955), metformin (est. 1995), acarbose (est. 1995), and thiazolidinediones (TZDs, est. 1996). The first incretin-targeted therapies, GLP-1 RA (exenatide) and DPP4 inhibitors (DPP4i, sitagliptin), were introduced in 2005 and 2006, respectively. The first SGLT2i, canagliflozin, debuted in 2013.[6] Interestingly and of major concern, although these agents were FDA-approved based on A1c-lowering effect and provided new glucose-lowering options with favorable side effect profiles, studies have shown that the percentage of patients reaching glycemic control targets did not improve from 2003 through 2014. Of further concern, there was a decline in achieving individualized targets from 69.8% to 63.8% between 2007 and 2014.[7,8]

Before 2008, antihyperglycemic agents were approved solely based on short-term glycemic effect and safety data, typically tested on younger individuals with recent onset of T2D and no CVD history. Multiple CVD risk metanalyses in the mid-2000s suggested an increase in CVD complications with rosiglitazone (myocardial infarction [MI] and death).[9] A later prospective trial with rosiglitazone that focused on CV safety of the medication did not confirm these findings.[10] Regardless, these findings led to the development of CV safety guidelines by the FDA for approval of diabetes drugs in development. This guidance stipulated the necessity for cardiovascular outcome trials (CVOTs). CVOTs were required to demonstrate the new medication had an upper limit of two-sided 95% confidence interval of the estimated HR of less than 1.8 for major adverse cardiac events (MACE).[9] Diabetes medications were therefore approved based on the demonstration of efficacy (glucose-lowering) and noninferiority in CV safety when compared to placebo.

In the series of prospectively performed trials, GLP-RAs, DPP4is, and SGLT2is demonstrated noninferiority to placebo and surprisingly, GLP-1 RAs and SGLT2is have both shown evidence of CV benefit for MACE. SGLT2is have also shown evidence of slowing renal failure progression in CKD and decreasing HF hospitalization.[9] With these findings, these classes of antihyperglycemic agents were established to provide additional benefits beyond glucose-lowering, drastically changing the landscape of diabetes treatment of high-risk individuals. At the same time, barriers, such as cost to the patient and the health care delivery system, provider familiarity with new therapies, and concerns regarding side effects, have contributed to slow uptake. The slowed uptake of evidence-based interventions has parallels in the early introduction of statins and angiotensin-converting enzyme inhibitors (ACEi). Statins and ACEi now have significant impact and penetrance for use in the optimal patient.[5] The messaging around the new evidence for GLP-1 RAs and SGLT2is needs to be clearly outlined to mold practice moving forward in the management of T2D. Overall, the individual with diabetes has many characteristics informing optimal treatment for their diabetes, and this new evidence base enhances well-informed patient-centered management of T2D.

Rapidly Evolving Treatment Guidelines

The 2018 Consensus Report by the American Diabetes Association (ADA) and the European Association for the Study of Diabetes (EASD) and its 2019 update call for a focus on patient-centered care (**Fig. 1**).[11,12] This emphasis includes evaluating for patient barriers, including cost, language, preference, and cultural beliefs, while taking into account comorbidities such as ASCVD, HF, and CKD, risk of hypoglycemia, body weight, and side effects.[13] These guidelines were the first step to the fundamental reframing of T2D management, beyond a focus on glucose-lowering and toward an emphasis on additional benefits gained from medications based on patient comorbidities.

Lifestyle measures

The foundation and structure of T2D treatment is lifestyle therapy, including medical nutrition therapy (MNT) and working toward meeting physical activity guidelines. Regardless of pharmacologic therapy, lifestyle measures should be addressed at *each visit*. The focus on MNT should include choosing nutrient-rich foods that are

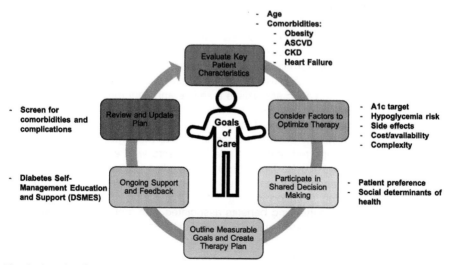

Fig. 1. A cycle of patient-centered care in type 2 diabetes.

balanced and promote glycemic control, target and maintain normal body weight (or permit weight loss), and improve overall health. There is no evidence for a single "diabetes diet" for people with T2D; therefore, the best practices are to meet an individual where they are, understand their current eating patterns, and encourage healthy eating patterns. Specifics that should be discussed include increasing nonstarchy vegetables and whole foods while decreasing added sugar and processed foods.[14] One strategy, used in the Diabetes Prevention Program, includes a food frequency questionnaire and working with the patient to identify foods that they may be willing to exclude from their diet and recommend replacements to add to their diet.[15] Most importantly, changes should be doable and acceptable to the patient. With regards to physical activity, people with T2D should work toward 150 minutes or more of moderate to vigorous intensity aerobic exercise every week with no more than 2 consecutive days without exercise, 2 to 3 sessions per week of resistance training on nonconsecutive days, and general increase in incidental physical activity coupled with decrease in sedentary time.[16] Here again it is critical to identify goals that are achievable to increase patient self-efficacy. Coaching patients through lifestyle goals is as critical as improving their medication adherence. Although barriers exist that may inhibit patients from achieving their lifestyle goals, providers should emphasize a regimen that their patients can carry out based on personal factors, including comorbidities, living situation, and cost. Research demonstrates that when the provider stresses the importance of MNT and physical activity, the likelihood of durable behavior change improves.[17]

Metformin

Metformin has consistent glycemic control efficacy, low cost, metabolic benefits, and safety profile, securing it as first-line pharmacologic therapy for people with uncomplicated T2D without established ACVD, stage 3 CKD or HF with reduced ejection fraction.[13] Metformin is an oral biguanide that is inexpensive, generally well-tolerated, and promotes improved A1c and weight loss.[13] It additionally carries the benefit of relative risk reduction for any diabetes-related outcome (including death), MI, and all-cause mortality.[18] It has also been associated with decreased incidence of dementia and decline in overall cognitive function.[19] The most common side effects of metformin therapy are gastrointestinal symptoms including bloating, diarrhea, and general discomfort. However, these side effects can be alleviated with a graduated increase in dosing over time and/or moving from an immediate release to an extended-release formulation.[20] Metformin can be associated with vitamin B12 deficiency in about 6% of people with T2D, which can be addressed with close monitoring of diet and B12 levels.[21,22] Lactic acidosis is a severe and very rare side effect that is mainly seen with medication overdose, acute renal failure (the drug is renally cleared), or in the setting of hemodynamic collapse.

Metformin was previously contraindicated in mild to moderate renal impairment. However, based on reported safety of use in patients with eGFR $\geq$ 30 mL/min/ 1.73 m^2, the FDA issued a revised label in 2016 expanding metformin's use to include those with mild and moderate impairment in kidney function, defined by glomerular filtration rate estimating equation (eGFR), rather than blood creatinine concentration.[23,24] Given the overwhelming benefits associated with metformin use and low-risk profile, it is ideal monotherapy for many patients with T2D. After initiation of metformin, additional medications should be added if the patient has established ASCVD, CKD, or HF, is at high risk for these outcomes, or has an A1c that is $\geq$1.5% above their individualized target.[13]

GLP-1 receptor agonists (GLP-1 RAs)

The indications for use of GLP-1 RAs have expanded because of their finding of prevention of ASCVD, propensity for weight loss, tolerable side effect profile, low risk of hypoglycemia, and efficacy in glucose lowering. When used as add-on therapy to metformin, GLP-1 RAs decrease A1c by 0.9% to 1.5%, making them highly efficacious. Hypoglycemia risk is low with these agents. They additionally have been shown to promote weight loss in this patient population, making them a beneficial adjunct to therapy in those with diabetes who are overweight/obese. In people with or at very high risk for ASCVD, these agents should be considered as first-line therapy. The most common side effect of GLP-1 RAs is nausea, particularly at the initiation of therapy, minimized with gradual dose increases.[25,26] Therefore, they are excellent agents for improving glycemic control with very tolerable side effects.

Multiple large randomized control trials have shown significant reductions in MACE with the use of GLP-1 RAs. Liraglutide, semaglutide, and dulaglutide are current GLP-1 RAs on the market that have exhibited cardiovascular benefit in trials and are indicated for secondary prevention of cardiac events in people with T2D and a history of ASCVD. Furthermore, the REWIND trial indicated that dulaglutide lowered CV events in those at high risk for ASCVD, suggesting it can also be used for primary prevention of ASCVD in high-risk patients with T2D.[27] Given the numerous patients with T2D at high risk for ASCVD or with a history of previous ASCVD, these agents have the potential to impact health outcomes beyond the effect of glucose lowering. In light of these cardioprotective data, most guidelines are now harmonized to state that GLP-1 RAs should be considered in people with ASCVD regardless of A1c or current metformin use.

The main drawbacks of GLP-1 RA therapy are its injectable delivery and its cost. Fear of needles, pain with injection, and inconvenience are barriers to adherence with injectables. Ease of use can be increased through the use of one of the once-weekly GLP-1 RAs (semaglutide, dulaglutide, exenatide XR) instead of daily or twice daily (liraglutide, exenatide, respectively). In addition, an oral formulation of semaglutide has been approved that has shown high efficacy for weight loss and A1c lowering and has a similar safety and tolerability profile as liraglutide.[28] In the CVOT, oral semaglutide did not meet statistical significance for superiority to placebo for the primary MACE endpoint (HR = 0.79 [0.52–1.11]).[29] This class of agents is still on patent, thus currently quite expensive both for third party payers and the patient. As such, high cost is an important barrier with a median monthly average wholesale price of ~$900 to $1100 for the 3 GLP-1 RAs with associated CV benefit.[13] This high cost makes it unattainable for many globally who would benefit from this class of medications.[11] Affordability of optimal patient-centered care is a crucial issue facing the health care system. As noted earlier, the current cost constraints may diminish with time as occurred with statins. As providers, we should advocate for access to life-saving therapeutics.

SGLT2 inhibitors (SGLT2i)

SGLT2i are effective therapy for many with T2D because of high efficacy and tolerable side effect profile with minimal hypoglycemia and weight loss. SGLT2i also offer additional benefits in reducing DM-associated adverse outcomes with regards to ASCVD, CKD progression, and HF hospitalization. They provide an average reduction in A1c of 0.5% to 0.9% when added to metformin with a low risk of hypoglycemia and promotion of weight loss.[26] Notable side effects include genitourinary infections, volume depletion, hypotension, and potential for euglycemic diabetic ketoacidosis (DKA), although this last side effect is rare in T2D, more commonly encountered in insulin-requiring T2D in the setting of significant decreases or omission of insulin dosing or during off-label use in type 1 diabetes (which is not recommended). The risk for DKA can be mitigated by optimal hydration, holding the medication during acute illness, holding the medication 3 days before elective surgery or fasting, and, in people on insulin, not holding insulin. As is common with newer patent agents, the major drawback to this therapy is currently cost. Although SGLT2i are generally less expensive than GLP-1 RA, their median average wholesale price ranges from ~$300 to $600, which is a limiting factor for many patients who may potentially benefit from SGLT2i initiation.[13]

SGLT2i have also demonstrated a reduction in MACE. Empagliflozin and canagliflozin have shown statistically significant CV event reduction in their CVOTs. Dapagliflozin showed a statistically significant reduction in CVD death. In addition, all SGLT2i studied have been found to reduce the risk of HF hospitalization in T2D patients with established ASCVD and at high risk for ASCVD. DECLARE-TIMI 58 showed a 27% reduction in HF hospitalizations in patients with or at risk for ASCVD who took dapagliflozin.[30] The DAPA-HF and EMPOROR-Reduced trials then showed that SGLT2i (dapagliflozin and empagliflozin, respectively) reduced the risk of HF hospitalization or CV death in patients with HF with reduced ejection fraction *with or without* T2D. Therefore, these agents have the potential to improve cardiac outcomes, regardless of glycemic control.

SGLT2i have also been shown to reduce the risk of CKD progression in established diabetic nephropathy (eGFR 30–60 mL/min/1.73 m^2 or urine albumin to creatinine ratio [UACR] $\geq$300 mg/g). A meta-analysis using the data generated from DAPA-HF and EMPEROR-Reduced trials demonstrated improved renal outcomes.[31] This led to trials evaluating SGLT2i in a population of patients with T2D and CKD. The Canagliflozin and Renal End points in Diabetes with Established Nephropathy Clinical Evaluation (CREDENCE) trial was stopped early after showing a 34% reduction in renal-specific composite of end-stage kidney disease, doubling of creatinine level, or renal death and a 32% risk reduction for ESRD development in those with UACR $\geq$ 300 mg/g Cr and mean eGFR 56 mL/min/1.73 m^2.[32] The Study to Evaluate the Effect of Dapagliflozin on Renal Outcomes and Cardiovascular Mortality in Patients with Chronic Kidney Disease (DAPA-CKD) demonstrated reduction in CV/renal death, renal disease progression, and HF hospitalization when dapagliflozin was given to people with CKD in addition to renin-angiotensin system blockade, regardless of diabetes status.[33] Based on this evidence, SGLT2i have a role in T2D similar to that of ACEi and angiotensin II receptor blockers (ARBs) in preventing worsening of renal function, particularly in those patients with significant microalbuminuria and low GFR. In light of these cardiorenal data, most guidelines are now harmonized to state that SGLT2i should be used in people with kidney disease (eGFR 30–60 mL/min/1.73 m^2) and HF with reduced ejection fraction regardless of A1c or current metformin use.

Thiazolidinediones

TZDs are a cost-effective next step in people failing to attain glycemic targets on metformin because of their low cost, low risk for hypoglycemia, and effective glucose lowering.[13] Pioglitazone is the currently available TZD in the United States. When used as add-on therapy to metformin, TZDs lower A1c by 1.0% to 1.2% with a low risk of hypoglycemia.[26] These agents are of great use in people with severe insulin resistance on high doses of insulin. Pioglitazone can be very effective at a dose of 15 mg.[34] Noteworthy side effects of TZDs include weight gain, edema, and increase in HF hospitalization rates in high-risk individuals.[13] Patients with overweight and obesity should be advised to use this agent with MNT to mitigate weight gain. In people with established HF, these agents should not be used.

Pioglitazone has been shown to have benefits in CVD and nonalcoholic fatty liver disease (NAFLD). The PROspective pioglitazone Clinical Trial In macroVascular Events (PROactive) study showed a reduction of the composite of all-cause mortality, nonfatal MI, and stroke in patients with T2D and evidence of macrovascular disease who took pioglitazone, but failed to reach to primary cardiovascular endpoint in this study.[35] In the Insulin Resistance Intervention after Stroke (IRIS) trial, people with insulin resistance (HOMA-IR score >3) who had a recent history of ischemic stroke or transient ischemic attack who took pioglitazone had reduced risk of stroke or MI compared with placebo.[36] In addition, pioglitazone has been shown to lead to a significant reduction of at least 2 points in NAFLD activity score in 2 histologic categories without worsening of fibrosis in people with nonalcoholic steatohepatitis and prediabetes or T2D.[37] These studies have shown potential additional benefit for patients with macrovascular disease and NAFLD beyond glucose lowering.

Sulfonylureas

In people with a low risk of hypoglycemia and where the cost of care presents a significant barrier, SUs are a useful tool for glucose lowering. SUs are inexpensive and efficacious but have a high risk of hypoglycemia, particularly if not taken with food or in a frail population. Glipizide and glimepiride have the least hypoglycemia and are the preferred SUs. The risk of hypoglycemia can be mitigated using these agents at lower doses and not using these agents if fasting or hospitalized. Patients should be educated on signs and symptoms of hypoglycemia and have glucose monitoring tools to test glucose if symptomatic. These agents increase insulin secretion and are associated with modest weight gain. With optimum education, including focus on lifestyle, weight gain and hypoglycemia can be minimal, and patients can reach glucose targets cost-effectively.[13] Studies with a first-generation SU performed in the 1970s suggested a possible increase in CV risk. A new trial, CAROLINA, compared glimepiride to linagliptin in a prospective CVOT. This study demonstrated that there is not an increased risk of CVD with the currently available SUs.[38]

DPP4 inhibitors

A second class of insulin secretagogues, DPP4i, augment glucose-dependent insulin secretion via prolonging circulating concentrations of endogenously secreted GLP-1. DPP4i have a low risk of hypoglycemia and are well tolerated. However, DPP4i are still on patent and thus expensive. DPP4i provide 0.5% to 0.8% A1c lowering either as monotherapy or as an add-on to metformin or SUs. These agents are weight neutral and do not cause hypoglycemia; insulin secretion is stimulated by glucose concentration.[13] The DPP4 class was noninferior to placebo in the CVOT programs (SAVOR,[39] EXAMINE,[40] TECOS,[41] CARMELINA,[42] CAROLINA[38]). An increase in HF hospitalization was reported in the saxagliptin CVOT (SAVOR-TIMI 53).[39,42] Therefore, these agents have CV safety, and their use is driven by patient characteristics, such as modest A1c lowering to achieve patient-directed goals or high risk of hypoglycemia (such as in the elderly).[13]

Insulin

Insulin is often needed for T2D control as the disease progresses; however, it is also sometimes necessary as initial therapy in T2D given that it has the greatest efficacy with regards to glucose lowering. As a provider caring for people living with T2D, it is critical to discuss insulin with people early in T2D management because it is common regardless of the good patient adherence to recommended therapy. As beta cell function declines over time in people with T2D, the need to use insulin to optimize glycemic control should be anticipated and *not considered a failure on the part of the patient*. Initiation of insulin is generally recommended when A1c $\geq$ 10%, blood glucose levels are consistently $\geq$ 300 mg/dL, or in the presence of catabolic symptoms (polyuria, polydipsia, weight loss) with hyperglycemia. Patients in these categories often do not respond to oral pharmacologic therapy. In people with severe hyperglycemia symptoms, insulin is often required to resolve their glucotoxicity. For many patients, once glycemic control improves, other antihyperglycemic agents can be added and insulin can be decreased or stopped.[13] Combination therapy with a TZD or SGLT2i can reduce the amount of insulin needed in those with poor control requiring large insulin doses.[13] Addition of GLP-1 RAs to basal insulin can lead to great improvements in glycemic control while minimizing weight gain and hypoglycemia often seen with basal-prandial insulin regimens.[43] Head-to-head comparison between prandial-basal insulin regimen compared to basal insulin plus GLP-1 demonstrate similar glucose lowering.[44,45]

Insulin initiation is often a barrier for both patients and providers because of its injectable form (fear of needles, low self-efficacy), preconceived fear that the use of insulin is associated with severe disease and complications, cost, and potential complexity of the regimen.[46] Initiation of basal insulin is a convenient starting point, but caution should be taken by providers to avoid over-reliance on basal insulin and initiate prandial insulin or other agents when appropriate.[47] Choice of basal and prandial insulin (human insulin vs analogs) should be driven by cost and lifestyle and patient engagement to maximize adherence with therapy.

DISCUSSION AND FUTURE DIRECTIONS

With the wealth of data available due to CVOTs, medications in the GLP-1 RA and SGLT2i classes can be considered dual efficacy with glucose lowering and cardiorenal benefits.

Notably, these agents have garnered FDA approval for weight loss (GLP-1 RA) and HF with reduced ejection fraction (SGLT2i) in people without diabetes. Given the CVD and renal benefits, these medications are becoming standard of care for individuals with cardiorenal comorbidities independent of glycemic control and metformin use, specifically in high-risk patients with established ASCVD (GLP-1 RAs and SGLT2is), stage 3 CKD (SGLT2is) or HF with reduced ejection fraction (SGLT2is). Given this overwhelming evidence, the 2019 European Society of Cardiology (ESC) guidelines on Diabetes, Prediabetes, and Cardiovascular Diseases recommend initiation of GLP-1 RA or SGLT2i in patients with T2D and CVD, regardless of glycemic control or metformin use.[48]

Table 1
Choice of add-on therapy based on patient factors

| Cost Concerns | A1c $\geq$ 10% | Hypoglycemia Risk | Weight Loss | Comorbidities: Regardless of A1c or Metformin Use | | |
				ASCVD	HF	CKD
SUs	Insulin	DPP4i	GLP-1 RAs	GLP-1RAs	SGLT2i	SGLT2i
TZDs	GLP-1 RAs	TZDs	SGLT2i	SGLT2i		GLP-1 RAs
		GLP-1 RAs				
		SGLT2i				

Cost remains a major factor in the management of diabetes, a disease that lasts a lifetime. The affordability of glucose-lowering medications needs to be woven into the overall management strategy for an individual. The overall cost and burden already associated with a diabetes diagnosis is beyond medication, such as visit co-pays, testing, and management of lipids, blood pressure, depression, and weight. Newer studies reveal that SGLT2i are cost-effective from the health care payer perspective in the United Kingdom, China, and United States, based on the reduction in complication costs and improvement in life expectancy, and weight loss, with the greatest benefit in high-risk groups.[49] Future steps include development of policies and removal of insurance and health system-related barriers to make these medications more accessible to most of the patients with T2D.

SUMMARY

The 21st century has brought multiple new pharmacologic options for T2D into the market. Previously, metformin and SUs were the main oral therapy options before initiation of insulin. Although metformin is still the first-line therapy for uncomplicated T2D, the addition of these new medication classes has led to a breadth of choices to achieve patient-centered goals (**Table 1**). A focus should be placed on patient barriers and circumstances to pick the best regimen for their lifestyle to enable durable glycemic control.

CLINICS CARE POINTS

- Diet and exercise is the ultimate combination therapy—the provider needs to convey this message.
- Metformin should be slowly titrated to improve tolerability.
- SUs should only be used at the lowest dose possible to minimize weight gain and the risk of hypoglycemia.
- GLP-1 RAs and SGLT1is should be used on all people with ASCVD, HF, or renal disease.

ACKNOWLEDGEMENT

LAA supported by American Diabetes Association grant #1-21-CMF-003. JEBR supported by R01-DK-124344, P30-DK-116073, UL1-TR-001082, R01-AG-066562, Department of Veterans Affairs BX002046, and CX001532, Ludeman Family Center for Women's Health Research.

DISCLOSURE

The authors have nothing to disclose.

REFERENCES

1. National diabetes Statistics Report. Atlanta, GA: Centers for Disease Control and Prevention; 2020.
2. Stokes A, Preston SH. Deaths Attributable to Diabetes in the United States: Comparison of Data Sources and Estimation Approaches. PLoS One 2017;12(1): e0170219.
3. Kannel WB, McGee DL. Diabetes and cardiovascular disease. The Framingham study. J Am Med Assoc 1979;241(19):2035–8.

4. Morrish NJ, Wang SL, Stevens LK, et al. Mortality and causes of death in the WHO Multinational Study of Vascular Disease in Diabetes. Diabetologia 2001; 44(Suppl 2):S14–21.

5. Arnold SV, de Lemos JA, Rosenson RS, et al. Use of Guideline-Recommended Risk Reduction Strategies Among Patients With Diabetes and Atherosclerotic Cardiovascular Disease. Circulation 2019;140(7):618–20.

6. White JR Jr. A Brief History of the Development of Diabetes Medications. Diabetes Spectr 2014;27(2):82–6.

7. Carls G, Huynh J, Tuttle E, et al. Achievement of Glycated Hemoglobin Goals in the US Remains Unchanged Through 2014. Diabetes Ther 2017;8(4):863–73.

8. Ali MK, Bullard KM, Saaddine JB, et al. Achievement of goals in U.S. diabetes care, 1999-2010. N Engl J Med 2013;368(17):1613–24.

9. Cefalu WT, Kaul S, Gerstein HC, et al. Cardiovascular Outcomes Trials in Type 2 Diabetes: Where Do We Go From Here? Reflections From a Diabetes Care. Expert Forum. Diabetes Care 2018;41(1):14–31.

10. Mahaffey KW, Hafley G, Dickerson S, et al. Results of a reevaluation of cardiovascular outcomes in the RECORD trial. Am Heart J 2013;166(2):240–9.e241.

11. Buse JB, Wexler DJ, Tsapas A, et al. 2019 Update to: Management of Hyperglycemia in Type 2 Diabetes, 2018. A Consensus Report by the American Diabetes Association (ADA) and the European Association for the Study of Diabetes (EASD). Diabetes Care 2020;43(2):487–93.

12. Davies MJ, D'Alessio DA, Fradkin J, et al. Management of Hyperglycemia in Type 2 Diabetes, 2018. A Consensus Report by the American Diabetes Association (ADA) and the European Association for the Study of Diabetes (EASD). Diabetes Care 2018;41(12):2669–701.

13. American Diabetes A. 9. Pharmacologic Approaches to Glycemic Treatment: Standards of Medical Care in Diabetes-2020. Diabetes Care 2020;43(Suppl 1): S98–110.

14. American Diabetes Association. 5. Facilitating Behavior Change and Well-being to Improve Health Outcomes: Standards of Medical Care in Diabetes-2020. Diabetes Care 2020;43(Suppl 1):S48–65.

15. Mayer-Davis EJ, Sparks KC, Hirst K, et al. Dietary intake in the diabetes prevention program cohort: baseline and 1-year post randomization. Ann Epidemiol 2004;14(10):763–72.

16. Colberg SR, Sigal RJ, Yardley JE, et al. Physical Activity/Exercise and Diabetes: A Position Statement of the American Diabetes Association. Diabetes Care 2016; 39(11):2065–79.

17. Powers MA, Bardsley J, Cypress M, et al. Diabetes Self-management Education and Support in Type 2 Diabetes: A Joint Position Statement of the American Diabetes Association, the American Association of Diabetes Educators, and the Academy of Nutrition and Dietetics. Clin Diabetes 2016;34(2):70–80.

18. Holman RR, Paul SK, Bethel MA, et al. 10-year follow-up of intensive glucose control in type 2 diabetes. N Engl J Med 2008;359(15):1577–89.

19. Samaras K, Makkar S, Crawford JD, et al. Metformin Use Is Associated With Slowed Cognitive Decline and Reduced Incident Dementia in Older Adults With Type 2 Diabetes: The Sydney Memory and Ageing Study. Diabetes Care 2020;43(11):2691–701.

20. Blonde L, Dailey GE, Jabbour SA, et al. Gastrointestinal tolerability of extended-release metformin tablets compared to immediate-release metformin tablets: results of a retrospective cohort study. Curr Med Res Opin 2004;20(4):565–72.

21. Aroda VR, Edelstein SL, Goldberg RB, et al. Long-term Metformin Use and Vitamin B12 Deficiency in the Diabetes Prevention Program Outcomes Study. J Clin Endocrinol Metab 2016;101(4):1754–61.
22. Reinstatler L, Qi YP, Williamson RS, et al. Association of biochemical B(1)(2) deficiency with metformin therapy and vitamin B(1)(2) supplements: the National Health and Nutrition Examination Survey, 1999-2006. Diabetes Care 2012; 35(2):327–33.
23. (FDA) USFDA. FDA Drug Safety Communication: FDA revises warnings regarding use of the diabetes medicine metformin in certain patients with reduced kidney function. 2017. Available at: https://www.fda.gov/drugs/drug-safety-and-availability/fda-drug-safety-communication-fda-revises-warnings-regarding-use-diabetes-medicine-metformin-certain. Accessed October 5, 2020.
24. Ekstrom N, Schioler L, Svensson AM, et al. Effectiveness and safety of metformin in 51 675 patients with type 2 diabetes and different levels of renal function: a cohort study from the Swedish National Diabetes Register. BMJ Open 2012;2(4).
25. Tran S, Retnakaran R, Zinman B, et al. Efficacy of glucagon-like peptide-1 receptor agonists compared to dipeptidyl peptidase-4 inhibitors for the management of type 2 diabetes: A meta-analysis of randomized clinical trials. Diabetes Obes Metab 2018;20(Suppl 1):68–76.
26. Cavaiola TS, Pettus JH. Management of type 2 diabetes: selecting amongst available pharmacological agents. In: Feingold KR, Anawalt B, Boyce A, et al, editors. Endotext. 2000. South Dartmouth (MA).
27. American Diabetes A. Cardiovascular Disease and Risk Management: Standards of Medical Care in Diabetes-2020. Diabetes Care 2020;43(Suppl 1):S111–34.
28. Pratley R, Amod A, Hoff ST, et al. Oral semaglutide versus subcutaneous liraglutide and placebo in type 2 diabetes (PIONEER 4): a randomised, double-blind, phase 3a trial. Lancet 2019;394(10192):39–50.
29. Husain M, Birkenfeld AL, Donsmark M, et al. Oral Semaglutide and Cardiovascular Outcomes in Patients with Type 2 Diabetes. N Engl J Med 2019;381(9): 841–51.
30. Wiviott SD, Raz I, Bonaca MP, et al. Dapagliflozin and Cardiovascular Outcomes in Type 2 Diabetes. N Engl J Med 2019;380(4):347–57.
31. Zannad F, Ferreira JP, Pocock SJ, et al. SGLT2 inhibitors in patients with heart failure with reduced ejection fraction: a meta-analysis of the EMPEROR-Reduced and DAPA-HF trials. Lancet 2020;396(10254):819–29.
32. Perkovic V, Jardine MJ, Neal B, et al. Canagliflozin and Renal Outcomes in Type 2 Diabetes and Nephropathy. N Engl J Med 2019;380(24):2295–306.
33. Heerspink HJL, Stefansson BV, Correa-Rotter R, et al. Dapagliflozin in Patients with Chronic Kidney Disease. N Engl J Med 2020;383(15):1436–46.
34. Miyazaki Y, Matsuda M, DeFronzo RA. Dose-response effect of pioglitazone on insulin sensitivity and insulin secretion in type 2 diabetes. Diabetes Care 2002; 25(3):517–23.
35. Dormandy JA, Charbonnel B, Eckland DJ, et al. Secondary prevention of macrovascular events in patients with type 2 diabetes in the PROactive Study (PROspective pioglitAzone Clinical Trial In macroVascular Events): a randomised controlled trial. Lancet 2005;366(9493):1279–89.
36. Kernan WN, Viscoli CM, Furie KL, et al. Pioglitazone after Ischemic Stroke or Transient Ischemic Attack. N Engl J Med 2016;374(14):1321–31.
37. Cusi K, Orsak B, Bril F, et al. Long-Term Pioglitazone Treatment for Patients With Nonalcoholic Steatohepatitis and Prediabetes or Type 2 Diabetes Mellitus: A Randomized Trial. Ann Intern Med 2016;165(5):305–15.

38. Rosenstock J, Kahn SE, Johansen OE, et al. Effect of Linagliptin vs Glimepiride on Major Adverse Cardiovascular Outcomes in Patients With Type 2 Diabetes: The CAROLINA Randomized Clinical Trial. J Am Med Assoc 2019;322(12): 1155–66.

39. Scirica BM, Bhatt DL, Braunwald E, et al. Saxagliptin and cardiovascular outcomes in patients with type 2 diabetes mellitus. N Engl J Med 2013;369(14): 1317–26.

40. Zannad F, Cannon CP, Cushman WC, et al. Heart failure and mortality outcomes in patients with type 2 diabetes taking alogliptin versus placebo in EXAMINE: a multicentre, randomised, double-blind trial. Lancet 2015;385(9982):2067–76.

41. Green JB, Bethel MA, Armstrong PW, et al. Effect of Sitagliptin on Cardiovascular Outcomes in Type 2 Diabetes. N Engl J Med 2015;373(3):232–42.

42. Rosenstock J, Perkovic V, Johansen OE, et al. Effect of Linagliptin vs Placebo on Major Cardiovascular Events in Adults With Type 2 Diabetes and High Cardiovascular and Renal Risk: The CARMELINA Randomized Clinical Trial. J Am Med Assoc 2019;321(1):69–79.

43. Maiorino MI, Chiodini P, Bellastella G, et al. Insulin and Glucagon-Like Peptide 1 Receptor Agonist Combination Therapy in Type 2 Diabetes: A Systematic Review and Meta-analysis of Randomized Controlled Trials. Diabetes Care 2017;40(4): 614–24.

44. Diamant M, Nauck MA, Shaginian R, et al. Glucagon-like peptide 1 receptor agonist or bolus insulin with optimized basal insulin in type 2 diabetes. Diabetes Care 2014;37(10):2763–73.

45. Riddle MC, Forst T, Aronson R, et al. Adding once-daily lixisenatide for type 2 diabetes inadequately controlled with newly initiated and continuously titrated basal insulin glargine: a 24-week, randomized, placebo-controlled study (GetGoal-Duo 1). Diabetes Care 2013;36(9):2497–503.

46. Sharma SK, Kant R, Kalra S, et al. Prevalence of Primary Non-adherence with Insulin and Barriers to Insulin Initiation in Patients with Type 2 Diabetes Mellitus - An Exploratory Study in a Tertiary Care Teaching Public Hospital. Eur Endocrinol 2020;16(2):143–7.

47. Cowart K. Overbasalization: Addressing Hesitancy in Treatment Intensification Beyond Basal Insulin. Clin Diabetes 2020;38(3):304–10.

48. Cosentino F, Grant PJ, Aboyans V, et al. 2019 ESC Guidelines on diabetes, prediabetes, and cardiovascular diseases developed in collaboration with the EASD. Eur Heart J 2020;41(2):255–323.

49. McEwan P, Bennett H, Khunti K, et al. Assessing the cost-effectiveness of sodium-glucose cotransporter-2 inhibitors in type 2 diabetes mellitus: A comprehensive economic evaluation using clinical trial and real-world evidence. Diabetes Obes Metab 2020;22(12):2364–74.

Continuous Glucose Monitoring for the Internist

Grace S. Lee, MD[a],*, Beatrice C. Lupsa, MD[b]

KEYWORDS

- Continuous glucose monitoring • Real-time continuous glucose monitoring
- Intermittently scanned glucose monitoring
- Continuous glucose monitoring interpretation • Self-monitoring of blood glucose
- Type 1 diabetes mellitus • Type 2 diabetes mellitus

KEY POINTS

- Continuous glucose monitoring (CGM) system is a wearable device that provides glucose readings from the interstitial fluid every few minutes, and most systems are approved to replace fingerstick glucoses for treatment decisions.
- Most CGM systems not only show glucose trends, but also have alerts and alarms to notify the patient about impending and current hypoglycemia, respectively.
- CGM data are reviewed and interpreted using the ambulatory glucose report (AGP), which provides the percentages of time in the target range, hyperglycemia, and hypoglycemia, and graphical representations of glycemic patterns.
- CGM systems can benefit patients with diabetes by improving hemoglobin A_{1c} and reducing hypoglycemia.

INTRODUCTION

Continuous glucose monitoring (CGM) system is a wearable device that provides glucose readings from the interstitial fluid every few minutes. The CGMs have revolutionized diabetes care and unlike traditional blood glucose measurement using a glucometer, which provides just a single glucose reading, these systems provide continuous, dynamic glucose information.

Currently, two different types of CGM systems are available on the market: real-time continuous glucose monitoring (rtCGM) systems and intermittently scanned continuous glucose monitoring (isCGM), also known as flash glucose monitoring systems.

[a] Section of Endocrinology, Department of Internal Medicine, Yale University School of Medicine, VA CT Healthcare System, 950 Campbell Avenue, Mc111, West Haven, CT 06516, USA;
[b] Section of Endocrinology, Department of Internal Medicine, Yale University School of Medicine, Yale-New Haven Hospital, 333 Cedar Street, FMP 107, PO Box 208020, New Haven, CT 06520, USA
* Corresponding author.
E-mail address: grace.lee@yale.edu

Med Clin N Am 105 (2021) 967–982
https://doi.org/10.1016/j.mcna.2021.06.004
0025-7125/21/Published by Elsevier Inc.

medical.theclinics.com

The rtCGM systems automatically transmit the glucose data continuously to the user's receiver or smart device and provide alerts and alarms. The isCGM system provides similar glucose data but requires the user to actively scan the sensor to show the glucose reading on the device display. The scans have to be performed at least every 8 hours to retain all of the glycemic data recorded by the system.

CGMs typically have three components:

- Sensor: Most CGMs have a glucose oxidase–based glucose sensor, which is inserted into the subcutaneous fat tissue and continuously measures glucose concentration in the interstitial fluid every few minutes. Eversense (Senseonics, Germantown, MD) sensor uses fluorescence-based technology to measure the glucose. The sensors are worn for 7 to 180 days, depending on the system. For most brands, users insert the sensor just under the skin using an automatic applicator. Eversense sensor is implanted under the skin by a medical provider.
- Transmitter: This is attached to the sensor and transfers the data to a receiver or a smart device app. The transmitters usually last for a few months. In the case of FreeStyle Libre (Abbott, Chicago, IL), there is no reusable transmitter; each transmitter is integrated with the sensor, which is discarded and replaced after 14 days of use.
- Receiver or smart device app: This displays real-time glucose level, indicates glucose trends (if glucose is trending up or down and the rate of change), allows a review of glucose history, and provides various statistical analyses. Most CGMs are compatible with smartphone apps for viewing data. Freestyle Libre and Dexcom (San Diego, CA) also offer handheld devices for people who do not use a smartphone. Some CGM devices send the glucose value to an insulin pump and some of these systems allow for real-time adjustments in the insulin delivery based on the glucose reading and predicted glucose trend.

As of this writing, four companies have personal CGM devices on the market: Abbott (FreeStyle Libre 14 day and Freestyle Libre 2, which replace the previous FreeStyle Libre CGM), Dexcom (G6; the previous models G4 and G5 were discontinued in June 2020), Medtronic (Guardian Connect using the Guardian Sensor 3, Minneapolis, MN), and Senseonics (Eversense).

Some companies provide professional CGMs, such as Freestyle Libre Pro and Dexcom G6 Pro and iPro 2. Professional CGM systems are devices provided by health care providers for patients to wear for short-term use (up to 2 weeks). Devices are worn "blinded" (no data available to the patient while wearing the device) or "unblinded." Patients are instructed to log their meals, exercise, and insulin administration. Patients return the equipment to the clinic, and data are downloaded and analyzed providing useful information about blood sugar patterns and the frequency of unrecognized hypoglycemia.

Table 1 outlines some of the key features of personal CGMs.

General Use

CGM system measures the glucose in the subcutaneous interstitial fluid. The CGM device displays a measurement result that is calculated by an algorithm based on tissue glucose and capillary blood glucose values used for calibration. The diffusion of glucose from the intravascular to the subcutaneous interstitial fluid compartment leads to a physiologic delay (around 7–8 minutes),[1] whereas the processing of the gained data results in a technological delay (around 4–6 minutes). The resulting total time delay accounts for the difference between concurrent CGM and fingerstick measurement values.[2–4]

Table 1
Key features of available personal CGM systems

	Dexcom G6	Freestyle Libre 14 d	Freestyle Libre 2	Medtronic Guardian 3	Eversense and Eversense XL
Manufacturer	Dexcom	Abbott	Abbott	Medtronic	Senseonics
CGM group	rtCGM	isCGM	isCGM	rtCGM	rtCGM
Sensor technology	Enzyme electrode	Enzyme electrode	Enzyme electrode	Enzyme electrode	Optical fluorescence
Fingerstick calibration	0 (factory calibrated)	0 (factory calibrated)	0 (factory calibrated)	2/d minimum	2/d minimum
Requires fingerstick confirmation	No	No	No	Yes	Yes
Approved for ages	2+ y	18+ y	4+ y	7+ y (with 670G pump) 14+ y with Guardian Connect	18+ y
Sensor application	Abdomen	Back of upper arm	Back of upper arm	Back of upper arm and abdomen	Upper arm (implanted)
Warm up	2 h	1 h	1 h	2 h	24 h
Wear length	10 d	14 d	14 d	7 d	90 d/180 d
Transmitter design	3-mo use transmitter separate from sensor	Fully disposable transmitter integrated with sensor patch	Fully disposable transmitter integrated with sensor patch	Rechargeable transmitter separate from sensor	Rechargeable, transmitter separate from sensor
Alarms for high and lows	Yes	No	Yes	Yes	Yes
Data Display	Receiver, Dexcom G6 app for Android, iPhone, smartwatches, Tandem t:slim X2 pump	Reader, FreeStyle LibreLink app for Android and iPhone	Reader (mobile app not yet available in United States)	630G or 670G pump, Guardian Connect app for Android and iPhone	Eversense app for Android and iPhone

(continued on next page)

Table 1
(continued)

	Dexcom G6	Freestyle Libre 14 d	Freestyle Libre 2	Medtronic Guardian 3	Eversense and Eversense XL
Software for analysis	Dexcom Clarity	FreeStyle Libre LibreView	FreeStyle Libre LibreView	Carelink	Eversense DMS
Remote monitoring	Dexcom Share	LibreLinkUp	LibreLinkUp	CareLink Connect	Eversense Now
Integration with pump	Tandem T:slim Control IQ and Basal IQ	No	No	The Guardian 3 is part of the 670G hybrid closed-loop insulin pump system	No

Continuous Glucose Monitoring Insertion

All sensors except for the Eversense sensor are inserted by the users themselves. Typical sensor application sites are upper arm and abdomen (see **Table 1**). The Eversense CGM is implanted by the medical practitioner under the skin of the upper arm. For accuracy, the sensors may only be used at the approved application sites.

Continuous Glucose Monitoring Calibration

Sensor calibration of CGM systems is necessary to convert the signal of the electric current into the corresponding glucose concentration. The calibration is performed during the manufacturing process, implemented by users themselves, or both. For factory-calibrated CGM systems, the sensitivity of the sensor is determined by a sensor code that is preprogrammed into its electronics memory. For CGMs that need calibration, the user needs to check the fingerstick using a glucometer and enter this value into the CGM device.[5] The accuracy of a CGM system depends on the accuracy of fingerstick value used and the time when the calibration is done (the accuracy is lower if the calibration is done when the blood glucose is low or when the glucose levels change rapidly).[6]

Visualization of Continuous Glucose Monitoring Data

Data from CGMs are visualized by using a receiver, or a smart device, such as a phone or watch. CGMs are reviewed by the health care provider using specific software provided by the manufacturers. Patients can share their real-time glucose readings with designated persons who are able to remotely monitor patient data from their compatible smart devices. The software and apps compatible with specific CGMs are summarized in **Table 1**.

Dexcom G6 and Medtronic Guardian 3 devices can be linked to insulin pumps, constituting the hybrid closed-loop systems.

Sensor Accuracy

The accuracy of CGM systems has significantly improved over the last two decades. The mean absolute relative difference (MARD) is often used to evaluate accuracy. MARD is calculated by averaging the absolute values of relative differences between CGM system results and corresponding comparison methods, mainly fingerstick results. An MARD of 10% or less for a CGM system is considered accurate enough for making insulin dosing decisions based on the CGM glucose reading without a confirmatory fingerstick.[7] Accuracy of early sensors of CGM systems showed an MARD of nearly 20%,[8] but this has much improved over the years and for the newer devices the MARD is generally less than 11%.[9–11] All CGM systems currently on the market, except for Medtronic Guardian 3, are approved by the Food and Drug Administration (FDA) to replace fingersticks for treatment decisions.

CGM systems are less accurate if the glucose is extremely low (<40 mg/dL) or high (>400 mg/dL). Also, CGMs are the least accurate on the first day of use. This is explained by the flow rate of glucose into the sensor that requires several hours to stabilize after insertion.[12]

Blood and interstitial fluid are closely connected, with interstitial fluid glucose lagging behind the blood glucose as glucose is transported from the blood to the cells. If glucose levels change rapidly in one compartment (eg, during exercise or postprandially), it will take some time for the change to be seen in the other compartment. Thus, during times of glucose variability, a discrepancy between the glucose measurement by CGM and fingerstick is not a measurement error.

Patients taking medications containing acetaminophen or treated with high-dose vitamin C may experience falsely elevated glucose values with some CGM devices. This is caused by the oxidation of acetaminophen by CGM electrodes and is dependent on the acetaminophen tissue levels.[13] There is also some evidence of CGM interference with lisinopril, albuterol, atenolol, and red wine.[14] In addition, the tetracycline class of medications may falsely lower the Eversense sensor glucose readings.[15]

Continuous Glucose Monitoring Features

Most CGMs have alerts, alarms, and trend arrows. The exception is the isCGM Freestyle Libre 14 day system, which does not have alerts and alarms.

Alarms and alerts are programmable features that warn the user of current or impending hypoglycemic or hyperglycemic events. This allows the user to be made aware of the rapidly changing glucose levels so that counteracting measures can be taken to prevent these events. For example, Dexcom G6 has an "Urgent Low Alarm," which notifies the user when the glucose is at or less than 55 mg/dL; an "Urgent Low Soon Alert," which notifies the user when the glucose will be at or less than 55 mg/dL within 20 minutes; and customizable alerts that notify the user if the glucose is less than or greater than the target glucose range established by the patient.

Trend arrows tell the user in what direction the glucose is going and allow patients to anticipate future glucose levels. Downward trend arrows indicate that the glucose level is decreasing, whereas upward arrows indicate that the level is rising. The user can adjust the insulin dose and food intake based on the direction of the trend arrows to prevent hypoglycemia or hyperglycemia. These trend arrows are not standardized among CGM systems made by different manufacturers and thus are not comparable because they can indicate different rates of rise or fall of glucose levels.

CLINICAL BENEFITS

Benefits of Real-Time Continuous Glucose Monitoring in Type 1 Diabetes Mellitus

There have been many clinical trials demonstrating the benefits of CGM systems in patients with type 1 diabetes mellitus (T1DM). These benefits have included an improvement in hemoglobin A_{1c} and a decrease in hypoglycemic events. We briefly review some of these salient trials.

In the 2008 Juvenile Diabetes Research Foundation trial, 322 adults and children with T1DM on either continuous subcutaneous insulin infusion (CSII) or at least three daily insulin injections were randomized to CGM or self-monitoring blood glucose (SMBG) using a glucometer. Adults who were 25 years of age or older were found to have a significant decrease in hemoglobin A_{1c} at 26 weeks (−0.53%; 95% confidence interval [CI], −0.71 to −0.35; $P<.001$).[16] In contrast, there was no significant improvement in hemoglobin A_{1c} for participants in the younger age groups.[16] The greater use of CGM in the oldest age group (6 or more days per week in most subjects 25 years old and older vs 30%–50% in the younger age groups) may help to explain why the hemoglobin A_{1c} benefit was not seen in the younger patients.[16]

In 2009, a randomized controlled trial including 129 adults and children with well-controlled T1DM on intensive insulin treatment showed that at 26 weeks, the duration of "time out of range" ($\leq$70 or >180 mg/dL) was significantly lower in the CGM group (377 vs 491 min/day; $P = .003$) than in the control group using SMBG at least four times a day.[17] The researchers also found that the median time of glucose less than or equal to 60 mg/dL was lower in the CGM group (18 min/day vs 35 min/day; $P = .05$), although the P value was borderline.[17] In these already well-controlled

T1DM subjects, a greater number of subjects in the CGM group had a hemoglobin A_{1c} improvement of greater than or equal to 0.3% (31% vs 5%; $P<.001$).[17]

CGM trials of longer duration have also been performed in patients with T1DM. In 2016, the Comparison of Different Treatment Modalities for Type 1 Diabetes, Including Sensor-Augmented Insulin Regimens (COMISAIR) study was a nonrandomized, prospective clinical trial that followed 65 subjects with T1DM over a period of 1 year.[18] Patients were analyzed in the following groups: CGM with CSII or multiple daily injections (MDI), SMBG with CSII, and SMBG with MDI. The COMISAIR collaborators found that the CGM group (with CSII or MDI) had a significant decrease in hemoglobin A_{1c} (-1.2%; $P<.0001$) when compared with baseline.[18] In addition, the study suggested that CGM can improve hemoglobin A_{1c} with either CSII or MDI because an improvement in hemoglobin A_{1c} was seen in both of these subgroups. There were also significant decreases in hemoglobin A_{1c} in the CGM group when compared with either SMBG group.[18] With regard to hypoglycemia, the CGM group had less incidence of hypoglycemia at 1 year (defined as ≤ 70 mg/dL; $8 \pm 4\%$ vs $6 \pm 3\%$; $P<.01$) when compared with baseline.[18]

The Sensing With Insulin Pump Therapy to Control Hemoglobin A1c (SWITCH) study was a randomized, controlled, crossover study in 77 adults and children that sought to determine the efficacy of adding CGM to CSII therapy in T1DM.[19] Subjects were randomized to a CGM on/off arm or a CGM off/on treatment sequence. The primary end point was difference in hemoglobin A_{1c} levels between study arms after 6 months.[19] The mean difference in hemoglobin A_{1c} was -0.43% showing benefit in the CGM on arm (8.04% vs 8.47%; 95% CI -0.32% to -0.55%; $P<.001$) and after discontinuation of CGM, the hemoglobin A_{1c} returned to baseline.[19] Another benefit was less time spent in hypoglycemia (<70 mg/dL) in the CGM on arm compared with the off arm (19 vs 31 min/day; $P = .009$).[19]

Trials have also been performed to determine the efficacy of CGM use specifically in patients with T1DM on MDI. The Multiple Daily Injections and Continuous Glucose Monitoring in Diabetes (DIaMonD) study was a randomized controlled trial designed to assess the effectiveness of CGM in adults with T1DM on MDI.[20] This study included 158 subjects who were randomized 2:1 to CGM or SMBG.[20] At 24 weeks, the CGM group showed a mean hemoglobin A_{1c} decrease that was greater than that seen in the control group (-1.0% vs -0.4%; $P<.001$).[20] The adjusted treatment-group difference in mean change in hemoglobin A_{1c} from baseline was -0.6% (95% CI, -0.8% to -0.3%; $P<.001$) and is similar to the degree of benefit seen in prior trials using CGM in T1DM patients with CSII.[16,19–21] The CGM group also had a lower median duration of hypoglycemia (defined as <70 mg/dL; 43 min/day vs 80 min/day; $P = .002$) and a greater number of minutes per day with glucose in the 70 to 180 target range (mean adjusted difference of 77 minutes; 99% CI, 6–147; $P = .005$).[20]

The GOLD trial was another study focusing on patients with suboptimally controlled T1DM on MDI; the investigators also found improvement in hemoglobin A_{1c} and less hypoglycemia.[22,23] In further analysis in the GOLD-3 study, CGM use also seemed to improve quality of life because patients reported feeling more confident doing the desired activities of their lives despite the risk of hypoglycemia.[24]

Benefits of Real-Time Continuous Glucose Monitoring in Type 2 Diabetes Mellitus

Compared with the evidence in patients with T1DM, there is less evidence about the use of CGM in patients with type 2 diabetes mellitus (T2DM). We briefly summarize the data available to support its use thus far.

Yoo and colleagues[25] conducted a randomized controlled trial in 65 subjects with poorly controlled T2DM on oral hypoglycemic agents or insulin. Subjects were randomized to CGM or SMBG (at least four times per week) for 3 months.[25] There was a greater reduction in hemoglobin A_{1c} in the CGM group (9.1 ± 1.0% to 8.0 ± 1.2%; P<.001) when compared with the control group (8.7 ± 0.7% to 8.3 ± 1.1%; P = .01).[25]

Ehrhardt and colleagues[26] conducted a prospective randomized trial in 100 subjects with T2DM whose treatment regimen did not include prandial insulin. Subjects were randomized to CGM or SMBG. At 12 weeks, the mean ± standard deviation (SD) decrease in hemoglobin A_{1c} was greater in the CGM group than in the SMBG group (−1.0 ± 1.1% vs −0.5 ± 0.8%, respectively; P = .006).[26] The subjects who used CGM for greater than or equal to 48 days had a greater hemoglobin A_{1c} decrease compared with those who used it less than 48 days (1.2 ± 1.1% vs 0.6 ± 1.1%, respectively; P = .003), which suggests that the frequency of CGM use is a significant predictor of hemoglobin A_{1c} improvement. This idea is consistent with what the Juvenile Diabetes Research Foundation noted in their 2008 study of patients with T1DM. In the Ehrhardt and colleagues[26] study, the hemoglobin A_{1c} improvement occurred without a net increase in number or dose of hypoglycemic medications.

Later, the DIaMonD Study Group conducted a randomized clinical trial in 158 adults with T2DM on MDI who were randomized to CGM or SMBG.[27] At 24 weeks, the CGM group had a greater decrease in mean hemoglobin A_{1c} with an adjusted difference in mean change of −0.3% (95% CI, −0.5% to 0.0%; P = .022).[27]

Benefits of Intermittently Scanned Continuous Glucose Monitoring in T1DM and T2DM

There are also limited data regarding the use of isCGM in patients with T1DM and T2DM. The data available thus far suggest that isCGM decreases time in hypoglycemia but has not demonstrated an improvement in hemoglobin A_{1c}.

Bolinder and colleagues[28] examined the effects of isCGM (Freestyle Libre) versus SMBG in a prospective randomized controlled trial of 241 adults with well-controlled T1DM. At 6 months, the investigators found that the isCGM group had a 38% greater decrease in time spent in hypoglycemia when compared with the SMBG group (−1.24 h/day; standard error, 0.239; P<.0001).[28] Haak and colleagues[29] reported on the effects of isCGM versus SMBG in a randomized controlled study in adults with T2DM on MDI. At 6 months, there was no effect on the primary outcome of change in hemoglobin A_{1c} between these groups.[29] They did, however, show that the frequency of hypoglycemia (<70 mg/dL) decreased by 28% (−0.16 ± 0.065; P = .0164) in the CGM group when compared with the SMBG group.[29]

Benefits of Continuous Glucose Monitoring in Pregnancy

At the time of this writing, CGM use is not FDA-approved to be used during pregnancy, although there is growing evidence for potential benefits of CGM in pregnant women with T1DM and T2DM.[30] In 2017, a randomized controlled trial by Feig and colleagues[31] looked at CGM use in women with T1DM who were pregnant or planning pregnancy and who were receiving intensive insulin therapy (MDI or CSII). The investigators randomized 325 women to CGM or SMBG and the primary outcome was change in hemoglobin A_{1c} from randomization to 34 weeks' gestation for pregnant women and to 24 weeks or conception in women planning pregnancy.[31] The CGM group spent a greater time in the target range (68% vs 61%; P = .0034) and had less hyperglycemia (27% vs 32%; P = .0279).[31] A small decrease in hemoglobin A_{1c} (mean difference, −0.19%; 95% CI, −0.34 to −0.03; P = .0207) at 34 weeks' gestation was also demonstrated.[31] There were additional benefits of decreased infants who were large for gestational age, decreased neonatal hypoglycemia, less admission to neonatal intensive care for more than 24 hours, and a 1-day shorter hospital stay seen in mothers in the CGM group during the first trimester.[31]

In 2018, in a multicenter randomized controlled trial by Voormolen and colleagues,[32] 300 pregnant women with T1DM, T2DM, or gestational diabetes mellitus were randomized to either intermittent retrospective CGM or SMBG.[32] Although no significant differences were observed in either hemoglobin A_{1c} or rates of macrosomia, CGM data were only intermittently assessed retrospectively by CGM for 5 to 7 days every 6 weeks.[32] Thus, the patients did not have continuous rtCGM throughout the entire duration of pregnancy, which may explain the lack of benefit in this study.

DOWNLOAD AND INTERPRETATION OF CONTINUOUS GLUCOSE MONITORING DATA

The ambulatory glucose profile (AGP) is the international standard report for glucose analysis and is used worldwide by medical providers and individuals with diabetes to review glucose monitoring results. Versions of the AGP report are available through the licensing partners, including CGM manufacturers.

The AGP report includes a glucose profile graph, glucose statistics, and glucose daily calendar graphs. The glucose profile graph converts all of the readings from the days the sensor was worn into a waveform over one period with a length of 24 hours. The waveform starts developing after 5 days of data collection but 14 days of data collection is considered ideal for accurate analysis of glucose patterns.[33] **Fig. 1**A shows the 14 daily glucose profiles collapsed to create a single AGP visual display. **Fig. 1**B shows the summary statistics including average glucose, glucose management indicator, SD, and time in range (TIR). TIR is the CGM metric most commonly used as a guide for diabetes management. The glucose target range for most patients is 70 to 180 mg/dL (importantly, including preprandial and postprandial readings), but there may be circumstances when the clinician or patient wants to set an alternative target. There are five categories to quantitate the time a patient is

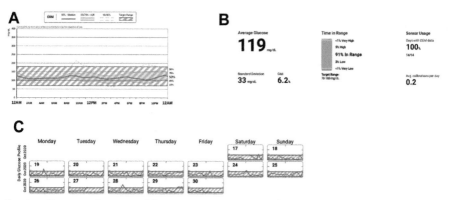

Fig. 1. AGP report (generated from Dexcom CLARITY software). (*A*) AGP. The *solid orange line* is the median or the 50th percentile line; half of all glucose values are greater than and half are less than this value. The 25th and 75th percentile curves shaded in *blue* represent the interquartile range, or 50% of all values, and are a good visual indicator of the degree of glucose variability. The *dashed outer lines* (the 10th to 90th percentile curves) indicate that 10% of glucose readings were greater than or less than these values over the 2-week period. (*B*) Glucose statistics including an overview of the percentage of time spent in specific ranges. (*C*) Daily glucose profiles. Each *box* represents a single day's glucose pattern and the target range is shown as the *shaded area*.

spending with glucose values that are greater than (high/very high), less than (low/very low), or in the target range. The primary goal is to increase the TIR while reducing the time below range. An increase in TIR of 10% (2.4 h/day) corresponds to a decrease in hemoglobin A_{1c} of approximately 0.5%.[34]

The percent coefficient of variation (%CV) and SD are measures of glucose variability. The %CV is less influenced by the mean glucose and is calculated by dividing the SD by the mean glucose and multiplying by 100. Ideally, the SD should be less than one-third of the mean glucose and %CV less than or equal to 36%.[35] The glucose management indicator indicates the average hemoglobin A_{1c} level that would be expected based on the CGM data available. The key CGM metrics are summarized in **Table 2**.

Daily glucose profiles are shown in **Fig. 1**C. Looking at individual days helps assess if high or low glucose events are clustered on certain days of the week (eg, weekends, days of increased physical activity).

By looking at the AGP, providers can determine the extent to which values are within the target range and the times of day when low or high glycemic patterns occur. **Figs. 2–5** exemplify the four glycemic patterns: daytime hyperglycemia, nighttime hyperglycemia, daytime hypoglycemia, and nighttime hypoglycemia. The overall management goal is to make the curve as narrow and flat as possible within the designated target range.

Some tips for effective review of the AGP report by the medical provider include the following:

1. Assess if there is enough data for review, including the percentage of time the patient is using the sensor.

Table 2
Key CGM metrics (glucose statistics and targets)

CGM Metrics	Comments
Dates and number of days in report	Recommended 14-d wear
Percent of time CGM is active	Represents hours the CGM collected data, divided by number of hours in report Recommended at least 70% of data from 14 d
Glucose ranges and targets	For most patients target is 70–180 mg/dL
Average glucose (mean)	Represents all glucose values added together, divided by number of readings
Glucose management indicator	Calculated from average glucose; estimates the A_{1c}
Glycemic variability (SD or %CV)	Indicates how wide the glucose excursions are Ideally the %CV should be ≤36%
Time in range	Shown in % of device readings and in h/min of a 24-h day
Time in range	Ideally, all/most glucose values are in target range
Time below range	Low glucose 54–69 mg/dL, very low glucose <54 mg/dL Goal is to have few very low or low values
Time above range	High glucose 181–250 mg/dL, very high glucose >250 mg/dL Goal is to have few very high or high values

Adapted from: http://www.agpreport.org/agp/agpreports

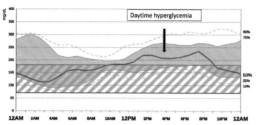

Fig. 2. Daytime hyperglycemia (generated from Dexcom CLARITY software).

2. Review the statistics: average glucose, TIR, percent low and high glucose readings, SD or %CV.
3. Look for patterns of low glucose readings (once low blood sugars events are identified, review the daily graphs to double check patterns of low glucose and see if they are clustered on certain days).
4. Look for patterns of high glucose readings (review the daily graphs to see if the hyperglycemic events are clustered on certain days or are caused by missed insulin doses).
5. Review the area shaded in blue (between the 25th and 75th percentile curves). The wider the area, the higher the glucose variability.
6. Compare current AGP and CGM metrics with those from last visit.
7. Make recommendations regarding changes in diabetes regimen: always treat hypoglycemia first, then address hyperglycemia.
8. Print a copy of the AGP for the patient and save the AGP in the patient's health record.

DISCUSSION

CGM systems offer patients with diabetes mellitus a convenient method of monitoring their glucose that can also help to improve glycemic control. The data that CGM provides are useful to patients and their providers, including primary care providers and specialists.

There is evidence to support the use of CGM systems in patients with T1DM and T2DM, regardless of the type of treatment regimen. CGM should be considered for patients on MDI, on insulin pumps, and for patients with recurrent hypoglycemia. In addition, improved accuracy of the newer CGM systems has permitted the development of a hybrid closed-loop pump system. This system uses a computer algorithm to adjust insulin delivery from an insulin pump in real time based on the CGM reading and the

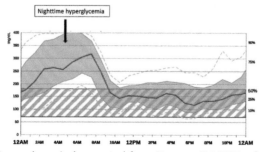

Fig. 3. Nighttime hyperglycemia (generated from Dexcom CLARITY software).

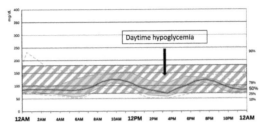

Fig. 4. Daytime hypoglycemia (generated from Dexcom CLARITY software).

predicted glucose trend. Another possible patient group that may benefit from CGM use is patients with steroid-induced hyperglycemia. One may also consider the short-term use of CGM in patients with adrenal insufficiency to detect unrecognized hypoglycemia, which could help to optimize glucocorticoid replacement therapy.[36] The use of CGM in pregnancy is also supported by some data but as of this writing, it is not FDA-approved for use in pregnancy.

After identifying an appropriate patient candidate for CGM, education and training regarding the CGM device insertion, receiver, and associated software can be provided by one's clinic staff or from a company representative manufacturing the chosen product. If the patient has any technical difficulties, the patient should contact the provider's office or company representative and use SMBG until the issue has been resolved.

When starting to use CGM with a patient, a collaborative approach is important for setting goals for glycemic control. Recommendations from the International Consensus on Time in Range emphasize that these goals should be individualized to meet the needs of each patient with diabetes.[34] Factors to consider include the patient's age, comorbidities, and risk for severe hypoglycemia.[34] The target range for most patients with T1DM and T2DM is 70 to 180 mg/dL, with a typical goal of greater than 70% of readings in that range.[34] High-risk patients include those with cognitive deficits, renal disease, osteoporosis, fracture, cardiovascular disease, and/or high fall risk.[34] For example, for patients with advanced age and cardiovascular disease, a conservative approach is recommended. This would mean having a primary goal of reducing hypoglycemia (time below range) and accepting higher glucoses. That being said, the time spent in the "very high" glucose range should be limited.[34] A more conservative approach may also be taken with patients with hypoglycemia unawareness.

Although hemoglobin A_{1c} remains the cornerstone of evaluating glycemic status, it does not provide information about glucose variability or the incidence and severity of hypoglycemia. CGM does provide this information and may thus be used in conjunction with hemoglobin A_{1c}. The additional data provided by CGM are reviewed using the

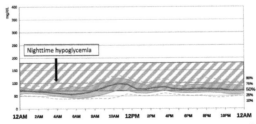

Fig. 5. Nighttime hypoglycemia (generated from Dexcom CLARITY software).

AGP report and help patients and providers better understand where glycemic control has been suboptimal. Review of this information can reveal patterns of hyperglycemia or hypoglycemia and by using this information, patient and provider can make therapeutic changes to help improve hemoglobin A_{1c} and reduce time spent in hypoglycemia. This can translate into improved patient confidence in managing hypoglycemia and thereby improve quality of life.

Although there are many benefits of CGM systems and these have technically improved over time, there are some limitations. Although the alerts and alarms are useful, false alarms for hypoglycemia can also occur from physical compression of tissue around the sensor.[37] Too many alarms can lead to "alarm fatigue" and lead a patient to silence or ignore them. Also, the patient may not be able to hear the alarms if the smart device is on "do not disturb/sleep" mode. Other inconveniences to the user include the need for a skin puncture each time the glucose sensor is inserted or a procedure to insert the implantable sensor. Also, it is burdensome to have to wear a device at all times. Technical issues may occur, such as transmission issues or sensor malfunction. For some patients, the sensor may fall off because of sweating. Adverse reactions that may occur are insertion site reactions or skin rashes because of the adhesive used to keep the sensor in place. Cost is also an issue because these CGM systems are expensive.[38]

In conclusion, the technology of CGM systems has been beneficial to patients with diabetes and evidence supports its use in patients with T1DM and T2DM. In clinical trials and in clinical practice, CGM has been effective at improving glucose control, reducing hypoglycemia, and improving quality of life. CGM may be used not only by specialists but also by primary care providers to help manage patients with poorly controlled diabetes or recurrent hypoglycemia.

SUMMARY

CGM system is a convenient wearable device that provides glucose readings from the interstitial fluid every few minutes. Patients with T1DM and T2DM, regardless of the type of treatment regimen, can benefit from CGM. CGM systems provide patients with diabetes and their providers with an ambulatory glucose report that summarizes and also gives graphical representations of the glucose data. This wealth of information helps to better understand patients' glycemic patterns, and thereby reduce hemoglobin A_{1c} and hypoglycemia.

CLINICAL CARE POINTS

- CGM systems provide glucose monitoring every few minutes and most CGM systems are approved to replace fingerstick glucoses for treatment decisions.

- CGM systems are less accurate if the glucose is extremely low (<40 mg/dL) or high (>400 mg/dL) and thus at these extremes, a fingerstick glucose should be performed.

- Providers can access and interpret the CGM data using the AGP report, which provides the percentages of time in the target range and the times of day when hyperglycemia or hypoglycemia occur. Looking for patterns of hypoglycemia and hyperglycemia can provide insight and help in adjusting the treatment regimen. Always treat hypoglycemia first, then address hyperglycemia.

- CGM systems can improve hemoglobin A_{1c} and hypoglycemia in patients with well-controlled and poorly controlled T1DM. CGM systems can improve hemoglobin A_{1c} in patients with T2DM.

DISCLOSURE

The authors have nothing to disclose.

G.S. Lee and B.C. Lupsa do not have any commercial or financial conflicts of interest.

REFERENCES

1. Basu A, Dube S, Veettil S, et al. Time lag of glucose from intravascular to interstitial compartment in type 1 diabetes. J Diabetes Sci Technol 2015;9(1):63–8.
2. Bailey TS, Chang A, Christiansen M. Clinical accuracy of a continuous glucose monitoring system with an advanced algorithm. J Diabetes Sci Technol 2015; 9(2):209–14.
3. Bailey T, Bode BW, Christiansen MP, et al. The performance and usability of a factory-calibrated flash glucose monitoring system. Diabetes Technol Ther 2015;17(11):787–94.
4. Schmelzeisen-Redeker G, Schoemaker M, Kirchsteiger H, et al. Time delay of CGM sensors: relevance, causes, and countermeasures. J Diabetes Sci Technol 2015;9(5):1006–15.
5. Wadwa R, Laffel L, Shah V, et al. Accuracy of a factory-calibrated, real-time continuous glucose monitoring system during 10 days of use in youth and adults with diabetes. Diabetes Technol Ther 2018;20(6):395–402.
6. Kamath A, Mahalingam A, Brauker J. Analysis of time lags and other sources of error of the DexCom SEVEN continuous glucose monitor. Diabetes Technol Ther 2009;11(11):689–95.
7. Kovatchev BP, Patek SD, Ortiz EA, et al. Assessing sensor accuracy for non-adjunct use of continuous glucose monitoring. Diabetes Technol Ther 2015; 17(3):177–86.
8. Gross TM, Bode BW, Einhorn D, et al. Performance evaluation of the MiniMed continuous glucose monitoring system during patient home use. Diabetes Technol Ther 2000;2(1):49–56.
9. Freckmann G, Link M, Kamecke U, et al. Performance and usability of three systems for continuous glucose monitoring in direct comparison. J Diabetes Sci Technol 2019;13(5):890–8.
10. Welsh JB, Gao P, Derdzinski M, et al. Accuracy, utilization, and effectiveness comparisons of different continuous glucose monitoring systems. Diabetes Technol Ther 2019;21(3):128–32.
11. Christiansen MP, Klaff LJ, Brazg R, et al. A prospective multicenter evaluation of the accuracy of a novel implanted continuous glucose sensor: PRECISE II. Diabetes Technol Ther 2018;20(3):197–206.
12. Castle JR, Ward WK. Amperometric glucose sensors: sources of error and potential benefit of redundancy. J Diabetes Sci Technol 2010;4(1):221–5.
13. Maahs DM, DeSalvo D, Pyle L, et al. Effect of acetaminophen on CGM glucose in an outpatient setting. Diabetes Care 2015;38(10):e158–9.
14. Basu A, Slama MQ, Nicholson WT, et al. Continuous glucose monitor interference with commonly prescribed medications: a pilot study. J Diabetes Sci Technol 2017;11(5):936–41.
15. Available at: https://www.eversensediabetes.com/. Accessed September 1, 2020.
16. Juvenile Diabetes Research Foundation Continuous Glucose Monitoring Study G, Tamborlane WV, Beck RW, et al. Continuous glucose monitoring and intensive treatment of type 1 diabetes. N Engl J Med 2008;359(14):1464–76.

17. Beck RW, Hirsch IB, Laffel L, et al. The effect of continuous glucose monitoring in well-controlled type 1 diabetes. Diabetes Care 2009;32(8):1378–83.

18. Soupal J, Petruzelkova L, Flekac M, et al. Comparison of different treatment modalities for type 1 diabetes, including sensor-augmented insulin regimens, in 52 weeks of follow-up: a COMISAIR study. Diabetes Technol Ther 2016;18(9): 532–8.

19. Battelino T, Conget I, Olsen B, et al. The use and efficacy of continuous glucose monitoring in type 1 diabetes treated with insulin pump therapy: a randomised controlled trial. Diabetologia 2012;55(12):3155–62.

20. Beck RW, Riddlesworth T, Ruedy K, et al. Effect of continuous glucose monitoring on glycemic control in adults with type 1 diabetes using insulin injections: the DIAMOND randomized clinical trial. JAMA 2017;317(4):371–8.

21. Bergenstal RM, Tamborlane WV, Ahmann A, et al. Effectiveness of sensor-augmented insulin-pump therapy in type 1 diabetes. N Engl J Med 2010; 363(4):311–20.

22. Lind M, Polonsky W, Hirsch IB, et al. Continuous glucose monitoring vs conventional therapy for glycemic control in adults with type 1 diabetes treated with multiple daily insulin injections: the GOLD randomized clinical trial. JAMA 2017; 317(4):379–87.

23. Seyed Ahmadi S, Westman K, Pivodic A, et al. The association between HbA(1c) and time in hypoglycemia during CGM and self-monitoring of blood glucose in people with type 1 diabetes and multiple daily insulin injections: a randomized clinical trial (GOLD-4). Diabetes Care 2020;43(9):2017–24.

24. Olafsdottir AF, Polonsky W, Bolinder J, et al. A randomized clinical trial of the effect of continuous glucose monitoring on nocturnal hypoglycemia, daytime hypoglycemia, glycemic variability, and hypoglycemia confidence in persons with type 1 diabetes treated with multiple daily insulin injections (GOLD-3). Diabetes Technol Ther 2018;20(4):274–84.

25. Yoo HJ, An HG, Park SY, et al. Use of a real time continuous glucose monitoring system as a motivational device for poorly controlled type 2 diabetes. Diabetes Res Clin Pract 2008;82(1):73–9.

26. Ehrhardt NM, Chellappa M, Walker MS, et al. The effect of real-time continuous glucose monitoring on glycemic control in patients with type 2 diabetes mellitus. J Diabetes Sci Technol 2011;5(3):668–75.

27. Beck RW, Riddlesworth TD, Ruedy K, et al. Continuous glucose monitoring versus usual care in patients with type 2 diabetes receiving multiple daily insulin injections: a randomized trial. Ann Intern Med 2017;167(6):365–74.

28. Bolinder J, Antuna R, Geelhoed-Duijvestijn P, et al. Novel glucose-sensing technology and hypoglycaemia in type 1 diabetes: a multicentre, non-masked, randomised controlled trial. Lancet 2016;388(10057):2254–63.

29. Haak T, Hanaire H, Ajjan R, et al. Flash glucose-sensing technology as a replacement for blood glucose monitoring for the management of insulin-treated type 2 diabetes: a multicenter, open-label randomized controlled trial. Diabetes Ther 2017;8(1):55–73.

30. Yu Q, Aris IM, Tan KH, et al. Application and utility of continuous glucose monitoring in pregnancy: a systematic review. Front Endocrinol (Lausanne) 2019; 10:697.

31. Feig DS, Donovan LE, Corcoy R, et al. Continuous glucose monitoring in pregnant women with type 1 diabetes (CONCEPTT): a multicentre international randomised controlled trial. Lancet 2017;390(10110):2347–59.

32. Voormolen DN, DeVries JH, Sanson RME, et al. Continuous glucose monitoring during diabetic pregnancy (GlucoMOMS): a multicentre randomized controlled trial. Diabetes Obes Metab 2018;20(8):1894–902.

33. Mazze RS, Strock E, Wesley D, et al. Characterizing glucose exposure for individuals with normal glucose tolerance using continuous glucose monitoring and ambulatory glucose profile analysis. Diabetes Technol Ther 2008;10(3):149–59.

34. Battelino T, Danne T, Bergenstal RM, et al. Clinical targets for continuous glucose monitoring data interpretation: recommendations from the international consensus on time in range. Diabetes Care 2019;42(8):1593–603.

35. Monnier L, Colette C, Wojtusciszyn A, et al. Toward defining the threshold between low and high glucose variability in diabetes. Diabetes Care 2017;40(7): 832–8.

36. Watanabe T, Ozawa A, Ishii S, et al. Usage of continuous glucose monitoring (CGM) for detecting an unrecognized hypoglycemia and management of glucocorticoid replacement therapy in adult patients with central hypoadrenalism. Endocr J 2018;65(5):547–56.

37. Rodbard D. Continuous glucose monitoring: a review of successes, challenges, and opportunities. Diabetes Technol Ther 2016;18(Suppl 2):S3–13.

38. Petrie JR, Peters AL, Bergenstal RM, et al. Improving the clinical value and utility of CGM systems: issues and recommendations: a joint statement of the European Association for the Study of Diabetes and the American Diabetes Association Diabetes Technology Working Group. Diabetologia 2017;60(12):2319–28.

Treating the Chronic Disease of Obesity

Mona Gossmann, MD[a], W. Scott Butsch, MD[b,c], Ania M. Jastreboff, MD, PhD[a,d],*

KEYWORDS

- Obesity • Anti-obesity medications • Obesity pharmacotherapy • Obesity treatment
- Weight management • Weight loss • Bariatric surgery

KEY POINTS

- Obesity is a treatable chronic disease, necessitating life-long care.
- Owing to the heterogeneity and complexity of obesity, an individualized approach is needed to match each patient with therapeutic modalities.
- Effective, safe, evidence-based treatments for obesity include intensive lifestyle interventions, antiobesity medications, and bariatric surgery.
- Consider obesity-related comorbidities in the assessment and treatment of patients.
- A comprehensive and compassionate approach is paramount in caring for patients with obesity.

THE MAGNITUDE OF OBESITY

The following statement speaks for itself: 1 in 2 Americans is projected to have obesity by 2030.[1] Globally 650 million adults have obesity (defined as a body mass index [BMI] ≥ 30 kg/m^2).[2] The obesity epidemic has increased rates of weight-related diseases, including type 2 diabetes (T2DM), cardiovascular (CV) disease, and certain types of cancer.[3] Currently, in the midst of the SARS-CoV-2 pandemic, obesity has emerged as a significant contributor to a more severe course of COVID-19,[4–9] underscoring the underlying biology of obesity[10] and the broad impact it has on health.[11]

[a] Department of Internal Medicine (Endocrinology & Metabolism), Yale University School of Medicine, New Haven, CT, USA; [b] Department of Surgery, Bariatric and Metabolic Institute, Cleveland Clinic, Cleveland, OH, USA; [c] Department of Internal Medicine and Geriatrics, Bariatric and Metabolic Institute, Cleveland Clinic, Cleveland, OH, USA; [d] Department of Pediatrics (Pediatric Endocrinology), Yale University School of Medicine, New Haven, CT, USA
* Corresponding author. Section of Endocrinology, Yale University School of Medicine, 2 Church Street South, Suite 201, New Haven, CT 06519.
E-mail address: ania.jastreboff@yale.edu

Med Clin N Am 105 (2021) 983–1016
https://doi.org/10.1016/j.mcna.2021.06.005
0025-7125/21/© 2021 Elsevier Inc. All rights reserved.

THE IMPORTANCE OF TREATING OBESITY AS A DISEASE

In the past, obesity was not accepted or understood as a disease. Patients were blamed, as if having obesity was a personal choice. Treatment focused largely on diet, exercise, and lifestyle. We now understand that perturbations in complex neurobiological mechanisms, precipitated by an obesogenic environment,[12] underlie the metabolic disease of obesity.[13] We increasingly recognize that to improve patient health outcomes, obesity must be approached and treated as a chronic disease[11,14] with therapies targeted to its pathophysiology.[10]

With a mirror to other chronic diseases, we will frame our discussion around several key concepts. First, obesity is heterogeneous; thus, significant individual variability is observed in response to interventions. Second, the underlying pathophysiology of obesity is complex often requiring combination therapeutic interventions. Third, obesity is a chronic condition and requires life-long treatment. Finally, it is critical to approach patients with obesity with compassion and reassurance with the understanding that their disease is not a lifestyle choice. We treat our patients with obesity with safe and effective therapies as we do patients with any other chronic disease.

IDENTIFYING BARRIERS TO TREATING OBESITY

Fortunately, effective treatments for obesity are available but, unfortunately, are significantly underutilized.[15] It is estimated that 46% of Americans meet treatment criteria for Federal Drug Administration (FDA)-approved obesity pharmacotherapy by having a BMI of ≥ 30 kg/m^2 or ≥ 27 kg/m^2 with a weight-related disease such as T2DM. Yet, only about 2% receive appropriate treatment with antiobesity medications.[15] The numbers are even lower for bariatric surgery, where an estimated less than 1% of eligible patients are treated.[16,17] Identifying barriers which contribute to undertreatment can help identify solutions to these challenges and hurdles.

The Awareness, Care, and Treatment in Obesity maNagement (ACTION) study[16] was conducted nationwide to investigate barriers to obesity care from the perspective of health care providers (HCPs) and patients. A key finding was that although most HCPs perceived obesity to be a disease, it was not treated as such. Providers reported that one of the most significant barriers to addressing obesity was lack of time during clinic visits.[16] Additionally, most patients believed it was their personal responsibility to lose weight and so they did not seek help from their HCPs.[16]

The perception that obesity is not a disease, coupled together with the misconception that treatment options are limited, ineffective, or unsafe, certainly pose significant barriers. There is a paucity of obesity education in medical schools[18] and residency training programs.[19] As such, the inadvertent lack of knowledge among providers about clinical practice guidelines (CPGs) for obesity treatment[20,21] perpetuate these misconceptions, creating an environment where effective strategies are not initiated because they are unknown.[12] Additionally, there exists the fear of causing harm given the history of antiobesity medications, such as fenfluramine (cardiac valvulopathy, 1997),[22] rimonabant (depression and suicidal ideation, 2007),[22] sibutramine (increased risk for CV events, 2010),[22] and, most recently, lorcaserin (potential increased risk for cancer, 2020), which have been taken off the market because of safety concerns.[23] Shame, bias, and stigma coupled with inadequate insurance present another significant barrier that limits access.[24] Patients with obesity receive less preventative care,[20] and overall health care delivery is not uniform.[25] Barriers to heath care access, limited access to healthy food, and reduced opportunities to be physically active are especially magnified among racial and ethnic minority communities, who already suffer higher rates of obesity,[26] which in turn further exacerbates health inequities.[27]

OVERVIEW OF THE CLINICAL APPROACH TO CARING FOR PATIENTS WITH OBESITY

As the frontline clinicians diagnosing, evaluating, treating, and referring patients who require more intensive obesity therapy, primary care providers have a key role in caring for patients with obesity.

Care begins with a comprehensive evaluation and development of an individualized weight-management plan. The first, and fundamental, step in this process is creating a nonjudgmental environment.[28] It is essential for providers and staff to approach patients with compassion. Using person-first language is a crucial and effective tool to avoid defining patients by their disease (eg, the "patient with obesity" rather than the "obese patient"). Pejorative terms (eg, morbid or fat) contribute to patients' shame and are highly detrimental to the patients' well-being. Additionally, even with effective treatments, such negative language undermines the effectiveness of obesity care.[24,29] A clinical environment with appropriate chairs, blood pressure cuffs, gowns, and scales (discreetly placed in private assessment areas) welcomes individuals of all sizes. Creating such a safe space is crucial for laying the foundation for a trusting relationship where engagement is an integral part of the care process.

An initial weight history includes onset and potential triggers of weight gain (eg, weight-gain promoting medications [**Table 1**], smoking cessation, pregnancy, stressors, and so forth) as well as previous attempts to lose weight. A 24-hour dietary recall helps elucidate diet composition and overall eating behaviors, while real-time food records can clarify details of food preferences, meal patterns, and timing of eating.[37,38] It is also important to screen and assess for disordered eating.[39,40] The level of physical activity and functional capacity should be assessed, as should sleep duration and patterns.[40] Screening for obstructive sleep apnea (OSA) using STOP-Bang,[41] a brief 8-item assessment tool, may help identify individuals who are at risk and need further evaluation. It is also important to assess mood conditions, life stressors, and psychosocial factors, such as limited access to healthful food or a built environment not conducive to physical activity.[12] Review of past medical history should focus on presence of, or risk for, weight-related medical conditions which add to morbidity and mortality [**Table 2**].[40] Mental health conditions, such as depression or anxiety, often co-occur with obesity[40]; thus, appropriate follow-up and care with mental health care professionals may be needed.

The initial physical examination gathers key data such as vital signs, height, weight, BMI, and waist circumference; with trends reviewed at every visit. Features such as adipose distribution (gynecoid, android, dystrophic), skin examination (acanthosis nigricans, skin tags, striae), thyroid (goiter), gastrointestinal, extremities (edema), and musculoskeletal (mobility) may point to secondary causes such as certain endocrinopathies (ie, hypothyroidism, polycystic ovarian syndrome, Cushing's disease).[40] Baseline laboratory test parameters include hemoglobin A1c (HbA1c), fasting glucose, fasting lipid panel, complete metabolic profile including liver enzymes, and Thyroid Stimulating Hormone (TSH). **Table 2** includes a list of assessments for targeted evaluation of additional weight-related diseases.

The patient-provider discussion sets weight goals and identifies potential health benefits. Notably, these goals will change over time depending on the patient's health and chosen treatment approach. Available treatment modalities are discussed within the context of set goals and available treatment approaches (ie, intensive lifestyle interventions [ILIs], meal replacement, antiobesity medications [**Table 3**], devices and endoscopic procedures for weight loss [**Table 4**], and bariatric and metabolic surgery [**Table 5**]).

Table 1
Weight-Promoting Medications and Alternatives[30-33]

Drug Class	Examples	Alternatives if Clinically Indicated
Glucocorticoids	**Prednisone, dexamethasone, hydrocortisone**	Use steroid-sparing treatments
Sulfonylureas	Glipizide, glimepiride, **glyburide**	GLP-1 receptor agonist, SGLT2 inhibitor, DPP4 inhibitor, metformin
Thiazolidinediones	Pioglitazone[a]	
Insulin		Basal insulin alone with oral or injectable diabetes medications instead of prandial insulin if not needed to maintain glycemic control
SSRIs	**Paroxetine, citalopram** Escitalopram[b], sertraline[b]	Fluoxetine
SNRIs	Duloxetine[b]	Venlafaxine, desvenlafaxine
Tricyclic antidepressants	**Amitriptyline, nortriptyline**	Imipramine SSRI/SNRI
Atypical antidepressants and mood stabilizers	**Mirtazapine** **Lithium**	Bupropion, trazodone
Antipsychotics	**Clozapine, olanzapine, quetiapine, risperidone, perphenazine**	Ziprasidone, aripiprazole, lurasidone
Anticonvulsants	Gabapentin, pregabalin, **valproic acid**, vigabatrin, **carbamazepine**	Felbamate, topiramate, zonisamide
Hormonal contraceptives	Depot medroxyprogesterone acetate[34]	Oral contraceptives, barrier methods
Beta blockers	Metoprolol, atenolol, propanolol[35]	ACE inhibitors, ARBs, calcium channel blockers If BB is required, carvedilol[36] has less associated weight gain

Bolded medications denote highest degree of weight gain.
Abbreviations: ACE, angiotensin-converting enzyme; ARB, angiotensin receptor blocker; BB, beta blocker; DPP4, dipeptidyl peptidase-4; GLP-1, glucagon-like peptide 1; SGLT2, sodium-glucose linked transporter 2; SNRI, selective norepinephrine reuptake inhibitors; SSRI, selective serotonin reuptake inhibitors.
[a] Weight distribution may be metabolically favorable.
[b] Associated with weight loss or weight neutral in acute treatment but weight gain with long term treatment.

Table 2
Assessment and screening for obesity-related conditions[39]

Obesity-Related Condition	Testing to Consider
Hypertension	• Systolic and diastolic sitting blood pressure • Screen for cardiovascular disease
Type 2 diabetes	Two abnormal test results: • Fasting plasma glucose ≥126 mg/dL (7.0 mmol/L) • HbA1c≥6.5% • 2-h plasma glucose > 200 mg/dL (11.1 mmol/L) with 75 gram glucose challenge • Diagnosis is also made if single plasma glucose≥200 mg/dL with symptoms of hyperglycemia
Prediabetes	• Fasting plasma glucose 100-125 mg/dL, or • HbA1c 5.7%-6.4%, or • 2-h plasma glucose 140-199 mg/dL with 75 gram glucose challenge
Metabolic syndrome	ATP III criteria (3 out of 5): • Waist circumference ≥40 in for men, ≥35 in for women • Blood pressure≥130/85 mm Hg • Triglycerides≥150 mg/dL • HDL-c<40 mg/dL in men or <50 mg/dL in women • Fasting glucose≥100 mg/dL
Dyslipidemia	• Lipid panel • Lipoprotein subclasses to further define risk
NAFLD	• Liver function tests • Diagnostic imaging (eg, elastography, ultrasound) • Liver biopsy as indicated
Obstructive sleep apnea (OSA)	• STOP-BANG questionnaire • Neck circumference • Polysomnography
PCOS	• Hormone level testing (androgen levels, LH, FSH, estradiol)
Male hypogonadism	• Hormone level testing (total and free testosterone, SHBG, LH, FSH, prolactin)
GERD	• Endoscopy, esophageal motility study
Vitamin D deficiency	• 25-hydroxy vitamin D level
Cancer (colon, endometrial, breast-postmenopausal, esophageal, rectal, renal, pancreatic, thyroid, gallbladder)	• Mammogram • Colonoscopy • Pap smear
Depression Anxiety Eating disorders Asthma Osteoarthritis Urinary incontinence Disability/mobility	• Review of symptom • Physical examination

Abbreviations: FSH, follicle-stimulating hormone; GERD, gastroesophageal reflux disease; HbA1c, hemoglobin A1c; HDL-c, high-density lipoprotein cholesterol; LH, luteinizing hormone; NAFLD, nonalcoholic fatty liver disease; PCOS, polycystic ovary syndrome; SHBG, sex hormone binding globulin; STOP-BANG, Snoring, Tiredness, Observed apnea, blood Pressure, BMI, Age, Neck circumference, Gender.

Table 3
FDA-approved antiobesity medications[30,39,42–44] (in alphabetical order)

Medication Mechanism of Action	Dosing	Common Side effects	Contraindications/Cautions	Monitoring/Considerations
Liraglutide 3 mg[45] GLP-1 receptor agonist avg TBWL 8.0% TBWL in excess of placebo 5.4%	Formulation: • SC injectable • Pen device with multiple doses Titrate up dose Q1-2 wk as side effects tolerated: Week 1: 0.6 mg SC QD Week 2: 1.2 mg SC QD Week 3: 1.8 mg SC QD Week 4: 2.4 mg SC QD Week 5 and on: 3.0 mg SC QD Max dose: 3.0 mg/d	• Nausea • Vomiting • Diarrhea • Constipation • Headache • Dyspepsia • Injection site reaction	• Personal or family history of medullary thyroid cancer or MEN2 • Pancreatitis • Untreated or acute gallbladder disease	Considerations: • If abdominal pain, evaluate for cholelithiasis and pancreatitis, check lipase • Insulin or antidiabetes medications (such as sulfonylureas) may require dose reduction • Discontinue DPP4 inhibitor with GLP-1 receptor agonist start • Slow up-titration of the medication to help mitigate side effects • $$$
Naltrexone/Bupropion SR[46,47] Opioid receptor antagonist (naltrexone) NE, DA reuptake inhibitor (bupropion) avg TBWL 6.4% TBWL in excess of placebo 5.2%	Formulation: • Tablet Naltrexone 8 mg/bupropion 90 mg Week 1: 1 tab QD Week 2: 1 tab BID Week 3: 2 tabs QAM & 1 tab QPM Week 4: 2 tabs BID Max dose: naltrexone 32 mg/bupropion 360 mg/d (in two divided doses)	• Nausea • Vomiting • Constipation • Diarrhea • Insomnia • Dizziness • Dry mouth • Increased HR and BP • Mood changes • Headache, worsening of migraines	• Uncontrolled HTN • Seizure disorder • Chronic opioid use • Untreated closed angle glaucoma • Bulimia nervosa • Anorexia nervosa • Uncontrolled anxiety, depression or bipolar disorder • Undergoing drug/alcohol withdrawal • MAOI use • Uncontrolled migraine disorder	Monitoring: BP, HR, LFTs (due to risk for liver injury with naltrexone) Considerations: • Watch for worsening depression, suicidal ideation • Can cause false positive urine test for amphetamine • Insulin or oral antidiabetes medications may require dose reduction • $$
Orlistat[48] Gastric and pancreatic lipase inhibitor avg TBWL 10.6 kg TBWL in excess of placebo 4.4 kg	Formulation: • OTC: 60-mg capsules • Prescription: 120-mg capsules Start 60 mg before meals up to TID Increase to 120 mg TID before meals as side effects tolerated Max dose: 360 mg/d (in three divided doses)	• Steatorrhea • Flatulence • Fecal urgency/incontinence • Cholelithiasis • Abdominal pain • Vitamin deficiency • Severe liver injury (rare)	• Malabsorptive disorders • Cholestasis • Oxalate nephrolithiasis Eating lower fat diet can help mitigate side effects	Monitoring: Vitamin D, LFTs Considerations: • Start multivitamin, to be taken at least 2 h after taking orlistat • Levothyroxine and orlistat should be taken at least 4 h apart (decreases absorption) • Decreases absorption of antiepileptics and cyclosporine • Increases absorption of warfarin • $$

Drug	Formulations/Dosing	Side Effects	Contraindications	Monitoring/Considerations
Phentermine[49] Sympathomimetic, releases NE, DA, 5-HT avg TBWL 7.4% (24 mo)	Formulations: 15-mg capsule 37.5-mg tablet 8-mg tablet Start 15 mg QAM or 18.75 mg (½ tablet of 37.5 mg) QAM If concern for side effects, can start with ¼ tab QD of 37.5-mg tablet and titrate up to ½ tablet QD Max dose: 37.5 mg/d can start with ½ tab (4 mg) or 1 tab (8 mg) BID-TID before meals Max dose: 24 mg/d	• Insomnia • Tachycardia • Increased BP • Anxiety • Restlessness • Agitation • Dry mouth • Constipation • Headache	• History of cardiovascular disease • History of stroke • Poorly controlled or labile HTN • Uncontrolled anxiety • MAOI use • Untreated closed angle glaucoma • Uncontrolled hyperthyroidism	Monitoring: BP and HR Considerations: • Watch for change in mood • Insulin/oral anti-DM medications may require reduction • FDA-approved for a few weeks of continuous use; longer term use based on local medical-legal guidance • $ Schedule IV controlled substance FDA-approved sympathomimetics less commonly used for obesity treatment include phendimetrazine and diethylpropion
Phentermine/ Topiramate ER[50] Sympathomimetic, releases NE, DA, 5-HT (phentermine) Modulates GABA release (topiramate) avg TBWL 10.9% TBWL in excess of placebo 9.3%	Formulation: Four different tablets with escalating doses of phentermine/topiramate: 3.75 mg/23 mg 7.5 mg/46 mg 11 mg/69 mg 15 mg/92 mg Start 3.75 mg/23 mg QAM, for 14 d, then increase to 7.5 mg/46 mg QAM If < 3% TBWL at 12 wk, then increase to 11 mg/69 mg QD for 14 d, then 15 mg/92 mg tab QD Max dose: 15 mg/92 mg per d	Phentermine: • as described above Topiramate: • Drowsiness • Dysgeusia • Mental fogginess • Word finding difficulty • Paresthesia • Constipation • Dry mouth • Hyperchloremic metabolic acidosis • Nephrolithiasis	Phentermine: • as described above Topiramate: • Uncontrolled depression • Untreated closed angle glaucoma • Nephrolithiasis Note: If medication is to be discontinued, it should be tapered to minimize risk for seizures	Monitoring: BP, HR, electrolytes, and creatinine Considerations: • Watch for worsening depression • Check pregnancy test before initiation and home test Qmonth • Use with alcohol or depressant drugs can worsen cognitive impairment • Risk for lactic acidosis in combination with metformin • See previous mentions for phentermine-specific considerations • $$

(continued on next page)

Table 3
(continued)

Medication Mechanism of Action	Dosing	Common Side effects	Contraindications/Cautions	Monitoring/Considerations
Semaglutide 2.4mg GLP-1 receptor agonist avg TBWL 14.9% TBWL in excess of placebo 12.5%	Formulation: SC injectable Pen-injector device with single dose Titrate up every 4 weeks as side effects tolerated: Week 1-4: 0.25mg SC QWeek Week 5-8: 0.5mg SC QWeek Week 9-12: 1.0mg SC QWeek Week 13-16: 1.7mg SC QWeek Week 17 and on: 2.4mg SC QWeek Max dose: 2.4mg/week	• Nausea • Vomiting • Diarrhea • Constipation • Headache • Dyspepsia • Injection site reaction	• Personal or family history of medullary thyroid cancer or MEN2 • Pancreatitis • Untreated or acute gallbladder disease	*Considerations:* If abdominal pain, evaluate for cholelithiasis and pancreatitis, check lipase Insulin or anti-diabetes medications (such as sulfonylureas) may require does reduction Discontinue DPP4 inhibitor with GLP-1 receptor agonist start Slow up-titrating of medication may help mitigate side effects $$$
Setmelanotide[51] Melancortin-4 receptor agonist avg TBWL 12.5%–25.6% compared to baseline	Formulation: 10 mg/1 mL vial for multiple doses Start 2 mg SC QD for 2 wk If tolerated, increase to 3 mg SC QD If 2 mg is not tolerated, decrease to 1 mg SC QD Max dose 3 mg/d	• Nausea • Diarrhea • Abdominal pain • Injection site reactions • Skin hyperpigmentation	• Spontaneous penile erection • Adverse sexual reactions in females have been reported • New or worsening depression and suicidal ideation have also been reported	Approved only for: POMC, PCSK1, LEPR deficiency (monogenic forms of obesity)

All the medications Table 3 are contraindicated in pregnancy and breastfeeding.

Cost: $ = low, $$ = medium, $$$ = high.

Abbreviations: 5-HT, serotonin; BID, twice daily; BP, blood pressure; DA, dopamine; HTN, hypertension; HR, heart rate; LFT, liver function test; LEPR, leptin receptor; MAOI, monoamine oxidase inhibitor; NE, norepinephrine; OTC, over the counter; PCSK1, proprotein convertase subtilisin/kexin type 1; POMC, proopiomelanocortin; QAM, daily in the morning; QD, daily; QPM, daily in the evening; SC, subcutaneous; TID, three times daily; TBWL, total body weight loss (at 1 y except where indicated).

Table 4
FDA-approved devices and endoscopic procedures for weight loss[52-56]

Procedure (TBWL)	BMI Indications	Description	Side Effects/Contraindications	Comments
Aspiration therapy (AspireAssist) 14.2 ± 9.8% aspiration 4.9 ± 7% control	BMI 35–55 kg/m²	Percutaneous gastrostomy tube placed, allowing for patient self-removal of food 20–30 min after a meal	• Stoma granulation, tissue formation • Stoma infection • Peritonitis • Gastric ulcer Contraindications: Prior gastrointestinal surgery, bulimia nervosa, recalcitrant gastric ulcers	• Change in eating behavior • 26% device removal rate in the first year • Unknown rate of stoma closure after removed
Space-occupying gastric balloon (Orbera) 10.2 ± 6.5% balloon 3.3 ± 5% control (Obalon) 6.5 ± 5% balloon 3.0 ± 5% control	BMI 30–40 kg/m²	Orbera Silicone balloon filled with saline (450–700 cc) placed in stomach Obalon gas-filled balloon (250 cc) swallowed in capsule form into stomach; up to 3 balloons can be swallowed sequentially	• Nausea • Vomiting • Abdominal pain • Balloon migration • Gastric perforation (rare) Contraindications: Prior gastrointestinal surgery, large hiatal hernia	• Delays gastric emptying • Increases fullness • Obera balloon removed at 6 mo (7.5%–19% early removal rate) – 10% SAE in clinical trial • Obalon balloon is removed endoscopically at 12–26 wk
Transpyloric Shuttle (BAROnova) 41% EBWL shuttle 25% EBWL control	BMI 35–40kg/m² or BMI 30–34.9kg/m² + obesity-related condition	Spherical balloon attached to smaller bulb, placed at the transpyloric position at the junction of stomach and duodenum	• Nausea • Vomiting • Abdominal Pain • Risk for gastric ulcers Contraindications: Prior gastrointestinal surgery	• Delays gastric emptying • In place for up to 12 mo

(continued on next page)

Table 4
(continued)

Procedure (TBWL)	BMI Indications	Description	Side Effects/Contraindications	Comments
Vagal Nerve-Blocking Device (MAESTRO) 9.2% device 6% control	BMI 40–45kg/m² or BMI 35–39.9 kg/m²+ obesity-related condition	Like a pacemaker, electrical stimulation intermittently block signals at the gastric branch of the vagus nerve Device is inserted subcutaneously, on for 12–15 h/d	• Pain at generator site • Nausea • Vomiting • Heartburn • Dysphagia • Belching Contraindications: Cirrhosis, portal HTN, esophageal varices	• No anatomic changes • Blocking the vagus nerve reduces hunger • Low complication rate • Device is incompatible with MRI
Oral Hydrogels (Plenity) 6.4% hydrogel 4.4% control	BMI 25–40 kg/m²	Capsule taken orally 20–30 min before a meal; multiple small hydrogel pieces swell after ingestion	• Diarrhea • Abdominal distension • Flatulence • Nasopharyngitis Contraindications: History of allergic reaction to citric acid, cellulose, sodium stearyl fumarate, gelatin, or titanium oxide	• Increases fullness • Capsules/hydrogel not absorbed

Abbreviations: BMI, Body Mass Index; EBWL, excess body weight loss; SAE, severe adverse effects.

INTENSIVE LIFESTYLE INTERVENTIONS

Lifestyle modifications work to target microenvironmental factors, such as dietary composition and intake, physical activity, sleep, and stress, in an effort to promote weight loss. Two trials, the Diabetes Prevention Program (DPP) and the Look Action for Health in Diabetes (AHEAD) trial, laid the foundation for the efficacy of ILIs.

The DPP was a large randomized clinical trial of 3234 participants with prediabetes who were randomly assigned to placebo, metformin 850 mg twice daily, or an intensive lifestyle-modification program. At baseline, participants had an average age of 50.3 years and average overall BMI of 34.0 kg/m^2.[59] The intensive lifestyle modification program consisted of a curriculum that instructed on diet, exercise, and behavioral changes with the goal to lose 7% of total body weight (TBW). Focused on achieving this predefined goal, the intervention involved close contact with "lifestyle coaches" who met with participants individually at least 16 times in the first 24 weeks and then every 2 months with at least 1 phone call in between.[60] The mean follow-up duration was 2.8 years, and average weight loss was 0.1 kg for placebo, 2.1 kg for metformin, and 5.6 kg for the lifestyle intervention group; the difference between groups was statistically significant. The cumulative incidence of diabetes was also significantly lower in the metformin and lifestyle groups than that in placebo. In a 10-year follow-up of the DPP trial, the lifestyle intervention group was observed to lose the most weight initially (up to an average of 7 kg by 1 year), but did gradually regained, although still weighed 2 kg less than their initial weight. In comparison, the metformin group lost a mean of 2.5 kg but was able to consistently maintain the weight lost,[61] thus demonstrating metformin's therapeutic benefit in longer term weight loss maintenance.

The Look AHEAD trial included 5145 participants with T2DM who were randomized to an ILI group or a diabetes support and education group (DSE) to assess whether ILI would decrease CV morbidity and mortality. Across both groups, the average age was 58.7 years, and average BMI 35 to 36 kg/m^2. ILI involved changes in diet and exercise and was modeled on the DPP program. There was similarly an aim to reach a certain percent total body weight loss (TBWL) (individual goal of 10%), and participants were seen weekly in the first 6 months of the trial and then every other week in the second 6 months. The meetings were led by a multidisciplinary team including dietitians, behavioral psychologists, and exercise specialists. In comparison, the DSE group was able to attend three additional sessions during the first year which discussed diet, exercise, and social support, but participants were not weighed at those sessions, and there was no counseling on behavioral modifications. After median follow-up of 9.6 years, the trial was terminated early based on futility analyses which found that ILI did not reduce CV events compared with DSE. However, participants in the ILI group did have a statistically significant amount of weight loss: At 1 year, they lost 8.6% of their initial weight compared with 0.7% in the DSE group.[62] Weight loss was maintained over 4 years,[63] and at the time the study was terminated, participants had a mean weight loss of 6.0%.[62] Patients in the ILI group also had decreases in mean HbA1c[64] levels which were sustained until the end of the study and lower systolic blood pressure.[62] Thus, although the primary outcome was negative, there were many beneficial effects of ILI including reduction in sleep apnea, depression, and physical function, in addition to glycemic improvement and weight loss.[62]

These types of behavioral interventions which focus on modifying diet and physical activity do so through self-monitoring, goal setting, and brief counseling. In addition to leading to weight loss, they have other health benefits and are recommended by the US Preventative Services Task Force to prevent obesity-related morbidity and mortality.[65] Despite the benefits of these interventions, it can be difficult for patients to have access to and engage with a team of trained dietitians, behavioral psychologists, exercise specialists, and coaches. In an effort to make this more accessible, the Young Men's Christian Association (YMCA) has partnered with the Center for Medicare & Medicaid Services which now provides coverage for an ILI that is modeled from DPP.[66,67] When able to be implemented, a high-intensity lifestyle program in the community can be very effective for obesity treatment. This was demonstrated in the Promoting Successful Weight Loss in Primary Care in Louisiana (PROPEL) study, which enrolled 803 participants, from underserved primary care clinics, randomized to an intensive 24-month lifestyle intervention or a usual-care group. At baseline, participants' mean age was 49.4 years, and mean BMI was 37.2 kg/m^2. The intensive lifestyle group lost significantly more weight than the usual-care group; 4.99% TBWL in the intervention group compared with 0.48% TBWL in the placebo group.[68]

As mentioned, diet is an integral part of intensive lifestyle modifications, and the question often asked is, what is the best diet? Extensive research on nutrition interventions (eg, low-fat, low-carbohydrate,[69] high-protein,[70] low-glycemic, and Mediterranean diets[71]) has been unable to identify an "optimal diet" to maximize health.[72] In terms of weight loss, the ideal diet for a specific patient is the one that he or she is able to adhere to long term.[73] For individuals who struggle with portion control, meal replacements (eg, meal bars, liquid meals, or calorie-controlled packaged meals) may be effective; for example, substituting one or two daily meals with meal replacements has been shown to be beneficial for weight loss and weight maintenance strategies.[74] Studies on physical activity show little additional benefit in terms of weight loss itself,[75] but the benefits of physical activity are far-reaching and include weight maintenance,[75] preservation of lean muscle mass,[76] improvement in metabolic health (mitigating insulin resistance),[77] and improvement in mood.[78]

When initiating discussion of lifestyle change, it may feel overwhelming (to the patient and provider) in the setting of a multitude of factors to be addressed. Thus, starting by focusing on one, gradual, yet enduring, lifestyle change can be a useful approach.[79] Attention can be paid to specific lifestyle factors (eg, increased stressors, sleep deprivation/fragmentation, low levels of physical activity) with implementation of a stepwise, targeted approach (eg, first stress reduction, then sleep hygiene, then increasing physical activity). This approach allows the clinician and patient to more easily assess progress while encouraging patient engagement. Depending on the area of lifestyle modification, additional referrals to a dietitian, psychologist, social worker, exercise specialist, and/or sleep medicine specialist may be required.

OBESITY PHARMACOTHERAPY
Overview of Obesity Pharmacotherapy

FDA-approved antiobesity medications are indicated for patients with a BMI ≥30 kg/m^2 or ≥27 kg/m^2 with weight-related diseases, including T2DM, hypertension (HTN), dyslipidemia, and OSA. Medications have varied effectiveness, so the amount of weight loss demonstrated in a study may not predict an individual's response. This is because there is not just one type of obesity but rather differing phenotypes of obesity; thus, response to therapy depends on the "type" of obesity.[80] Trials generally report average efficacy; this makes the assumption that obesity is a single disease entity. In reality, treatment with any one specific antiobesity medication may result in some individuals losing no weight, some losing 5% to 10% TBW, and others losing in excess of 10% to 20% TBW.[80] With no predictive biomarkers to guide therapy, the choice of agent is often tailored according to risks, benefits, cost, and other clinical considerations. Medications are commonly titrated up slowly to mitigate potential side effects as weight loss response is assessed. Moreover, as with most other chronic diseases, multiagent therapy, added sequentially over time, is often required. Finally, to maintain therapeutic benefit, antiobesity medications need to be continued long term so that the weight loss is maintained.[81]

Federal Drug Administration-Approved Antiobesity Medications

Table 3 details each of the FDA-approved antiobesity medications (listed alphabetically) and includes information on dosing, prescribing, common side effects, contraindications, and considerations. Additional information is described about each medication in the following sections.

Liraglutide

Glucagon-like peptide 1 (GLP-1) is an incretin hormone secreted from the ileum in response to food ingestion which amplifies glucose-dependent insulin secretion.[82] Weight loss effects are primarily through central action that promotes satiety with GLP-1 receptors being abundant in multiple regions of the brain.[83] Liraglutide is a GLP-1 receptor agonist which was initially approved for the treatment of T2D with a maximum dose of 1.8 mg per day. In 2014, liraglutide was FDA-approved for obesity treatment at a higher maximal dose of 3 mg per day.[84] Liraglutide is a daily subcutaneous injectable medication which is titrated up to its maximum tolerated dose over several weeks. The Satiety and Clinical Adiposity - Liraglutide Evidence (SCALE) trial included 3731 participants with an average age of 45.1 years and average BMI 38.3 kg/m^2 who were randomly assigned to liraglutide 3.0 mg or placebo. After 1 year, there was a TBWL of 8.0% with liraglutide 3 mg compared with 2.6% TBWL with placebo.[45] Additionally, improvement in HbA1c, fasting glucose, and lipid profile were observed. Side effects of liraglutide are mainly gastrointestinal and include nausea, vomiting, constipation, and diarrhea. These gastrointestinal side effects can be mitigated by slow uptitration of the medication dose, advising patients not to eat past the point of fullness, to eat smaller amounts at any given time, and to eat fewer foods which may trigger their side effects (eg, fatty or spicy foods). There is an increased risk for cholelithiasis and a small increased risk for pancreatitis. Notably, liraglutide has also been shown to have beneficial CV side effects.[85] The Liraglutide Effect and Action in Diabetes: Evaluation of Cardiovascular Outcome Results (LEADER) trial randomized 9340 participants with T2DM and high CV risk (average age 64.3 years, mean BMI 32.5 kg/m^2) to liraglutide 1.8 mg or placebo. After a median follow-up of 3.8 years, patients in the liraglutide group were significantly less likely to suffer from the primary outcome (first occurrence of death from CV causes, nonfatal myocardial infarction, or nonfatal stroke). The rate of death from CV causes (hazard ratio 0.78 [95% confidence interval 0.66 - 0.93]) or any cause of death (0.85 [0.74 - 0.97]) was also significantly lower in the liraglutide group.[85] Notably, GLP-1 receptor agonists as a class of medications have demonstrated benefits in terms of weight loss, glycemic control, and secondary CV risk reduction,[86,87] thus an intriguing class of medications to consider for patients given their potential to address obesity itself as well as weight-related diseases.

Naltrexone/Bupropion

Naltrexone/bupropion is a combination antiobesity medication comprised of an opioid receptor antagonist (naltrexone, commonly used for treating opiate use/overdose) with a norepinephrine and dopamine reuptake inhibitor (bupropion, commonly used for the treatment of depression and smoking cessation).[30] Bupropion also stimulates pro-opiomelanocortin (POMC) neurons which promote satiety.[30] This effect is further enhanced by the addition of naltrexone which potentiates the release of feedback inhibition on POMC that bupropion mediates.[30] In the Contrave Obesity Research (COR)-I trial, 1742 participants were randomized to 16 mg of naltrexone plus bupropion, 32 mg of naltrexone plus bupropion, or placebo. Average BMI across all three groups was 36.2 kg/m², and median age was 45 years. At 1 year, TBWL was 5.0% in the lower dose group, 6.1% in the higher dose group, and 1.3% in the placebo group.[46] The subsequent COR-II trial randomized 1496 participants with an average age of 44.3 years and BMI 36.1 kg/m² to the 32-mg naltrexone/360-mg bupropion dose versus placebo and found TBWL of 6.4% in the medication group versus TBWL of 1.2% in the placebo group.[47] In patients with T2DM, treatment with bupropion/naltrexone resulted in significantly lower HbA1c (−0.6%) than placebo as well as improvements in triglycerides and high-density lipoprotein (HDL) levels.[88] Side effects primarily include nausea, vomiting, constipation, dizziness, dry mouth, and headache; these side effects can be mitigated by titrating up the dose of medication slowly. As bupropion is known to decrease seizure threshold, its use should be avoided in patients with pre-existing seizure disorder as well as in patients with bulimia or anorexia nervosa who purge as these patients are also at risk for seizure.[42] In addition, due to its noradrenergic activity, bupriopion can also increase blood pressure and heart rate, it can increase blood pressure and heart rate (HR), but this generally is on the order of less than 1 mm Hg increase in blood pressure and less than 1 bpm increase in HR and thus most commonly is not clinically significant.[46,47,89,90] Given that each of the two components in this medication has been used for other indications for several decades, potential adverse effects have been established. Notably though, as for antidiabetes medications,[91,92] as of 2012, the FDA[93] requires CV safety be established for antiobesity medications, to rule out "prespecified unacceptable level of CV risk." If a medication does not have an identifiable risk signal, a cardiovascular outcomes trial (CVOT) may not be required by the FDA. Given naltrexone/bupropion's effect on blood pressure, the Light Study, a CVOT, was under way (2012–2013) and included 8910 individuals with obesity randomized to naltrexone/bupropion (32 mg/360 mg) versus placebo.[90] Unfortunately, the trial was terminated after "public release of confidential interim data by the sponsor," and thus, noninferiority could not be established.[90]

Orlistat

Orlistat inhibits lipases in the gastrointestinal lumen thereby reducing absorption of fatty acids.[30] At maximum dose (120 mg three times per day with meals), about 30% of triglycerides that are ingested are malabsorbed and excreted.[30] Orlistat is also available over the counter at a lower (60 mg) dose. The XENical in the prevention of diabetes in obese subjects (XENDOS) trial included 3305 participants, average BMI 37.3 to 37.4 kg/m² and average age 43 years,[48] who were randomly assigned to ILI plus orlistat (120 mg three times per day) or ILI plus placebo. At 1 year, mean TBWL was 10.6 kg in the orlistat + ILI group versus 6.2 kg in the placebo + ILI group. Thus, in the orlistat group, there was a significant mean weight loss of 4.4 kg in excess of placebo after 1 year which remained significantly higher at the end of 4 years; specifically, 5.8 kg in the orlistat group and 3.0 kg in the placebo group at 4 years.[48] Orlistat has also been shown to reduce the incidence of T2DM over 4 years.[48] Orlistat is not systemically absorbed, so most of its effects are gastrointestinal, including steatorrhea, flatulence, fecal urgency, and cholelithiasis.[30] In the setting of orlistat treatment, there is decreased absorption of fat-soluble vitamins, thus patients should be started on a multivitamin and vitamin D supplementation with appropriate monitoring.[30] Although gastrointestinal side effects may deter patients from using this medication, consideration should be given to adding on orlistat to patients' existing obesity pharmacotherapy regimens, especially in patient who may have developed constipation from other antiobesity medications.

Phentermine

Approved in 1959, phentermine has been used as an antiobesity medication for over 6 decades. It is a sympathomimetic agent which increases release of norepinephrine primarily, as well as dopamine and serotonin.[94] Given its mechanism of action, side effects that are CV, including increased HR or blood pressure; therefore, it should be avoided in patients with a history of CV disease, stroke, or uncontrolled HTN. Side effects also include tachycardia, increase in blood pressure, anxiety, insomnia, headache, dry mouth, and, rarely, glaucoma.[30] Phentermine is contraindicated for use with monoamine oxidase inhibitors given a risk for hypertensive crisis.[30] Phentermine is available as a tablet or capsule that can be taken once daily. A lower dose formulation of phentermine is also available and can be taken up to 3 times per day before meals. This latter option provides flexibility for patients to minimize dose by timing the medication with meals when most food is consumed.

Phentermine is only FDA-approved for continuous use for a "few weeks"; longer term treatment is considered off-label, and most trials are less than 12 weeks long.[49] Given that obesity is a life-long disease, it stands to reason that interventions are use chronically; when considering longer term treatment with phentermine some local prescribing laws regulate utilization of phentermine beyond 3 months and thus should also be consulted. Unfortunately, long-term prospective CV safety data with phentermine are lacking. In one study, electronic health record data were retrospectively reviewed for 13,972 individuals (average age 43.5 years, average BMI 37.8 kg/m^2) who were prescribed phentermine. The study found that individuals who were prescribed phentermine for a short term (~3 months) had a TBWL of 2.7% at 6 months, 1.4% at 12 months, and 0% at 24 months, whereas individuals who were continuously prescribed phentermine for greater than 1 year had a TBWL of 7.5% at 24 months compared with baseline.[49] In this retrospective study, CV risk outcome was assessed with a composite measure (which included incident myocardial infarction, stroke, angina, coronary artery bypass grafting, carotid artery intervention, or death), with 0.3% (41 out of 13,972) individuals meeting criteria in the cohort; no increase in incident CV events or death was observed with continuous long-term phentermine use over 3 years of follow-up.[49] There are no CV data beyond 3 years, and no prospective long-term data; RCTs of long-term phentermine use are needed.

Phentermine/Topiramate

In 2012, the FDA approved a combination that added topiramate to phentermine. The mechanism by which topiramate, an antiseizure medication, affects weight is not entirely known. Topiramate modulates gamma-aminobutyric acid (GABA) release, reduces glutamate release by blocking voltage-gated Na channels, and inhibits carbonic anhydrase.[95] In the EQUIP trial, 1267 participants with obesity (average BMI 42.0 kg/m^2, average age 42.7 years) were randomized to phentermine 3.75 mg/topiramate 23 mg (3.75/23, low-dose group), phentermine 15 mg/topiramate 92 mg (15/92, high-dose group), and placebo. At the end of 1 year, TBWL was 5.1% in the low-dose (3.75/23) group and 10.9% in the high-dose (15/92) group, with 1.6% in the placebo group.[50] With 2 years of treatment in the SEQUEL trial, TBWL was 9.3% with phentermine 7.5 mg/topiramate 46 mg (7.5/46, mid-dose group) and 10.5% in the high-dose (15/92) group, with 1.8% in the placebo group.[96] The CONQUER trial included patients who had T2DM or prediabetes, HTN, or dyslipidemia and demonstrated TBWL of 7.8% in the mid-dose (7.5/46) group, 9.8% in the high-dose (15/92) group, and 1.2% in the placebo group.[97] Additionally, there were significant improvements in blood pressure, lipids levels, and HbA1c[97]; thus, phentermine/topiramate demonstrates beneficial effect in terms of both obesity treatment as well as weight-related diseases such as HTN, dyslipidemia, and T2DM.

Side effects of phentermine/topiramate primarily include insomnia, dysgeusia, paresthesias, anxiety, depression, and constipation. Additionally, cognitive side effects may be observed including changes in attention or memory. Because of its phentermine component, HR should be monitored after initiation of therapy. To assess CVOT for phentermine/topiramate (15/92), the A Qsymia CardiovascuLAr morbIdity and Mortality (AQCLAIM) trial was designed and authorized by the European Medicines Agency (EMA) in 2013,[98] but the trial was never started, therefore long-term CV safety data are currently lacking.[92] Topiramate can also cause hypokalemia and nephrolithiasis because of its action as a carbonic anhydrase inhibitor; thus, serum chemistry should be monitored before starting treatment and periodically thereafter. Phentermine/topiramate is considered pregnancy category X as the topiramate component is associated with increased risk of cleft lip and cleft palate in the first trimester of pregnancy. Therefore, it is recommended that women of childbearing age have a pregnancy test completed before starting phentermine/topiramate and monthly thereafter in addition to using effective contraception. Of note, topiramate can cause changes in the metabolism of oral contraceptives that may lead to spotting but is not anticipated to decrease the contraceptive's efficacy at the doses in the phentermine/topiramate combination. Owing to its teratogenic effects, providers are required to sign up for the Risk Evaluation and Mitigation Strategy program to prescribe phentermine/topiramate in combination.[43] If the decision is made to stop the medication, it should be tapered to avoid potentially triggering seizures.[43]

Semaglutide

Ushering in a new generation of more efficacious anti-obesity medication, semaglutide 2.4mg taken once weekly was recently granted FDA-approval for the treatment of obesity in June 2021. Semaglutide is a long acting GLP-1 receptor agonist, requiring subcutaneous injection once per week, rather once per day as with liraglutide. Like liraglutide, semaglutide was initially FDA-approved at a lower maximal dose (1.0 mg weekly) for the treatment of T2DM before its recent approval for obesity treatment at the higher maximal dose of 2.4mg weekly. Semaglutide is titrated up to its maximum tolerated dose over several months given that it is a weekly medication. Weight loss effects with semaglutide are also primarily through central action. The Semaglutide Treatment Effect in People with Obesity (STEP 1) trial included 1,961 individuals with obesity without T2DM, with an average age of 46 years and average BMI of 37.9 kg/m^2, who were randomized to receive semaglutide 2.4 mg or placebo, plus lifestyle intervention. After 68 weeks, participants who received the 2.4mg once weekly dose of semaglutide, had an average weight loss of 15.3 kg (14.9% TBWL), whereas weight loss in the placebo group was 2.6kg (2.4% TBWL)[84]. Additionally, 32% of individuals had >20% TBWL. Such a degree of weight loss response has not previously been observed with any single antiobesity medication. Additional studies with semaglutide 2.4mg weekly have demonstrated its higher efficacy to reduce body weight, including in the STEP 2 trial (participants with T2DM, semaglutide 2.4mg versus 1.0mg versus placebo, with TBWL at 68 weeks of 9.64%, 6.99% and 3.42%, respectively) and the STEP 3 trial (participants with obesity who all received intensive lifestyle intervention with semaglutide 2.4 mg weekly versus with placebo, with TBWL at 68 weeks of 16% versus 5.7%, respectively). Finally, the STEP 4 trial dramatically demonstrated the effect of continuing treatment with semaglutide compared to stopping treatment (switching to placebo). After a 20-week run-in period titrating to semaglutide 2.4mg, 803 participants (who on average demonstrated 10.6% TBWL at 20 weeks) were randomized to either continue taking semaglutide 2.4mg weekly or switch to placebo. During the subsequent 48 week, participants randomized to continued taking semaglutide demonstrated an additional 7.9% TBWL where as individuals randomized to stop semaglutide and switch to placebo gained 6.9% TBW.

As with other GLP-1 receptor agonists, the side effects of semaglutide 2.4mg are mainly gastrointestinal (including nausea, vomiting, constipation, and diarrhea) and can be mitigated by slow up titration of the medication dose, advising patients not to eat past the point of fullness, to eat smaller amounts at any given time, and to eat fewer foods which may trigger their side effects. There is an increased risk for cholelithiasis. Semaglutide has also been shown to have beneficial cardiovascular side effects. The Trial to Evaluate Cardiovascular and Other Long-term Outcomes with Semaglutide in Subjects with Type 2 Diabetes (SUSTAIN-6) randomized 3,297 participants with T2DM and high cardiovascular risk (average age 64.6 years, mean body weight of 92.1 kg) to semaglutide 1.0mg or placebo. After a median follow up of 2.1 years, patients in the semaglutide group were significantly less likely to suffer from the primary outcome (first occurrence of death from cardiovascular causes, nonfatal myocardial infarction, or nonfatal stroke), with a hazard ratio of 0.74 (95% confidence interval 0.58 to 0.95). Currently on going, the Semaglutide Effects on Heart Disease and Stroke in Patients with Overweight or Obesity (SELECT) trial is the first trial which will assess whether a GLP-1 receptor agonist decreases secondary CV risk in individuals with obesity but without T2DM[85]. Taken together, semaglutide 2.4mg weekly is currently the most efficacious FDA-approved antiobesity medication demonstrating the highest degree of weight reduction in individuals with obesity, with the additional benefits of glycemic control and secondary CV risk reduction and glycemic control in individuals with T2DM[86,87].

Setmelanotide

Recently, in December 2020, the FDA approved an antiobesity medication which targets treatment of several monogenic forms of obesity. This medication, setmelanotide, is a melanocortin-4 (MC4) receptor agonist. The melanocortin pathway is instrumental in energy and weight regulation.[51] Briefly, leptin, a hormone made in adipose tissue, binds to leptin receptor (LEPR) which is present on neurons in the hypothalamus that express POMC.[51] When in the fed state, leptin stimulates increases in POMC, which is then processed into α-melanocyte-stimulating hormone (α-MSH) and β-MSH which then activate MC4R and thereby serve to decrease food intake.[51] POMC is processed into these two melanocortins by proprotein convertase subtilisin and kexin type 1.[51] Defects in LEPR, POMC, or proprotein convertase subtilisin/kexin type 1 (PCKS1) result in rare forms of monogenic obesity marked by hyperphagia and early onset obesity.[51] An open-label, single-arm trial of ten patients with POMC or PCKS1 deficiency and 11 patients with LEPR deficiency resulted in a 25.6% decrease in body weight compared with baseline in the former group and a 12.5% decrease in body weight compared with baseline in the latter group.[51] Thus, setmelanotide is now FDA-approved for treatment of patients who have deficiency in POMC, PCKS1, or LEPR.[99] Phase 2 and 3 trials are currently underway to assess efficacy for other forms of monogenic obesity. Notably, this medication is the first monogenic obesity target-specific therapy.

Choosing antiobesity medications

Given the heterogeneity of obesity and lack of informative treatment biomarkers, the following stepwise process can be considered:

1. Consider *contraindications*; if a patient, for example, has a history of CV disease, stroke, or uncontrolled HTN, phentermine would not be chosen.
2. Evaluate for *dual-benefit*; if a patient has history of T2DM or prediabetes, a GLP-1 receptor agonist, SGLT2 inhibitor, or metformin may be preferred.
3. Assess *patient preference* and anticipate adherence through shared decision-making; a once or twice daily tablet may be preferred over a once weekly injection, or vice versa.
4. Consider *cost* to the patient; if insurance does not cover the cost of a branded antiobesity medication, a generic alternative can be considered.
5. Consider *potential efficacy*; as described, this may be difficult to predict given variability in response owing to heterogeneity of obesity.

At the outset, it is helpful for patients to know that treatment will be progressive with sequential, step-up therapy added to achieve health and weight goals. Patients must be made aware that treatment will need to be continued indefinitely if weight loss is to be maintained (**Fig. 1**). Importantly, discussing a long-term, comprehensive plan with patients instills hope and confidence.

Implementing obesity pharmacotherapy

A schematic (see **Fig. 1**) for initiating obesity pharmacotherapy outlines interval assessment for side effects and response. Notably, if there is clinically meaningful weight loss with an antiobesity medication, the antiobesity medication is continued indefinitely for the weight loss to be maintained. Once a weight plateau is reached with the first antiobesity medication, sequentially adding another antiobesity

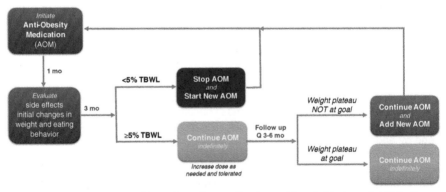

Fig. 1. Obesity treatment with antiobesity medications. After initiation of AOM, the patient returns in ~1 month to evaluate for side effects and assess for any changes in weight and eating behavior. If the patient is tolerating the AOM, a subsequent follow-up visit at 3 months evaluates percent change in weight from initiation of AOM. If TBWL is <5%, then the patient is not responding to first AOM and should be switched to a different AOM. If TBWL is ≥5%, the AOM should be continued and the dose adjusted, and potentially increased as needed and tolerated. Notably, if a patient responds to (loses weight with) a specific AOM, that AOM should be continued indefinitely to maintain the weight lost while taking that AOM. Additionally, while taking a given AOM, patients will plateau at a particular weight (more specifically, body fat mass set point), at that time another AOM can be added to the obesity treatment regimen if weight is not yet at goal. AOM, antiobesity medication; Q, every; TBWL, total body weight loss.

medication has the potential to lower the weight plateau further. As such, antiobesity medications are added stepwise to achieve health and weight goals. Provider visits at regular intervals are scheduled as they are for any other chronic disease. Initially, more frequent visits may be required when an antiobesity medication is initiated so that side effects and weight response can be assessed, but visits can eventually be spaced out to 3 or even 6 months as a stable regimen is set. It is pragmatic to schedule additional visits with key team members (including dieticians, exercise specialists, and so forth); to maximize healthful eating, physical activity, and behavior change; and to optimize continued adherence and engagement. Similar to standard practice in managing other chronic diseases, it is important to have regular follow-up visits with patients with obesity. Additionally, creating an environment where patients feel comfortable and welcome to schedule interval appointments, especially when weigh gain occurs, normalizes the chronicity of this disease, the ebbs and flows of weight change, and creates a safe medical care space where patients can find comfort, reassurance, and hope.

Additional considerations for antiobesity pharmacotherapy in clinical practice

Owing in part to barriers in access, availability, and cost of branded FDA-approved antiobesity medications, off-label use of other medications for obesity treatment has been followed over the years. One of the medications which is used off-label is metformin. A meta-analysis of 31 RCTs conducted to assess metformin effects on metabolic measures, as well as incidence of new diabetes, found that metformin reduced BMI by 5.3% in addition to improving fasting glucose, fasting insulin, insulin resistance, and triglyceride, low-density lipoprotein, and HDL levels and reduced the incidence of new-onset diabetes.[100] There is a notable variability in weight response, ranging from weight stability to some degree of weight loss, which may be due to differences in dose of metformin, degree of insulin resistance,[101,102] as well as the heterogeneity of obesity. Notably, as described in the DPP outcomes study, participants in the metformin group not only lost a mean of 2.5 kg but were also able to consistently maintain the weight lost with 10-year follow-up[61]; this demonstrated metformin's therapeutic benefit in longer term weight loss maintenance. Finally, as metformin has a long-standing track record of safety and potential additional benefits which are being explored,[103] it is not surprising that it is used off label for obesity treatment.

Sodium-glucose cotransporter 2 inhibitors (SGLT2i) are approved for diabetes treatment and have also shown promising weight benefit (1.5- to 2-kg weight loss in excess of placebo, sustained up to 4 years.)[104] This effect has also been demonstrated in patients without diabetes.[105,106] Additionally, SGLT2i have demonstrated CV[86] and renal benefits[107] in patients with T2DM, and there is emerging evidence of these benefits in individuals without T2DM.[108,109] Because SGLT2i lead to energy loss through glucosuria, there is a compensatory increase in appetite that may attenuate the weight loss benefit. As a result, there is on-going interest in pairing SGLT2i with other agents such as GLP-1 receptor agonists, which decrease food intake, to attain synergistic weight loss benefit.[104,110]

In addition to liraglutide 3.0mg and semaglutide 2.4mg, as a class, GLP-1 receptor agonists result in significant weight reduction[87]; thus, although these medications were initially developed for the treatment of T2DM, they are often used off-label for obesity treatment. Liraglutide at the 1.8mg dose is FDA-approved for T2DM and resulted in an average weight loss of 5.0kg in patients with T2DM. The 1.0-mg weekly dose of semaglutide is FDA-approved for T2DM; in this population, average weight loss with the 1.0-mg dose has been in the range of 4.5 to 6.5 kg[111] compared with baseline. Oral semaglutide is also approved for the treatment of patients with T2DM and with the highest currently available oral dose of 14mg resulted in 4.3kg weight loss in this population.[112] Additionally, recently published results of the Assessment of Weekly Administration of LY2189265 [dulaglutide] in Diabetes-11 (AWARD-11) trial in individuals with T2DM, demonstrated that a higher dose of dulaglutide, a weekly injectable GLP-1 analogue, resulted in 5.0kg of weight loss at 36 weeks; this new higher dose of dulaglutide (4.5mg weekly) was recently approved by the FDA for treatment of T2DM[113]. In addition to the medication-class effects on glycemic control, weight reduction, and potentially renal benefit[114], the GLP-1 receptor agonist class of medications has also demonstrated secondary CV risk reduction[86,87] in individuals with T2DM[86,115,116]. As this class of medications addresses obesity as well as weight-related diseases, it is not surprising that multiple agents with a GLP-1 backbone or paired with other compounds are currently under development for obesity treatment[117,118]. Several such agents undergoing phase 2/3 clinical trials for obesity and/or diabetes include cagrilintide-semaglutide (an amylin analogue with GLP-1 analogue), tirzepatide (a dual glucose-dependent insulinotropic polypeptide and GLP-1 receptor agonist), and danuglipron (an oral small-molecule GLP-1 receptor agonist). No doubt an exciting time in the field of obesity medicine with the anticipation of increasingly efficacious pharmacotherapeutics to come.

Other medications have demonstrated weight loss benefit and are used off-label for obesity treatment, including an antidiabetes medication, pramlintide,[119] and an anticonvulsant, zonisamide.[120] Additionally, to mitigate cost, several of the component agents of the FDA-approved antiobesity medications can be prescribed individually; for example, phentermine and topiramate[121,122] can be initiated individually, and bupropion can also be used alone without combination with naltrexone.[123] With careful, close monitoring, providers may use combinations of various medications to achieve greater cumulative weight reduction for obesity treatment.[124–127]

BARIATRIC AND METABOLIC SURGERY

Currently, bariatric and metabolic surgery is the most effective obesity treatment for moderate to severe obesity; however, just as with antiobesity medications, given the heterogeneity of obesity, there is a broad range of responses to surgical interventions.[128] Surgery can be considered for patients who have a BMI ≥ 40 kg/m^2 or a BMI ≥ 35 kg/m^2 with associated comorbidities, such as T2DM, HTN, OSA, and fatty liver disease. There are four main surgical interventions (detailed in **Table 5**) including Roux-en-Y gastric bypass (RYGB), vertical sleeve gastrectomy (VSG), adjustable gastric banding (AGB), and biliopancreatic diversion (BPD); all are predominantly preformed via laparoscopic approach. Each procedure has particular benefits, risks, and contraindications, and although safety has been a concern, current data indicate that the perioperative mortality rates range from 0.03% to 0.2%, which has substantially improved over the last 2 decades.[129] VSG is currently the most commonly performed bariatric procedure in the United States, accounting for nearly 60% of procedures conducted in 2019, a significant increase from 17.8% in 2011. RYGB procedures now make up about 18%, down from 36.7% in 2011.[130] AGB and BPD make up about 1% each of annual bariatric procedures, with revisions and other procedures making up the remaining 20%. In the Longitudinal Assessment of Bariatric Surgery (LABS) study, patients who underwent RYGB and gastric banding were followed up for 7 years. After 7 years, mean weight loss in the RYGB group was 38.2 kg (28.4% of baseline body weight lost) with a mean weight regain of 3.9% of baseline weight between years 3 to 7. Seven years after laparoscopic gastric banding, mean weight loss was 18.8 kg (14.9% of baseline body weight lost) with 1.4% weight regain.

Dyslipidemia was found to be less prevalent after 7 years, whereas diabetes and HTN prevalence were lower only in the RYGB group.[131]

Bariatric surgery specifically refers to the surgical treatment of obesity. As with medications, bariatric surgery has multiple beneficial metabolic effects and is now commonly referred to as "bariatric *and* metabolic surgery." As with obesity pharmacotherapy, longitudinal prospective studies have shown improvement or resolutions of many of the obesity-related diseases, including lowering HbA1c levels or even remission of T2DM for some period of time, as well as reduced incidence of microvascular and macrovascular complications of T2DM.[132,133] Notably in the Surgical Therapy And Medications Potentially Eradicate Diabetes Efficiently (STAMPEDE) trial, the addition of bariatric surgery to medical therapy for patients with T2DM significantly improved HbA1c levels with more patients achieving a HbA1c level of ≤6.0% after 5 years compared with medical therapy alone. In the surgical intervention group, triglycerides were also lower, HDL levels higher, insulin treatment was decreased, and patients reported improved quality of life.[134] Additionally, bariatric and metabolic surgery has beneficial effects on HTN,[135,136] CV disease and major adverse cardiovascular effects (MACE),[137] nonalcoholic steatohepatitis,[138] OSA,[139] improvements in gonadal function in men and women,[140] osteoarthritis and other musculoskeletal complaints,[141] and urinary incontinence.[142] A retrospective cohort study of 2500 patients who underwent bariatric surgery (74% RYGB) and the large prospective, nonrandomized (due to ethical considerations) Swedish Obesity Subject Study have also found significant decrease in mortality over 20 years of follow-up, especially related to a lower risk of death due to CV disease and cancer.[143,144]

Close monitoring is recommended for patients who undergo bariatric surgery, specifically every 3 months in the first year after surgery and annually thereafter.[52] Patients should continue life-long micronutrient supplementation and be screened annually for deficiencies with adjustments to supplementation as needed.[52] Nutrient deficiencies after bariatric surgery can be significant and include deficiencies in vitamin B1 (thiamine), B12, folate, vitamins A, D, E, K, calcium, iron, copper, and zinc (**Table 6**). Dumping syndrome as well as insulin-mediated hypoglycemia can also occur after bariatric surgery. Additionally, there is increased bone loss after surgery, possibly related to unloading, changes in vitamin D/calcium homeostasis, or changes in gut hormones as well as gonadal hormones.[145] It is therefore recommended that patients undergo dual-energy X-ray absorptiometry evaluation within 2 years of procedure.[145] Rapid weight loss leads to an increased risk of gallstones.[146] The risk for calcium oxalate kidney stones is also increased after bariatric surgery, primarily driven by hyperoxaluria, low urine volume, and hypocituria.[147] Nonsteroidal anti-inflammatory drugs (NSAIDs) should be avoided after bariatric surgery as there is concern for risk of ulcers. However, a recent retrospective study of 421 patients who underwent VSG suggests that for sleeve gastrectomy, NSAIDs may not pose as a significant risk.[148] In summary, bariatric and metabolic surgery has multiple beneficial effects in addition to weight loss although patients must be monitored for certain long-term side effects.

Although beyond the scope of this review, FDA-approved devices and endoscopic therapies are commercially available but have faced challenges in obtaining insurance coverage. These interventions have also been shown to be effective for obesity treatment and are in continued development (detailed in **Table 4**).

PUTTING IT ALL TOGETHER

The treatment approach for patients with obesity is not limited to any one single therapy discussed previously. Rather, owing to the mechanistic complexity of obesity, a

Table 5
Bariatric and metabolic surgery[52,57,58]

Procedure, %TBWL	Benefits	Risks
Adjustable gastric banding 15%–25%	• Reversible, no anastomosis • No nutritional deficiencies • Lower indication: BMI 30–40 kg/m²	• Band migration, erosion, infection • Pouch enlargement • Esophageal dilation • Esophageal dysmotility • GERD/esophagitis • Port infections/dislocation • Band explantation (5%–20%) • Conversion to other bariatric surgical procedure (up to 20%)[146] • Long term, weight loss not well sustained • Contraindications: previous weight loss surgery, portal HTN with varices, chronic steroid use
Vertical sleeve gastrectomy 20%–25%	• No anastomosis needed • Fewer complications • Fewer nutritional deficiencies	• Recurrent GERD • Gastric leaks • Gastric bleeding • Selective micronutrient deficiencies (Vitamin B12, folate, iron) • Contraindications: severe GERD, portal HTN with varices
Roux-en-Y gastric bypass 30%–35%	• Improvement in GERD • Beneficial metabolic effects with rapid improvement in glucose control • Significant weight loss benefit	• Anastomotic leak and ulcers • Internal hernias • Selected micronutrient deficiencies • Gastrointestinal and gastrojejunal stenosis/strictures • Gallstones • Bacterial overgrowth • Hyperinsulinemic hypoglycemia • Dumping syndrome • Contraindications: Class C cirrhosis, portal HTN with varices
Biliopancreatic diversion with duodenal switch 35%–45%	• Significant, sustained weight loss • Beneficial metabolic effects with rapid improvement in glucose control • Effective for patients with higher BMI, can be used as second stage after VSG	• Selected micronutrient (in particular fat-soluble vitamins) and macronutrient deficiencies • Internal hernia • Bile acid colitis • Bacterial overgrowth • Nephrolithiasis/renal failure • Osteoporosis • Need for surveillance endoscopy • Contraindications: Class C cirrhosis, portal HTN with varices

Abbreviation: GERD, gastroesophageal reflux disease; HTN, hypertension; %TBWL, percent total body weight loss; VSG, Vertical sleeve gastrectomy.

Table 6
Monitoring for micronutrient deficiencies after bariatric surgery[52]

Nutrient	Clinical Symptoms/Findings	Preventative Supplementation
Vitamin A	• Night blindness • Follicular hyperkeratosis	5000–10,000 IU/d
Vitamin B1 (thiamine)	• Confabulation, ataxia (Wernicke-Korsakoff) • Cardiomegaly, CHF (wet beriberi) • Peripheral neuropathy, paresthesias (Dry Beriberi)	50–100 mg PO QD from B-complex or high-potency multivitamin
Vitamin B9 (folate)	• Stomatitis • Glossitis • Diarrhea	400–800 μg PO QD from multivitamin 800–1000 μg PO QD (women of child-bearing age)
Vitamin B12 (cobalamin)	• Neuropathy, paresthesias, gait unsteadiness • Delusions	350–1000 μg PO QD, or 1000 μg IM or SQ monthly
Vitamin D	• Secondary hyperparathyroidism • Osteomalacia (bone pain, proximal muscle weakness) or rickets in children • Osteoporosis	3000 IU daily, adjust to goal level >30 ng/mL
Vitamin E	• Hemolytic anemia • Neuromuscular dysfunction • Changes in vision	15 mg/d
Vitamin K	• Excessive bleeding or bruising	90–120 μg/d (BPD/DS: 300 μg/d)
Calcium	• Secondary hyperparathyroidism • Osteomalacia (bone pain, proximal muscle weakness) • Osteoporosis	1200–1500 mg/d (BPD/DS 1800–2400 mg/d) Give in divided doses Calcium carbonate should be taken with meals
Copper	• Microcytic anemia • Progressive sensory ataxia • Myelopathy with spastic gait	200% of RDA, about 2 mg/d (BPD/DS, RYGB) 100% of RDA, about 1 mg/d (VSG, AGB) 1 mg of copper is recommended for every 8–15 mg of elemental zinc given to prevent copper deficiency Copper gluconate or sulfate is preferred
Iron	• Anemia • Pica	18 mg PO QD from multivitamin (males, no anemia) 45–60 mg elemental iron PO QD (menstruating females following RYGB, VSG, BPD/DS)
Zinc	• Impaired taste and smell • Poor wound healing • Dry, scaly skin, acrodermatitis enteropathica	200% of RDA, about 16–22 mg/d (BPD/DS) 100%–200% of RDA, about 8–22 mg/d (RYGB) 100% of RDA, about 8–11 mg/d (VSG, AGB)

Abbreviations: AGB, Adjustable gastric banding; BPD/DS, Biliopancreatic diversion with duodenal switch; CHF, congestive heart failure; IM, intramuscular; IU, international units; PO, oral; QD, daily; RDA, recommended daily allowance; RYGB, Roux-en-Y gastric bypass; SQ, subcutaneous; VSG, Vertical sleeve gastrectomy.

Screening should be conducted annually except for iron and B12 deficiency, which should be conducted every 3 mo for the first 1 y. Screen vitamin E and K only if symptomatic.

comprehensive approach with combination therapy may often be required.[39] For instance, a patient may require treatment with one or multiple antiobesity medications, followed by surgical intervention, and then followed again by different or additional anti-obesity medications all in the context of maximizing lifestyle changes. Implementing individualized combinations of various therapeutic modalities are key to effective care.

Additional guidance for the management of patients with obesity is detailed in several CPG referenced throughout this review. Each CPG focuses on a unique aspect of care for patients with obesity. The Endocrine Society CPG focuses on obesity pharmacotherapy,[30] guidelines from the American Society for Metabolic and Bariatric Surgery focus on surgery interventions and perioperative care[52], and the American Association of Clinical Endocrinology/American College of Endocrinology guidelines review comprehensive care of patients with obesity detailing all available treatment modalities.[39] The Academy of Nutrition and Dietetics has also published a position article with a focus on nutritional interventions.[149] Finally, consideration for younger patients (although not the focus of this review) should be included given that one in five adolescents in the United States has obesity.[150] The American Academy of Pediatrics developed a Position Statement on the use of bariatric and metabolic surgery in children and adolescents with severe obesity,[151,152] and the Endocrine Society developed a CPG for pediatric obesity[153]; with current FDA-approved antiobesity medications including liraglutide 3.0 mg and orlistat for use in adolescents aged $\geq$ 12 years[154] and phentermine in adolescents older than 16 years.[155] These CPGs are important resources for all practitioners who care for patients with obesity, and additionally, several new CPGs are currently in development.

SUMMARY

The primary care provider is essential on the frontline: diagnosing, evaluating, and treating patients with obesity. Additionally, primary care providers may need to coordinate an interdisciplinary team including covisits or internal/external referrals to dietitians, psychologists, and exercise specialists. The field of obesity medicine continues to evolve rapidly with novel therapies including increased-efficacy antiobesity medications such as the recently approved Semaglutide 2.4mg[111] and others[156–159] Clinicians clearly have an increasingly strengthened tool box to delve into in the care of their patients with obesity.

Obesity should be treated with the seriousness and rigor afforded to any other chronic disease. We need to continue translational research to differentiate subtypes of obesity, identify biomarkers, and elucidate pathophysiology, thus enabling development of mechanism-based targeted therapies to inform evidence-based clinical guidelines. Obesity education should be expanded at all levels of health care curricula, including the promotion of formal training in obesity medicine fellowships. Finally, we should advocate on behalf of our patients, both to ensure appropriate health care coverage for all available therapies for patients with obesity as well as to help support the urgently needed transformation of our current obesogenic environment into one which promotes health and well-being for all. These efforts in research, education, and advocacy are paramount to supporting comprehensive and compassionate care for all individuals with obesity.

CLINICS CARE POINTS

- Obesity is a chronic disease necessitating life-long treatment.

- A compassionate, comprehensive approach is paramount when caring for patients with obesity; individualize care and consider include combinations of available treatments based on patient needs, including intensive lifestyle interventions, antiobesity medications, devices and endoscopic procedures, and bariatric-metabolic surgery.
- As obesity is a heterogenous disease, variability in response to different interventions is to be expected, as is the case for any complex disease.
- Assess for weight-related diseases and tailor treatment as is appropriate.
- Always approach patients with obesity in a caring, compassionate, non-judgmental manner; create a safe environment, instilling confidence and hope.
- Treat obesity as you would any other chronic disease; with evidence-based interventions, persistence and escalation of therapy as is needed, and a focus on optimizing life-long health.

ACKNOWLEDGMENTS

The authors thank Richard Kibbey, MD, PhD for his editorial input.

DISCLOSURE

A.M. Jastreboff serves as a consultant for Boehringer Ingelheim, Eli Lilly, Novo Nordisk, Intellihealth, Scholar Rock, and Pfizer, and receives research support from the American Diabetes Association, Eli Lilly, Novo Nordisk, and NIH/NIDDKR01DK099039.

REFERENCES

1. Finkelstein EA, Khavjou OA, Thompson H, et al. Obesity and severe obesity forecasts through 2030. Am J Prev Med 2012;42(6):563–70.
2. WHO. Obesity and overweight 2020. Available at: https://www.who.int/newsroom/fact-sheets/detail/obesity-and-overweight. Accessed March 25, 2021.
3. Ogden CL, Carroll MD, McDowell MA, et al. Obesity among adults in the United States–no statistically significant change since 2003-2004. NCHS Data Brief 2007;(1):1–8.
4. Kim L, Garg S, O'Halloran A, et al. Risk Factors for Intensive Care Unit Admission and In-hospital Mortality Among Hospitalized Adults Identified through the US Coronavirus Disease 2019 (COVID-19)-Associated Hospitalization Surveillance Network (COVID-NET). Clin Infect Dis 2021;72(9):e206–14.
5. Al-Sabah S, Al-Haddad M, Al-Youha S, et al. COVID-19: impact of obesity and diabetes on disease severity. Clin Obes 2020;10(6):e12414.
6. Pettit NN, MacKenzie EL, Ridgway JP, et al. Obesity is associated with increased risk for mortality among hospitalized patients with COVID-19. Obesity (Silver Spring) 2020;28(10):1806–10.
7. Kalligeros M, Shehadeh F, Mylona EK, et al. Association of obesity with disease severity among patients with coronavirus disease 2019. Obesity (Silver Spring) 2020;28(7):1200–4.
8. Nakeshbandi M, Maini R, Daniel P, et al. The impact of obesity on COVID-19 complications: a retrospective cohort study. Int J Obes (Lond) 2020;44(9):1832–7.
9. Tartof SY, Qian L, Hong V, et al. Obesity and mortality among patients diagnosed with COVID-19: results from an integrated health care organization. Ann Intern Med 2020;173(10):773–81.

10. Bray GA, Heisel WE, Afshin A, et al. The science of obesity management: an endocrine society scientific statement. Endocr Rev 2018;39(2):79–132.

11. Jastreboff AM, Kotz CM, Kahan S, et al. Obesity as a disease: the obesity society 2018 position statement. Obesity (Silver Spring) 2019;27(1):7–9.

12. Brownell K, Horgen KB. Food fight: the inside story of the food industry, America's obesity Crisis, and what we can do about it. New York: McGraw-Hill; 2004.

13. Schwartz MW, Seeley RJ, Zeltser LM, et al. Obesity pathogenesis: an endocrine society scientific statement. Endocr Rev 2017;38(4):267–96.

14. Recognition of obesity as a disease. In: Association AM, editor. Resolution: 420 (A-13). American Medical Association; 2013.

15. Thomas CE, Mauer EA, Shukla AP, et al. Low adoption of weight loss medications: a comparison of prescribing patterns of antiobesity pharmacotherapies and SGLT2s. Obesity 2016;24(9):1955–61.

16. Kaplan LM, Golden A, Jinnett K, et al. Perceptions of barriers to effective obesity care: results from the national ACTION study. Obesity 2018;26(1):61–9.

17. English WJ, DeMaria EJ, Hutter MM, et al. American Society for Metabolic and Bariatric Surgery 2018 estimate of metabolic and bariatric procedures performed in the United States. Surg Obes Relat Dis 2020;16(4):457–63.

18. Butsch WS, Kushner RF, Alford S, et al. Low priority of obesity education leads to lack of medical students' preparedness to effectively treat patients with obesity: results from the U.S. medical school obesity education curriculum benchmark study. BMC Med Educ 2020;20(1):23.

19. Butsch WS, Robison K, Sharma R, et al. Medicine residents are unprepared to effectively treat patients with obesity: results from a U.S. internal medicine residency survey. J Med Educ Curric Dev 2020;7. 2382120520973206.

20. Wee CC, McCarthy EP, Davis RB, et al. Screening for cervical and breast cancer: is obesity an unrecognized barrier to preventive care? Ann Intern Med 2000;132(9):697–704.

21. Dietz WH, Baur LA, Hall K, et al. Management of obesity: improvement of healthcare training and systems for prevention and care. Lancet 2015;385(9986): 2521–33.

22. Coulter AA, Rebello CJ, Greenway FL. Centrally acting agents for obesity: past, present, and future. Drugs 2018;78(11):1113–32.

23. Sharretts J, Galescu O, Gomatam S, et al. Cancer risk associated with lorcaserin — The FDA's review of the CAMELLIA-TIMI 61 trial. N Engl J Med 2020;383(11): 1000–2.

24. Puhl RM, Phelan SM, Nadglowski J, et al. Overcoming weight bias in the management of patients with diabetes and obesity. Clin Diabetes 2016;34(1):44–50.

25. Hebl MR, Xu J. Weighing the care: physicians' reactions to the size of a patient. Int J Obes Relat Metab Disord 2001;25(8):1246–52.

26. Hales CM, Carroll MD, Fryar CD, et al. Prevalence of obesity among adults and youth: United States, 2015-2016. NCHS Data Brief 2017;(288):1–8.

27. Baker EA, Schootman M, Barnidge E, et al. The role of race and poverty in access to foods that enable individuals to adhere to dietary guidelines. Prev Chronic Dis 2006;3(3):A76.

28. Phelan SM, Burgess DJ, Yeazel MW, et al. Impact of weight bias and stigma on quality of care and outcomes for patients with obesity. Obes Rev 2015;16(4): 319–26.

29. Remmert JE, Convertino AD, Roberts SR, et al. Stigmatizing weight experiences in health care: associations with BMI and eating behaviours. Obes Sci Pract 2019;5(6):555–63.

30. Apovian CM, Aronne LJ, Bessesen DH, et al. Pharmacological management of obesity: an endocrine society clinical practice guideline. J Clin Endocrinol Metab 2015;100(2):342–62.
31. Gill H, Gill B, El-Halabi S, et al. Antidepressant medications and weight change: a narrative review. Obesity (Silver Spring). 2020;28(11):2064–72.
32. Musil R, Obermeier M, Russ P, et al. Weight gain and antipsychotics: a drug safety review. Expert Opin Drug Saf 2015;14(1):73–96.
33. Malone M. Medications associated with weight gain. Ann Pharmacother 2005; 39(12):2046–55.
34. Dianat S, Fox E, Ahrens KA, et al. Side effects and health benefits of depot medroxyprogesterone acetate: a systematic review. Obstet Gynecol 2019;133(2): 332–41.
35. Sharma AM, Pischon T, Hardt S, et al. Hypothesis: beta-adrenergic receptor blockers and weight gain: a systematic analysis. Hypertension 2001;37(2): 250–4.
36. Messerli FH, Bell DSH, Fonseca V, et al. Body weight changes with β-blocker use: results from GEMINI. Am J Med 2007;120(7):610–5.
37. O'Neil PM. Assessing dietary intake in the management of obesity. Obes Res 2001;9(Suppl 5):361S–6S [discussion 373S-374S].
38. Trepanowski JF, Kroeger CM, Barnosky A, et al. Effect of alternate-day fasting on weight loss, weight maintenance, and cardioprotection among metabolically healthy obese adults: a randomized clinical trial. JAMA Intern Med 2017;177(7): 930–8.
39. Garvey WT, Mechanick JI, Brett EM, et al. American Association of Clinical Endocrinologists and American College of Endocrinology comprehensive clinical practice guidelines for medical care of patients with obesity. Endocr Pract 2016;22(Suppl 3):1–203.
40. Butsch WS. Evaluation of overweight and obesity. In: Goroll A, Mulley A, editors. Primary care medicine. 8th edition. Philadelphia, PA: Wolters Kluwer; 2020.
41. Adesanya AO, Lee W, Greilich NB, et al. Perioperative management of obstructive sleep apnea. Chest 2010;138(6):1489–98.
42. FDA. Contrave® (naltrexone HCl and bupropion HCl) Prescribing Information. Available at: https://www.accessdata.fda.gov/drugsatfda_docs/label/2014/200063s000lbl.pdf. Accessed April 11, 2021.
43. FDA. Qysmia™ (phentermine and topiramate extended-release) Prescribing Information. Available at: https://www.accessdata.fda.gov/drugsatfda_docs/label/2012/022580s000lbl.pdf. Accessed April 11, 2021.
44. FDA. Phentermine Prescribing Information. Available at: https://www.accessdata.fda.gov/drugsatfda_docs/label/2012/085128s065lbl.pdf. Accessed April 11, 2021.
45. Pi-Sunyer X, Astrup A, Fujioka K, et al. A randomized, controlled trial of 3.0 mg of liraglutide in weight management. N Engl J Med 2015;373(1):11–22.
46. Greenway FL, Fujioka K, Plodkowski RA, et al. Effect of naltrexone plus bupropion on weight loss in overweight and obese adults (COR-I): a multicentre, randomised, double-blind, placebo-controlled, phase 3 trial. Lancet 2010; 376(9741):595–605.
47. Apovian CM, Aronne L, Rubino D, et al. A randomized, phase 3 trial of naltrexone SR/bupropion SR on weight and obesity-related risk factors (COR-II). Obesity (Silver Spring) 2013;21(5):935–43.
48. Torgerson JS, Hauptman J, Boldrin MN, et al. XENical in the prevention of diabetes in obese subjects (XENDOS) study: a randomized study of orlistat as an

adjunct to lifestyle changes for the prevention of type 2 diabetes in obese patients. Diabetes Care 2004;27(1):155–61.

49. Lewis KH, Fischer H, Ard J, et al. Safety and effectiveness of longer-term phentermine use: clinical outcomes from an electronic health record cohort. Obesity 2019;27(4):591–602.

50. Allison DB, Gadde KM, Garvey WT, et al. Controlled-release phentermine/topiramate in severely obese adults: a randomized controlled trial (EQUIP). Obesity 2012;20(2):330–42.

51. Clément K, van den Akker E, Argente J, et al. Efficacy and safety of setmelanotide, an MC4R agonist, in individuals with severe obesity due to LEPR or POMC deficiency: single-arm, open-label, multicentre, phase 3 trials. Lancet Diabetes Endocrinol 2020;8(12):960–70.

52. Mechanick JI, Apovian C, Brethauer S, et al. Clinical practice guidelines for the perioperative nutrition, metabolic, and nonsurgical support of patients undergoing bariatric procedures - 2019 update: cosponsored by American Association of Clinical Endocrinologists/American College of Endocrinology, The Obesity Society, American Society for Metabolic and Bariatric Surgery, Obesity Medicine Association, and American Society of Anesthesiologists. Obesity (Silver Spring) 2020;28(4):O1–58.

53. Sullivan S, Edmundowicz SA, Thompson CC. Endoscopic bariatric and metabolic therapies: new and emerging technologies. Gastroenterology 2017; 152(7):1791–801.

54. Bazerbachi F, Vargas Valls EJ, Abu Dayyeh BK. Recent clinical results of endoscopic bariatric therapies as an obesity intervention. Clin Endosc 2017;50(1): 42–50.

55. Abu Dayyeh BK, Eaton LL, Woodman G, et al. 444 a randomized, multi-center study to evaluate the safety and effectiveness of an intragastric balloon as an adjunct to a behavioral modification program, in comparison with a behavioral modification program alone in the weight management of obese subjects. Gastrointest Endosc 2015;81(5):AB147.

56. Greenway FL, Aronne LJ, Raben A, et al. A randomized, double-blind, placebo-controlled study of Gelesis100: a novel nonsystemic oral hydrogel for weight loss. Obesity 2019;27(2):205–16.

57. Corcelles R, Daigle CR, Schauer PR. Management of endocrine disease: metabolic effects of bariatric surgery. Eur J Endocrinol 2016;174(1):R19–28.

58. O'Brien PE, MacDonald L, Anderson M, et al. Long-term outcomes after bariatric surgery: fifteen-year follow-up of adjustable gastric banding and a systematic review of the bariatric surgical literature. Ann Surg 2013;257(1):87–94.

59. Reduction in the incidence of Type 2 diabetes with lifestyle intervention or metformin. N Engl J Med 2002;346(6):393–403.

60. The Diabetes Prevention Program (DPP). Description of lifestyle intervention. Diabetes Care 2002;25(12):2165–71.

61. Diabetes Prevention Program Research G. 10-year follow-up of diabetes incidence and weight loss in the diabetes prevention program outcomes study. Lancet 2009;374(9702):1677–86.

62. Wing RR, Bolin P, Brancati FL, et al. Cardiovascular effects of intensive lifestyle intervention in type 2 diabetes. N Engl J Med 2013;369(2):145–54.

63. Wing RR. Long-term effects of a lifestyle intervention on weight and cardiovascular risk factors in individuals with type 2 diabetes mellitus: four-year results of the look AHEAD trial. Arch Intern Med 2010;170(17):1566–75.

64. Pi-Sunyer X, Blackburn G, Brancati FL, et al. Reduction in weight and cardiovascular disease risk factors in individuals with type 2 diabetes: one-year results of the look AHEAD trial. Diabetes Care 2007;30(6):1374–83.
65. Curry SJ, Krist AH, Owens DK, et al. Behavioral weight loss interventions to prevent obesity-related morbidity and mortality in adults: US preventive services task force recommendation statement. JAMA 2018;320(11):1163–71.
66. YMCA's diabetes prevention program. 2021. Available at: https://www.ymca.net/diabetes-prevention/about.html. Accessed April 13, 2021.
67. CDC. Medicare Diabetes Prevention Program (MDPP) expanded model - home page. 2018. Available at: https://nationaldppcsc.cdc.gov/s/article/Medicare-Diabetes-Prevention-Program-MDPP-Expanded-Model-Home-Page. Accessed May 5, 2021.
68. Höchsmann C, Dorling JL, Martin CK, et al. Effects of a 2-year primary care lifestyle intervention on cardiometabolic risk factors: a cluster-randomized trial. Circulation 2021;143(12):1202–14.
69. Gardner CD, Trepanowski JF, Del Gobbo LC, et al. Effect of low-fat vs low-carbohydrate diet on 12-month weight loss in overweight adults and the association with genotype pattern or insulin secretion: the DIETFITS Randomized Clinical Trial. JAMA 2018;319(7):667–79.
70. Bray GA, Smith SR, de Jonge L, et al. Effect of dietary protein content on weight gain, energy expenditure, and body composition during overeating: a randomized controlled trial. JAMA 2012;307(1):47–55.
71. Estruch R, Ros E, Salas-Salvadó J, et al. Primary prevention of cardiovascular disease with a mediterranean diet. N Engl J Med 2013;368(14):1279–90.
72. Sacks FM, Bray GA, Carey VJ, et al. Comparison of weight-loss diets with different compositions of fat, protein, and carbohydrates. N Engl J Med 2009;360(9):859–73.
73. Johnston BC, Kanters S, Bandayrel K, et al. Comparison of weight loss among named diet programs in overweight and obese adults: a meta-analysis. JAMA 2014;312(9):923–33.
74. Heymsfield SB. Meal replacements and energy balance. Physiol Behav 2010;100(1):90–4.
75. Catenacci VA, Wyatt HR. The role of physical activity in producing and maintaining weight loss. Nat Clin Pract Endocrinol Metab 2007;3(7):518–29.
76. Jakicic JM, Marcus BH, Lang W, et al. Effect of exercise on 24-month weight loss maintenance in overweight women. Arch Intern Med 2008;168(14):1550–9 [discussion 1559-1560].
77. Magkos F, Fraterrigo G, Yoshino J, et al. Effects of moderate and subsequent progressive weight loss on metabolic function and adipose tissue biology in humans with obesity. Cell Metab 2016;23(4):591–601.
78. Park HS, Lee JM, Cho HS, et al. Physical exercise ameliorates mood disorder-like behavior on high fat diet-induced obesity in mice. Psychiatry Res 2017;250:71–7.
79. Savoye-DeSanti M. The 1 thing diet. Denver, CO: Outskirts Press, Inc; 2012.
80. Acosta A, Camilleri M, Abu Dayyeh B, et al. Selection of antiobesity medications based on phenotypes enhances weight loss: a pragmatic trial in an obesity clinic. Obesity 2021;29(4):662–71.
81. Rubino D, Abrahamsson N, Davies M, et al. Effect of Continued Weekly Subcutaneous Semaglutide vs Placebo on Weight Loss Maintenance in Adults With Overweight or Obesity: The STEP 4 Randomized Clinical Trial. JAMA 2021;325(14):1414–25.
82. Sun EW, de Fontgalland D, Rabbitt P, et al. Mechanisms controlling glucose-induced GLP-1 secretion in human small intestine. Diabetes 2017;66(8):2144–9.

83. Kanoski SE, Hayes MR, Skibicka KP. GLP-1 and weight loss: unraveling the diverse neural circuitry. Am J Physiol Regul Integr Comp Physiol 2016;310(10):R885–95.

84. FDA. SAXENDA (liraglutide [rDNA origin] injection), solution for subcutaneous use, prescribing information. 2014. Available at: https://www.accessdata.fda.gov/drugsatfda_docs/label/2014/206321Orig1s000lbl.pdf. Accessed April 11, 2021.

85. Marso SP, Daniels GH, Brown-Frandsen K, et al. Liraglutide and cardiovascular outcomes in type 2 diabetes. N Engl J Med 2016;375(4):311–22.

86. Cardiovascular benefits of SGLT2 inhibitors and GLP-1 receptor agonists in type 2 diabetes. JAMA 2019;321(17):1720–1.

87. Madsbad S. Review of head-to-head comparisons of glucagon-like peptide-1 receptor agonists. Diabetes Obes Metab 2016;18(4):317–32.

88. Hollander P, Gupta AK, Plodkowski R, et al. Effects of naltrexone sustained-release/bupropion sustained-release combination therapy on body weight and glycemic parameters in overweight and obese patients with type 2 diabetes. Diabetes Care 2013;36(12):4022–9.

89. Wadden TA, Foreyt JP, Foster GD, et al. Weight loss with naltrexone SR/bupropion SR combination therapy as an adjunct to behavior modification: the COR-BMOD trial. Obesity (Silver Spring) 2011;19(1):110–20.

90. Nissen SE, Wolski KE, Prcela L, et al. Effect of naltrexone-bupropion on major adverse cardiovascular events in overweight and obese patients with cardiovascular risk factors: a randomized clinical trial. JAMA 2016;315(10):990–1004.

91. FDA. Guidance for industry on diabetes Mellitus-evaluating cardiovascular risk in new antidiabetic therapies to treat type 2 diabetes. 2008. Available at: https://www.federalregister.gov/documents/2008/12/19/E8-30086/guidance-for-industry-on-diabetes-mellitus-evaluating-cardiovascular-risk-in-new-antidiabetic. Accessed May 5, 2021.

92. Wilding JPH, Jacob S. Cardiovascular outcome trials in obesity: a review. Obes Rev 2021;22(1):e13112.

93. Hiatt WR, Goldfine AB, Kaul S. Cardiovascular risk assessment in the development of new drugs for obesity. JAMA 2012;308(11):1099–100.

94. Melmed S, Koenig R, Rosen CJ, et al, editors. Williams textbook of endocrinology. 14th edition. Philadelphia: Elsevier; 2020. xiv, 1,777.

95. Halpern B, Mancini MC. Safety assessment of combination therapies in the treatment of obesity: focus on naltrexone/bupropion extended release and phentermine-topiramate extended release. Expert Opin Drug Saf 2017;16(1):27–39.

96. Garvey WT, Ryan DH, Look M, et al. Two-year sustained weight loss and metabolic benefits with controlled-release phentermine/topiramate in obese and overweight adults (SEQUEL): a randomized, placebo-controlled, phase 3 extension study. Am J Clin Nutr 2011;95(2):297–308.

97. Gadde KM, Allison DB, Ryan DH, et al. Effects of low-dose, controlled-release, phentermine plus topiramate combination on weight and associated comorbidities in overweight and obese adults (CONQUER): a randomised, placebo-controlled, phase 3 trial. Lancet 2011;377(9774):1341–52.

98. Register ECT. A Qsymia™ CardiovascuLAr morbIdity and Mortality (AQCLAIM) Study in subjects with documented cardiovascular disease. 2013. Available at: https://www.clinicaltrialsregister.eu/ctr-search/search?query=AQCLAIM. Accessed April 18, 2021.

99. FDA approves first treatment for weight management for people with certain rare genetic conditions. Available at: https://www.fda.gov/drugs/drug-safety-and-

availability/fda-approves-first-treatment-weight-management-people-certain-rare-genetic-conditions. Accessed April 11, 2021.

100. Salpeter SR, Buckley NS, Kahn JA, et al. Meta-analysis: metformin treatment in persons at risk for diabetes mellitus. Am J Med 2008;121(2):149–57, e142.
101. Golay A. Metformin and body weight. Int J Obes 2008;32(1):61–72.
102. Levri KM, Slaymaker E, Last A, et al. Metformin as treatment for overweight and obese adults: a systematic review. Ann Fam Med 2005;3(5):457–61.
103. Rea PAT, Anderson Y. Metformin: out of Backwaters and into the mainstream. In: American scientist, vol. 105. Research Triangle Park, NC: Sigma Xi; 2017. p. 102–11.
104. Pereira MJ, Eriksson JW. Emerging role of SGLT-2 inhibitors for the treatment of obesity. Drugs 2019;79(3):219–30.
105. Bays HE, Weinstein R, Law G, et al. Canagliflozin: effects in overweight and obese subjects without diabetes mellitus. Obesity (Silver Spring) 2014;22(4): 1042–9.
106. Ramírez-Rodríguez AM, González-Ortiz M, Martínez-Abundis E. Effect of dapa-gliflozin on insulin secretion and insulin sensitivity in patients with prediabetes. Exp Clin Endocrinol Diabetes 2020;128(8):506–11.
107. Giorgino F, Vora J, Fenici P, et al. Renoprotection with SGLT2 inhibitors in type 2 diabetes over a spectrum of cardiovascular and renal risk. Cardiovasc Diabetol 2020;19(1):196.
108. Heerspink HJL, Stefánsson BV, Correa-Rotter R, et al. Dapagliflozin in patients with chronic kidney disease. N Engl J Med 2020;383(15):1436–46.
109. McMurray JJV, Solomon SD, Inzucchi SE, et al. Dapagliflozin in patients with heart failure and reduced ejection fraction. N Engl J Med 2019;381(21): 1995–2008.
110. Lundkvist P, Sjöström CD, Amini S, et al. Dapagliflozin once-daily and exenatide once-weekly dual therapy: a 24-week randomized, placebo-controlled, phase II study examining effects on body weight and prediabetes in obese adults without diabetes. Diabetes Obes Metab 2017;19(1):49–60.
111. Aroda VR, Ahmann A, Cariou B, et al. Comparative efficacy, safety, and cardio-vascular outcomes with once-weekly subcutaneous semaglutide in the treatment of type 2 diabetes: Insights from the SUSTAIN 1–7 trials. Diabetes Metab 2019;45(5):409–18.
112. Wilding JPH, Batterham RL, Calanna S, et al. Once-weekly semaglutide in adults with overweight or obesity. N Engl J Med 2021;384(11):989–1002.
113. Frias JP, Bonora E, Nevarez Ruiz L, et al. Efficacy and safety of Dulaglutide 3.0 mg and 4.5 mg versus Dulaglutide 1.5 mg in metformin-treated patients with type 2 diabetes in a randomized controlled trial (AWARD-11). Diabetes Care 2021;44(3):765–73.
114. Mosterd CM, Bjornstad P, van Raalte DH. Nephroprotective effects of GLP-1 re-ceptor agonists: where do we stand? J Nephrol 2020;33(5):965–75.
115. Varin EM, McLean BA, Lovshin JA. Glucagon-like peptide-1 receptor agonists in adult patients with type 2 diabetes: review of cardiovascular outcome trials. Can J Diabetes 2020;44(1):68–77.
116. Ryan DH, Lingvay I, Colhoun HM, et al. Semaglutide effects on cardiovascular outcomes in people with overweight or obesity (SELECT) rationale and design. Am Heart J 2020;229:61–9.
117. Brandt SJ, Kleinert M, Tschöp MH, et al. Are peptide conjugates the golden ther-apy against obesity? J Endocrinol 2018;238(2):R109–19.

118. Pilitsi E, Farr OM, Polyzos SA, et al. Pharmacotherapy of obesity: Available medications and drugs under investigation. Metabolism 2019;92:170–92.

119. Smith SR, Aronne LJ, Burns CM, et al. Sustained weight loss following 12-month pramlintide treatment as an adjunct to lifestyle intervention in obesity. Diabetes Care 2008;31(9):1816–23.

120. Gadde KM, Kopping MF, Wagner HR 2nd, et al. Zonisamide for weight reduction in obese adults: a 1-year randomized controlled trial. Arch Intern Med 2012; 172(20):1557–64.

121. Verrotti A, Scaparrotta A, Agostinelli S, et al. Topiramate-induced weight loss: a review. Epilepsy Res 2011;95(3):189–99.

122. Kramer CK, Leitão CB, Pinto LC, et al. Efficacy and safety of topiramate on weight loss: a meta-analysis of randomized controlled trials. Obes Rev 2011; 12(5):e338–47.

123. Anderson JW, Greenway FL, Fujioka K, et al. Bupropion SR enhances weight loss: a 48-week double-blind, placebo- controlled trial. Obes Res 2002;10(7): 633–41.

124. Gadde KM, Yonish GM, Foust MS, et al. Combination therapy of zonisamide and bupropion for weight reduction in obese women: a preliminary, randomized, open-label study. J Clin Psychiatry 2007;68(8):1226–9.

125. Aronne LJ, Halseth AE, Burns CM, et al. Enhanced weight loss following coadministration of pramlintide with sibutramine or phentermine in a multicenter trial. Obesity (Silver Spring) 2010;18(9):1739–46.

126. Toplak H, Hamann A, Moore R, et al. Efficacy and safety of topiramate in combination with metformin in the treatment of obese subjects with type 2 diabetes: a randomized, double-blind, placebo-controlled study. Int J Obes (Lond) 2007; 31(1):138–46.

127. Hollander P, Bays HE, Rosenstock J, et al. Coadministration of canagliflozin and phentermine for weight management in overweight and obese individuals without diabetes: a randomized clinical trial. Diabetes Care 2017;40(5):632–9.

128. Manning S, Pucci A, Carter NC, et al. Early postoperative weight loss predicts maximal weight loss after sleeve gastrectomy and Roux-en-Y gastric bypass. Surg Endosc 2015;29(6):1484–91.

129. Arterburn DE, Telem DA, Kushner RF, et al. Benefits and risks of bariatric surgery in adults: a review. JAMA 2020;324(9):879–87.

130. ASMBS. Estimate of bariatric surgery numbers, 2011-2019. 2021. Available at: https://asmbs.org/resources/estimate-of-bariatric-surgery-numbers. Accessed April 12, 2021.

131. Courcoulas AP, King WC, Belle SH, et al. Seven-year weight trajectories and health outcomes in the longitudinal assessment of bariatric surgery (LABS) study. JAMA Surg 2018;153(5):427–34.

132. Sjöström L, Peltonen M, Jacobson P, et al. Association of bariatric surgery with long-term remission of type 2 diabetes and with microvascular and macrovascular complications. JAMA 2014;311(22):2297–304.

133. Müller-Stich BP, Senft JD, Warschkow R, et al. Surgical versus medical treatment of type 2 diabetes mellitus in nonseverely obese patients: a systematic review and meta-analysis. Ann Surg 2015;261(3):421–9.

134. Schauer PR, Bhatt DL, Kirwan JP, et al. Bariatric surgery versus intensive medical therapy for diabetes — 5-year outcomes. N Engl J Med 2017;376(7): 641–51.

135. Schiavon CA, Bersch-Ferreira AC, Santucci EV, et al. Effects of bariatric surgery in obese patients with hypertension: the GATEWAY randomized trial (Gastric

Bypass to Treat Obese Patients With Steady Hypertension). Circulation 2018; 137(11):1132–42.

136. Wilhelm SM, Young J, Kale-Pradhan PB. Effect of bariatric surgery on hypertension:a meta-analysis. Ann Pharmacother 2014;48(6):674–82.

137. Aminian A, Zajichek A, Arterburn DE, et al. Association of metabolic surgery with major adverse cardiovascular outcomes in patients with type 2 diabetes and obesity. JAMA 2019;322(13):1271–82.

138. Lassailly G, Caiazzo R, Ntandja-Wandji LC, et al. Bariatric surgery provides long-term resolution of nonalcoholic steatohepatitis and regression of fibrosis. Gastroenterology 2020;159(4):1290–301, e1295.

139. Sarkhosh K, Switzer NJ, El-Hadi M, et al. The impact of bariatric surgery on obstructive sleep apnea: a systematic review. Obes Surg 2013;23(3):414–23.

140. Escobar-Morreale HF, Santacruz E, Luque-Ramírez M, et al. Prevalence of 'obesity-associated gonadal dysfunction' in severely obese men and women and its resolution after bariatric surgery: a systematic review and meta-analysis. Hum Reprod Update 2017;23(4):390–408.

141. Peltonen M, Lindroos AK, Torgerson JS. Musculoskeletal pain in the obese: a comparison with a general population and long-term changes after conventional and surgical obesity treatment. Pain 2003;104(3):549–57.

142. Kuruba R, Almahmeed T, Martinez F, et al. Bariatric surgery improves urinary incontinence in morbidly obese individuals. Surg Obes Relat Dis 2007;3(6): 586–90.

143. Arterburn DE, Olsen MK, Smith VA, et al. Association between bariatric surgery and long-term survival. JAMA 2015;313(1):62–70.

144. Carlsson LMS, Sjöholm K, Jacobson P, et al. Life expectancy after bariatric surgery in the swedish obese subjects study. N Engl J Med 2020;383(16):1535–43.

145. Stein EM, Silverberg SJ. Bone loss after bariatric surgery: causes, consequences, and management. Lancet 2014;2(2):165–74.

146. Coupaye M, Castel B, Sami O, et al. Comparison of the incidence of cholelithiasis after sleeve gastrectomy and Roux-en-Y gastric bypass in obese patients: a prospective study. Surg Obes Relat Dis 2015;11(4):779–84.

147. Gonzalez RD, Canales BK. Kidney stone risk following modern bariatric surgery. Curr Urol Rep 2014;15(5):401.

148. Begian A, Samaan JS, Hawley L, et al. The use of nonsteroidal anti-inflammatory drugs after sleeve gastrectomy. Surg Obes Relat Dis 2021;17(3):484–8.

149. Raynor HA, Champagne CM. Position of the academy of nutrition and dietetics: interventions for the treatment of overweight and obesity in adults. J Acad Nutr Diet 2016;116(1):129–47.

150. CDC. Childhood obesity facts 2021. Available at: https://www.cdc.gov/obesity/data/childhood.html. Accessed April 11, 2021.

151. Armstrong SC, Bolling CF, Michalsky MP, et al. Pediatric metabolic and bariatric surgery: evidence, barriers, and best practices. Pediatrics 2019;144(6): e20193223.

152. Bolling CF, Armstrong SC, Reichard KW, et al. Metabolic and bariatric surgery for pediatric patients with severe obesity. Pediatrics 2019;144(6):e20193224.

153. Styne DM, Arslanian SA, Connor EL, et al. Pediatric obesity—assessment, treatment, and prevention: an endocrine society clinical practice guideline. J Clin Endocrinol Metab 2017;102(3):709–57.

154. Kelly AS, Auerbach P, Barrientos-Perez M, et al. A randomized, controlled trial of liraglutide for adolescents with obesity. N Engl J Med 2020;382(22):2117–28.

155. Cardel MI, Atkinson MA, Taveras EM, et al. Obesity treatment among adolescents: a review of current evidence and future directions. JAMA Pediatr 2020; 174(6):609–17.

156. AstraZeneca. AstraZeneca Pipeline. Available at: https://www.astrazeneca.com/our-science/pipeline.html. Accessed April 11, 2021.

157. Company ELa. Lilly Pipeline 2020. 2021. Available at: https://www.lilly.com/discovery/clinical-development-pipeline#/. Accessed April 11, 2021.

158. Opko. About oxyntomodulin. Available at: https://www.opko.com/what-we-do/our-research/opk88003-oxyntomodulin-analog. Accessed April 11, 2021.

159. Nordisk N. Novo Nordisk R&D pipeline. Available at: https://www.novonordisk.com/science-and-technology/r-d-pipeline.html. Accessed April 11, 2021.

Current Evaluation of Thyroid Nodules

Elizabeth H. Holt, MD, PhD

KEYWORDS

- Thyroid • Nodule • Cancer • Fine needle aspiration biopsy • Molecular testing
- Ultrasound

KEY POINTS

- Thyroid nodules are very common and carry a low risk of malignancy.
- Selection of thyroid nodules for biopsy should take place after imaging with ultrasound by an experienced practitioner.
- Fine needle aspiration biopsy on select thyroid nodules provides diagnostic information in most cases.
- For cytologically indeterminate thyroid nodules, molecular testing may provide additional information about likelihood of malignancy.
- Monitoring of thyroid nodules that do not undergo surgery should take place by ultrasound.

INTRODUCTION

Thyroid nodules are very common in adults. Most are benign. Of those that are malignant, many exhibit indolent behavior. Nevertheless, familiarity with evaluation of thyroid nodules is valuable for practitioners in many specialties. This article delineates the steps in evaluation and management of thyroid nodules.

EPIDEMIOLOGY OF THYROID NODULES AND THYROID CANCER

Although up to 20% of individuals will have palpable thyroid nodules on physical examination, about half the adult population will have incidental thyroid nodules evident on imaging.[1] Risk of malignancy in these nodules ranges from 7% to 15%, depending on a variety of risk factors (see later discussion).[2]

Most cases of thyroid cancer, about three-quarters, occur in women.[3] Thyroid cancer had been on a rapid increase in the United States between 1995 and 2008, primarily driven by an increase in the diagnosis of papillary thyroid cancers. During that time, it was the fastest increasing type of cancer among women in the United States and

Department of Internal Medicine, Section of Endocrinology, Diabetes and Metabolism, Yale Medical School, PO Box 208020, New Haven, CT 06520-8020, USA
E-mail address: elizabeth.holt@yale.edu

Med Clin N Am 105 (2021) 1017–1031
https://doi.org/10.1016/j.mcna.2021.06.006
0025-7125/21/© 2021 Elsevier Inc. All rights reserved.

other countries.[3] It is now the seventh most common cancer among women in the United States.[4] Thyroid cancer incidence is now leveling off,[5] and between 2008 and 2017, age-adjusted rates for new thyroid cancer diagnoses were stable. However, overall, there has been a slight increase of 0.6% per year in the age-adjusted death rate from thyroid cancer from 2009 to 2017.[5]

In part, the increased incidence in thyroid cancer is thought to be due to incidental detection of small cancers on other imaging studies. Other risk factors that have contributed to the increase include childhood exposure to ionizing radiation, smoking, and possibly, obesity.[3]

EVALUATION OF THE PATIENT WITH A THYROID NODULE: INITIAL OFFICE ASSESSMENT

Thyroid nodules may be discovered in a variety of ways. Some will present with compressive symptoms. Others will be discovered on a routine physical examination. In many cases, the nodules are found incidentally on imaging studies such as computed tomography (CT), MRI, carotid Doppler, or fluorodeoxyglucose (FDG)-PET scan. Therefore, thyroid nodules are commonly encountered by endocrinologists, but also by practitioners in many other specialties, including internal medicine. Familiarity with the importance of evaluating these nodules, as well as how to perform the workup, is essential.

The initial patient interview should begin with a query about symptoms related to thyroid function. Symptoms of hypothyroidism raise the possibility of benign thyroid nodularity owing to Hashimoto disease, whereas symptoms of hyperthyroidism suggest the thyroid nodule may be autonomously functioning. Symptoms of compression of surrounding tissues by the nodule should then be elicited. Because of the proximity of the thyroid gland to the trachea and esophagus, difficulty swallowing solid food or large tablets may be present. Nodules that cause tracheal narrowing may cause cough, dyspnea, or stridor. Involvement of the recurrent laryngeal nerve or growth directly into laryngeal cartilage is seen with aggressive thyroid cancers and will lead to hoarse or breathy voice or cough.

Risk factors for thyroid cancer are many, some better delineated than others.

Radiation Exposure

Radiation exposure, particularly in childhood, is a well-documented risk factor for thyroid cancer. Radiation exposure must be significant to increase the risk of thyroid cancer. One source of radiation exposure is external beam radiation therapy to the head and neck area. In the 1940s and 1950s, when radiation treatments first became available, treatment of benign conditions, such as acne, ringworm, and thymic enlargement, was common in pediatric patients and resulted in an increased risk of thyroid nodules and cancer in subsequent decades.[6] Although these practices have long been abandoned, patients who receive radiation to the neck area for other malignancies are also at risk. How these individuals should be monitored for thyroid cancer has not been determined.[6] In the aftermath of the Chernobyl nuclear accident in Ukraine in 1986, there was an increased incidence of thyroid cancer in younger individuals.[7]

Whether radiation from dental x-rays is a risk factor for thyroid cancer is controversial. A recent meta-analysis of all published studies of thyroid cancer and dental x-ray exposure concluded that there was evidence for an increased risk.[1] However, the investigators note that the studies evaluated did not uniformly control for amount of radiation exposure. In addition, since 1970, thyroid shielding during dental x-rays has been standard. Also, with the advent of digital x-ray imaging in dentistry in 2011, the amount of radiation exposure required for imaging has been reduced by 90% compared with that required for film images,[8] so study of patients imaged with current methods may show a lower risk of thyroid cancer.

Family History

Familial forms of nonmedullary thyroid cancer (FMNTC) (thyroid cancers derived from thyroid follicular cells, including papillary and follicular cancers) are relatively rare, constituting less than 10% of all thyroid cancers.[9] Nevertheless, a higher index of suspicion should be present in first-degree relatives of those with these tumors. FMNTC is considered to be present if the cancer is present in 3 or more first-degree relatives of the patient.[9] Medullary thyroid cancer (MTC) is associated with multiple endocrine neoplasia type 2 (MEN-2) syndromes, so a family history of MTC or other MEN-2-associated tumors should be elicited.

Iodine Deficiency

In areas of the world where iodine deficiency exists, risk of follicular thyroid cancer is increased. Table salt in the United States has been supplemented with iodine since the 1920s, so iodine deficiency is extremely rare today in Americans. However, diets in many parts of the world outside the Americas remain iodine deficient, including in Russia, Iraq, and Morocco, among many others. Updated information is available at the Iodine Global Network Web site (https://www.ign.org).[10] A history of living in one of these areas may be pertinent when evaluating the patient with thyroid nodular disease.

Metabolic Factors

Observational studies have linked increased thyroid cancer risk to obesity. However, a more recent Mendelian randomization study failed to show a connection with obesity but did show that type 2 diabetes is a risk factor for thyroid cancer.[11] Given the growing epidemic of obesity and type 2 diabetes around the world, the incidence of thyroid cancer may continue to increase if this correlation holds true.

Examination of the patient with a thyroid nodule should begin with the patient sitting up, facing the examiner. (Some examiners prefer to palpate the thyroid from behind the patient, whereas others prefer to do the examination face to face.) Firm pressure should be applied to the base of the anterior neck to adequately palpate the gland. Having the patient sip water will help the thyroid rise and fall with deglutition, in order to evaluate whether the thyroid is mobile (in the presence of substernal goiter or invasive cancer it may not be). For large nodules, the cervical portion of the trachea should be palpated to see if it is deviated laterally. Cervical nodes should be palpated to determine whether adenopathy is present.

EVALUATION OF THE PATIENT WITH A THYROID NODULE
Laboratory Studies

Thyrotropin measurement
The next step in evaluating patients with a thyroid nodule is to obtain a thyrotropin (TSH) level (**Fig. 1**). Although this step is a surprise to many clinicians, it is essential as a branch-point in the evaluation algorithm. Although patients with a normal or high TSH may go directly to ultrasound imaging, those with low TSH should proceed next to thyroid scintigraphy. The rationale for this is explained in the next section.

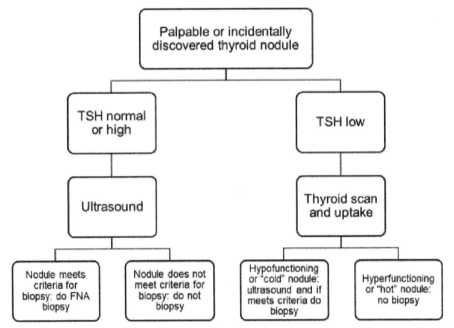

Fig. 1. Algorithm for initial evaluation of thyroid nodules.

Tumor markers

Thyroglobulin, a protein unique to the thyroid that is an intermediate in thyroid hormone synthesis, is used to monitor differentiated thyroid cancer (papillary, follicular). However, in patients with an intact thyroid, this marker is of little value, as its level in the blood will be primarily derived from the normal portions of the thyroid and can fluctuate widely. Therefore, thyroglobulin measurement is of no utility and should not be performed in the initial evaluation of thyroid nodules.

Calcitonin is a hormone produced by the C cells of the thyroid, from which MTC is derived. Monitoring of calcitonin levels in MTC is a standard part of surveillance. Whether calcitonin testing ought to be performed on all patients with thyroid nodules is controversial.[2] A recent meta-analysis concluded that serum calcitonin testing for all patients with a thyroid nodule was not definitely of use in diagnosis, nor was it shown that it would improve prognosis.[12] It is worth noting that only 0.3% of thyroid nodules are MTCs, so it is the rare patient with a thyroid nodule for whom this test would be relevant.

Imaging

Ultrasound

Ultrasound is the preferred next step for imaging thyroid nodules in patients with normal or high TSH (see **Fig. 1**; **Fig. 2**, **Table 1**). In addition to being safe and inexpensive, it provides detailed information about nodule size, morphology, pattern of echogenicity, and proximity to surrounding tissues. These findings are essential in determining the need for biopsy. Currently, there are several guidelines to aid in deciding which nodule to biopsy based on ultrasound criteria. Two commonly used guidelines in the United States are those provided by the American Thyroid Association (ATA)[2] and a committee under the auspices of the American College of Radiology,[13] known as the Thyroid Imaging, Reporting and Data System (TIRADS), criteria. Their ultrasound criteria for thyroid

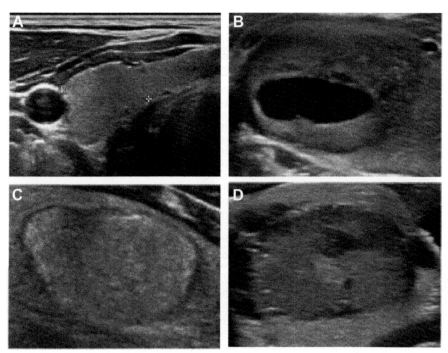

Fig. 2. Representative thyroid ultrasound images. (*A*) Transverse view of a normal thyroid lobe with no nodules (2.2 cm). (*B*) Mixed cystic and solid nodule with tiny bright foci of comet-tail artifact (a benign finding) (1.7 cm). Biopsy was benign. (*C*) Solid isoechoic nodule with irregular hypoechoic border (3.6 cm). Biopsy was indeterminate but surgical pathology showed a follicular carcinoma. (*D*) Solid and hypoechoic nodule with irregular margin and punctate, peripheral echogenic foci suggestive of calcifications (1.8 cm). Biopsy showed papillary thyroid cancer.

biopsy and some sample nodule images are shown in **Table 1**. Although the approaches to decision making in the 2 sets of guidelines are slightly different, both agree on the findings that should raise concern (hypoechoic lesions, punctate calcifications, irregular borders, taller-than-wide morphology), and those that are less worrisome (hyperechoic lesions, simple cysts). The TIRADS classification is simpler to use in that each aspect of the nodule (echogenicity, shape, echogenic foci) is scored separately. ATA guidelines are also notable for recommending biopsy at a smaller size threshold: although ATA recommends biopsy of intermediate risk nodules at 1.0 cm or larger, TIRADS recommends biopsy of similar nodules if 1.5 cm or larger. For lower-risk nodules, ATA recommends biopsy at 1.5 cm or larger, whereas TIRADS does not recommend biopsy unless the nodule is 2.5 cm or larger. In addition, many practitioners are hesitant to follow the TIRADS recommendations that smaller nodules do not require follow-up, which per TIRADS includes mildly suspicious lesions measuring less than 1.5 cm. As with all guidelines, the recommendations need to be interpreted for the clinical situation at hand and based on the clinician's own knowledge and experience, as well as the patient's comfort with some uncertainty.

Nuclear thyroid scan and uptake
Patients whose initial evaluation reveals a low TSH should proceed to thyroid scan and uptake before ultrasound. The purpose of this step is to determine if the nodule in

Table 1
ATA vs TIRADS Classification-

A. American Thyroid Association Recommendations for Thyroid Nodule Biopsy by Ultrasound Criteria (ref,[2] Adapted from Table 6).

Suspicion Level	Risk of Malignancy	Features	FNA if
High	70%–90%	Solid hypoechoic nodule or solid hypoechoic component of a partially cystic nodule **with** one or more of the following features: irregular margins (infiltrative, microlobulated), microcalcifications, taller than wide shape, rim calcifications with small extrusive soft tissue component, evidence of ETE	≥1 cm
Intermediate	10–20	Hypoechoic solid nodule with smooth margins **without** microcalcifications, ETE, or taller than wide shape	≥1 cm
Low	5–10	Isoechoic or hyperechoic solid nodule, or partially cystic nodule with eccentric solid areas, **without** microcalcification, irregular margin or ETE, or taller than wide shape.	≥1.5 cm
Very Low	<3	Spongiform or partially cystic nodules **without** any of the sonographic features described in low, intermediate, or high suspicion patterns	Consider FNA at ≥2 cm Observation without FNA is also a reasonable option
Benign	<1	Purely cystic nodules (no solid component)	No biopsy

B. TIRADS Recommendations for Thyroid Nodule Biopsy by Ultrasound Criteria (ref,[16] Adapted from Figure 1).

Ultrasound Feature	Composition	Echogenicity	Shape	Margin	Echogenic Foci
Findings and Assigned Points	Cystic or almost completely cystic = 0 Spongiform = 0 Mixed cystic and solid = 1 Solid or almost completely solid = 2	Anechoic = 0 Hyperechoic or isoechoic = 1 Hypoechoic = 2 Very hypoechoic = 3	Wider than tall = 0 Taller than wide = 3	Smooth = 0 Ill-defined = 0 Lobulated or irregular = 2 Extrathyroidal extension = 3	None or large comet tail artifacts = 0 Macrocalcifications = 1 Peripheral (rim) calcifications = 2 Punctate echogenic foci = 3

Total Points	0	2	3	4–6	7
TIRADS Level	1	2	3	4	5
Interpretation	Benign	Not suspicious	Mildly suspicious	Moderately suspicious	Highly suspicious
Management	No FNA	No FNA	FNA if ≥ 2.5 cm Follow if ≥ 1.5 cm	FNA if ≥ 1.5 cm Follow if ≥ 1 cm	FNA if ≥ 1 cm Follow if ≥ 0.5 cm

Table 1B. For each ultrasound feature, one finding and associated points are chosen and total points for all features and their findings are tallied to give total points. Total points, their TIRADS levels with interpretation and management are shown in the bottom panel.

question is hyperfunctioning or "hot." Many institutions use Tc99-pertechnetate for thyroid scans because of lower cost, but this isotope will give a false negative result for hyperfunctioning nodules in some patients. Therefore, if an index of suspicion for a hyperfunctioning nodule is high, a scan with Iodine 123 should be requested. Hyperfunctioning nodules are considered to have a very low incidence of malignancy and therefore are not usually recommended for biopsy.[2] However, this recommendation may change in light of recent data, including a meta-analysis showing that risk of malignancy is reduced by 55% in hyperfunctioning nodules, but notably is not zero.[14] Thyroid scintigraphy should therefore be incorporated in decision making when triaging nodules for biopsy that meet criteria for biopsy based on ultrasound findings.[15] At the present time, there are no specific guidelines for when to biopsy hyperfunctioning nodules. Biopsy with cytopathology and molecular testing would be appropriate before treatment with radioactive iodine (RAI) because findings of thyroid cancer would require surgical removal instead of RAI.

Role of other imaging modalities: computed tomography, MRI, fluorodeoxyglucose-PET

CT and MRI rarely have a role in the initial evaluation of thyroid nodules. Unenhanced CT of the neck and chest may be of value in assessing the degree of tracheal compression caused by a large nodule or goiter. CT and MRI are useful in evaluating the extent of known thyroid cancers, such as invasion of surrounding structures and degree of lymph node involvement. FDG-PET has a limited role in the initial evaluation of thyroid cancers, as many differentiated thyroid cancers and MTCs are not FDG avid. Thyroid nodules also may be found incidentally on FDG-PET imaging. These nodules have a higher risk of malignancy (10%–24% in some series) than incidentally discovered nodules on other forms of imaging, but notably most of these lesions will turn out to be benign.[16,17]

BIOPSY AND MICROSCOPY
Fine Needle Aspiration Biopsy

Fine needle aspiration (FNA) biopsy of a thyroid nodule is best performed with simultaneous ultrasound guidance to ensure correct needle placement. A 25- to 27-gauge needle is used. Sampling from the outer portion of the lesion as opposed to the center may yield more viable cells. Cells are placed on glass slides for microscopy and in solutions for cell block or molecular testing (see later discussion). A cytopathology technician who is present at the procedure can stain representative slides to determine if an adequate sample has been obtained for diagnosis, reducing the need to have the patient return on another date for a repeat procedure.

Results of Fine Needle Aspiration Biopsy

Most cytopathologists around the world report thyroid FNA results according to the 2017 Bethesda System for Reporting Thyroid Cytopathology.[18] This system reports

FNA results as unsatisfactory/nondiagnostic (Bethesda I), benign (Bethesda II), and malignant (Bethesda VI). In between benign and malignant are the so-called cytologically indeterminate designations, including atypia of undetermined significance or follicular lesion of undetermined significance (Bethesda III), follicular neoplasm or suspicious for follicular neoplasm (including Hurthle cell neoplasm) (Bethesda IV), and suspicious for malignancy (Bethesda V). These indeterminate diagnoses comprise about 15% of nodule FNA results.[18] They do not reflect a failure to obtain an adequate biopsy sample, but rather represent nodules for which a definitive diagnosis of benign versus malignant cannot be made on cytologic evaluation. Risks of malignancy in categories III, IV, and V are as high as 30%, 40%, and 75%, respectively[18]; however, each institution's pathology department will have statistics for their own risks of malignancy in each of these categories. In the past, many indeterminate thyroid nodules were removed surgically to obtain definitive pathology. Today, thanks to the advent of molecular testing (see later discussion), these lesions can be further classified regarding their risk of malignancy, allowing many patients to avoid unnecessary surgery.

The Role for Core Needle Biopsy

Most thyroid nodules are best evaluated by FNA with cytopathology. There are rare situations whereby a core needle biopsy with a wider gauge needle (18- to 21-gauge) is recommended. This includes rebiopsy of nodules in patients in whom FNA has not yielded adequate material on repeat sampling, and evaluation of patients with suspected thyroid lymphoma, whereby a larger amount of material needs to be collected for flow cytometry and surgical pathology.[19]

Limitations of Fine Needle Aspiration Results in Large Nodules

Biopsy of thyroid nodules has on average a 3% to 5% false negative rate,[20,21] but error rates may be higher in larger nodules. There is concern that biopsy of larger thyroid nodules (typically defined as those nodules measuring ≥4 cm) is more likely to yield false negative results and/or that these nodules are more likely to be malignant than their smaller counterparts. These questions have been examined by numerous investigators, with conflicting results. Some studies whereby surgical pathology was compared with biopsy cytopathology for nodules measuring 3 to 4 cm or larger have actually not shown an increased risk of missed malignancy for these larger nodules.[22–31] In contrast, other investigators found that larger nodules were more likely to yield false negative results on FNA than were smaller ones,[32–36] with the likelihood of false negative results as high as 10% to 20%.

A related question is whether larger nodules are more likely to be cancerous just based on their size. Some investigators found no association between nodule size and risk of malignancy.[24,25,30,37] Other investigators found large nodules were more likely to harbor malignancy. For example, Carrillo and colleagues[31] found that in their cohort of 61 nodules with malignant surgical pathology, 63.9% were ≥4 cm in diameter. Kuru and colleagues[24] found an incidence of thyroid cancer in nodules ≥4 cm of 24% versus 12% for smaller nodules. McCoy and colleagues[32] found thyroid cancer in 26% of thyroid nodules measuring ≥4 cm. Finally, Wharry and colleagues[30] found an incidence of malignancy in thyroid nodules ≥4 cm of 22%.

The investigators who found a higher false negative rate for FNA in larger nodules, and those that found a higher risk of thyroid cancer in larger nodules, recommended surgery for thyroid nodules measuring 4 cm or greater. In contrast, those investigators who found no relationship between size and false negative biopsy or malignancy risk have not advised routine surgery for these larger lesions. With the numbers of studies relatively equal on the 2 sides of this debate, the right approach is unclear and should be individualized. Shin and colleagues[36] performed a large review with statistical analysis of 15 studies including 13,180 patients. Their conclusion was that larger nodules have a higher pretest probability of malignancy and cited a reduced accuracy of biopsy for nodules measuring 3 to 4 cm or larger. They concluded that surgery is a reasonable approach for nodules greater than 3 cm in diameter. The current ATA guidelines[2] concluded that based on available evidence it is uncertain currently whether nodules ≥4 cm with benign cytology are more likely to be malignant and need to be managed differently than their smaller counterparts. Counseling patients with large nodules regarding this controversy is appropriate, so that they may decide whether to pursue surgery if it fits with their approach to medical care and risk tolerance.

EVALUATION OF THE PATIENT WITH A CYTOLOGICALLY INDETERMINATE THYROID NODULE: MOLECULAR TESTING

As noted above, approximately 15% of thyroid nodules will be cytologically indeterminate (Bethesda III, IV, or V) on FNA.[18] Before the advent of molecular testing, these lesions were often removed surgically to allow the entire nodule to be evaluated for the presence of capsular, vascular, or lymphatic invasion, which would indicate malignancy. Most patients would ultimately be found to have benign lesions, and surgical removal would therefore turn out to have been unnecessary. In recent years, molecular testing for these cytologically indeterminate lesions has become common and has prevented many patients from undergoing unnecessary surgery. Typically, at the time FNA biopsy, when samples are collected for cytopathology, an additional sample is collected in a special solution for molecular testing. This sample is processed only if the cytologic diagnosis is in fact indeterminate. There are several commercially available molecular testing platforms today that evaluate nodule DNA and RNA to create a risk profile for malignancy.[38,39] Typically, lesions with low (~3%–5%) risk of malignancy by molecular testing (which is comparable to the risk of malignancy in a cytologically "benign" nodule) can undergo periodic surveillance. Nodules with higher risks of malignancy should be considered for surgery. Decision making regarding surgical referral on the basis of molecular testing results should take into account the risk of malignancy, patient's age, overall health, and risk tolerance.

PREOPERATIVE MANAGEMENT OF MALIGNANT THYROID NODULES
Preoperative Cervical Lymph Node Mapping

Patients with biopsy-proven thyroid malignancy should undergo preoperative cervical lymph node mapping. Although nodes posterior to the thyroid are difficult to assess by imaging before surgery, ultrasound or CT can readily evaluate lymph nodes in the lateral neck. Nodes that appear abnormal by ultrasound criteria should be sampled by FNA with samples sent for cytopathology. A rinse of the biopsy needle in 1 cc normal saline for thyroglobulin testing is also recommended by the ATA,[2] as the measurement of thyroglobulin in the aspirate would strongly suggest lymph node metastases in cases whereby cytopathology is unrevealing. Yhe presence of metastatic disease in the lateral neck is an indication to perform a modified radical cervical lymph node dissection at the time of thyroidectomy.

Active Surveillance Instead of Surgery for Small Papillary Thyroid Cancers

Papillary thyroid cancer is typically a very indolent lesion. Studies on outcomes for select patients with small (≤1.0 cm) papillary thyroid cancers who undergo active surveillance instead of surgery have been very promising, with a very low risk of progression to metastatic disease.[2] Patients who are chosen for surveillance instead of surgery should have lesions that are not adjacent to the recurrent nerve or trachea and do not appear aggressive by imaging or pathologic criteria. They should have radiologic and cytologic evidence of metastatic disease excluded. Evidence of progression on serial imaging should prompt referral for surgery.[2] This approach is appropriate for patients who prefer to avoid loss of thyroid function and are able to accept the notion that they have a cancer that is not being removed. It is also a useful approach for individuals with short life expectancy or for whom surgery is deemed too risky. In these cases, the available data supporting the safety of active surveillance can provide reassurance to the patient and their family that this approach is sound.

Medullary Thyroid Cancer Patients

Patients whose nodule is found to be an MTC should have a preoperative calcitonin drawn, as this will provide information about extent of disease which will guide selection of imaging studies for staging. MTC may be seen as part of MEN-2 syndromes, which also include pheochromocytomas. Therefore, all MTC patients must be screened for pheochromocytoma before surgery, as the consequences of subjecting a patient with undiagnosed pheochromocytoma to general anesthesia can be dire. The simplest method is with a test of plasma-free metanephrines, which is a highly sensitive and specific test. This test also has a high false positive rate, so a positive result should be followed with a 24-hour urine test for catecholamines, metanephrines, and creatinine. Reviewing the patient's medication list for agents that cause false positives in these assays is recommended before testing. MEN-2A is also associated with parathyroid hyperplasia and resultant primary hyperparathyroidism, so screening for hyperparathyroidism before thyroidectomy is also recommended, so that any necessary parathyroid surgery may be performed at the same time. Patients with MTC should also be referred for genetic counseling and consider testing for the causative RET protooncogene.[40]

Referral to a High-Volume Thyroid Surgeon

Once the above preoperative studies have been performed, it is recommended that patients be referred to an experienced thyroid surgeon. Many studies have shown that thyroid cancer surgical outcomes include fewer complications[41] and lower risk of local recurrence[42] in the hands of a high-volume surgeon.

LONGITUDINAL MONITORING OF PATIENTS WITH BENIGN NODULES WHO DO NOT UNDERGO SURGERY

As noted above, it is estimated that cytologic evaluation of thyroid nodules has on average a 4% to 5% false negative rate[43,44] overall. Monitoring of cytologically benign thyroid nodules by ultrasound surveillance is therefore a common practice, and one recommended by the ATA[2] and TIRADS.[13] The goal of surveillance is to detect an increase in size of the nodule, or a change in the nodule's ultrasound appearance that renders it more suspicious in appearance. Nodules that grow significantly or become more suspicious in appearance are recommended for rebiopsy (see later discussion). In longitudinal follow-up studies, benign thyroid nodules grow significantly during several years' surveillance 10% to 50% of the time.[45–47] As noted in the current ATA guidelines,[2] there are no long-term surveillance studies for thyroid nodules beyond 5 years, so there is little to guide how long to monitor thyroid nodules after a benign cytologic diagnosis beyond 5 years. A surveillance regimen starting with 6- to 12-month follow-up ultrasounds, with less frequent intervals as stability is documented, is reasonable. Per ATA guidelines, repeat FNA is recommended for nodules that grow more than 20% in at least 2 nodule dimensions with a minimal increase of 2 mm or more than a 50% change in volume.[2] They recommend that for nodules with very low suspicion pattern, such as spongiform nodules, the utility of follow-up ultrasound for growth is limited, and repeat ultrasound can be done at 24 months.[2] After 5 years, lower-risk nodules with benign biopsy results and lack of growth can be considered for discontinuation of surveillance. For lesions having suspicious features but benign biopsy results and lack of growth, a longer period of surveillance, perhaps out to 10 years, may be appropriate.

Repeat FNA has been studied by many investigators[43,44,48–57] with the majority finding a new diagnosis of malignancy in 1% to 5% of patients, consistent with published reports of false negative rate for cytopathology. The current ATA guidelines state that high-suspicion ultrasound appearance rather than growth of the nodule is a better predictor of malignancy. They therefore recommend that for cytologically benign nodules with suspicious ultrasound appearance a repeat ultrasound and biopsy be performed within 12 months.

At follow-up visits, patients with benign nodules should also be asked about worsening compressive symptoms, which will sometimes prompt them to request surgery for relief of symptoms, regardless of ultrasound and FNA findings. Development of cosmetic concerns are also a reason patients may ask to be referred for surgery.

SUMMARY

Thyroid nodules are very common in adults. They may be discovered in a variety of ways. Risk of malignancy in these lesions is low, but this does not obviate further evaluation. A thorough history and physical examination and laboratory studies should be the first steps. Hyperthyroid patients should undergo thyroid scintigraphy. Ultrasound is the best imaging method for triaging thyroid nodules for FNA biopsy. Cytology on FNA material can provide a highly accurate diagnosis in about 85% of nodules, with the remainder requiring molecular testing for further risk-stratification. Patients with malignant lesions will need additional laboratory studies and imaging before referral to a surgeon. Outcomes for complications and recurrence of disease are better in the hands of high-volume surgeons. Individuals whose nodules are benign should undergo surveillance with periodic ultrasound, with consideration for repeat biopsy if ultrasound findings warrant.

CLINICS CARE POINTS

- Obtain a thorough history from each patient with nodules to determine risk factors for malignancy.
- Physical examination may provide evidence of malignancy.
- Thyrotropin testing will determine if scintigraphy is needed.
- Ultrasound of the thyroid will help determine the need for biopsy of a nodule.
- Cytology should be performed on all fine needle aspirations, with molecular testing on cytologically indeterminate nodules.
- Patients with benign nodules have a low risk of unrecognized malignancy and should continue surveillance with history and physical examination and ultrasound periodically.

DISCLOSURE

The author has nothing to disclose.

REFERENCES

1. Nguyen XV, Job J, Fiorillo LE, et al. Thyroid incidentalomas: practice considerations for radiologists in the age of incidental findings. Radiol Clin North Am 2020;58(6):1019–31.
2. Haugen BR, Alexander EK, Bible KC, et al. 2015 American Thyroid Association Management Guidelines for adult patients with thyroid nodules and differentiated thyroid cancer: the American Thyroid Association Guidelines Task Force on Thyroid Nodules and Differentiated Thyroid Cancer. Thyroid 2016;26(1): 1–133.
3. Kitahara CM, Sosa JA. The changing incidence of thyroid cancer. Nat Rev Endocrinol 2016;12(11):646–53.
4. American Cancer Society. Cancer facts and figures 2021. Available at: https://www.cancer.org/content/dam/cancer-org/research/cancer-facts-and-statistics/annual-cancer-facts-and-figures/2021/cancer-facts-and-figures-2021.pdf. Accessed April 12, 2021.
5. National Cancer Institute. Surveillance Epidemiology and End Results Program. Cancer Stat Facts: thyroid cancer. Available at: https://seer.cancer.gov/statfacts/html/thyro.html. Accessed April 12, 2021.
6. Shulan JM, Vydro L, Schneider AB, et al. Role of biomarkers in predicting the occurrence of thyroid neoplasms in radiation-exposed children. Endocr Relat Cancer 2018;25(4):481–91.
7. Jargin SV. Chernobyl-related thyroid cancer. Eur J Epidemiol 2018;33(4):429–31.
8. American Dental Association. Oral health topics. X-rays/radiographs. Available at: https://www.ada.org/en/member-center/oral-health-topics/x-rays. Accessed April 11, 2021.
9. Peiling Yang S, Ngeow J. Familial non-medullary thyroid cancer: unraveling the genetic maze. Endocr Relat Cancer 2016;23(12):R577–95.
10. Iodine Global Network. Global iodine nutrition scorecard and map. Available at: https://www.ign.org/scorecard.htm. Accessed April 11, 2021.
11. Fussey JM, Beaumont RN, Wood AR, et al. Does obesity cause thyroid cancer? A Mendelian randomization study. J Clin Endocrinol Metab 2020;105(7):e2398–407.
12. Verbeek HH, de Groot JWB, Sluiter WJ, et al. Calcitonin testing for detection of medullary thyroid cancer in people with thyroid nodules. Cochrane Database Syst Rev 2020;3(3):CD010159.
13. Grant EG, Tessler FN, Hoang JK, et al. Thyroid ultrasound reporting lexicon: White Paper of the ACR Thyroid Imaging, Reporting and Data System (TIRADS) Committee. J Am Coll Radiol 2015;12(12 Pt A):1272–9.
14. Lau LW, Ghaznavi S, Frolkis AD, et al. Malignancy risk of hyperfunctioning thyroid nodules compared with non-toxic nodules: systematic review and a meta-analysis. Thyroid Res 2021;14(1):3.
15. Noto B, Eveslage M, Pixberg M, et al. Prevalence of hyperfunctioning thyroid nodules among those in need of fine needle aspiration cytology according to ATA 2015, EU-TIRADS, and ACR-TIRADS. Eur J Nucl Med Mol Imaging 2020; 47(6):1518–26.
16. Abdel-Halim CN, Rosenberg T, Bjørndal K, et al. Risk of malignancy in FDG-avid thyroid incidentalomas on PET/CT: a prospective study. World J Surg 2019; 43(10):2454–8.
17. Kamakshi K, Krishnamurthy A, Karthik V, et al. Positron emission tomography-computed tomography-associated incidental neoplasms of the thyroid gland. World J Nucl Med 2020;19(1):36–40.

18. Cibas ES, Ali SZ. The 2017 Bethesda system for reporting thyroid cytopathology. J Am Soc Cytopathol 2017;6(11):217–22.
19. Pantanowitz L, Thompson LDR, Jing X, et al. Is thyroid core needle biopsy a valid compliment to fine-needle aspiration? J Am Soc Cytopathol 2020;9(5):383–8.
20. Amrikachi M, Ramzy I, Rubenfeld S, et al. Accuracy of fine-needle aspiration of thyroid. Arch Pathol Lab Med 2001;125:484–8.
21. Gharib H. Fine-needle aspiration biopsy of thyroid nodules: advantages, limitations, and effect. Mayo Clin Proc 1994;69:44–9.
22. Bohacek L, Milas M, Mitchell J, et al. Diagnostic accuracy of surgeon-performed ultrasound-guided fine-needle aspiration of thyroid nodules. Ann Surg Oncol 2012;19:45–51.
23. Kamran SC, Marqusee E, Kim MI, et al. Thyroid nodule size and prediction of cancer. J Clin Endocrinol Metab 2013;98:564–70.
24. Kuru B, Gulcelik NE, Gulcelik MA, et al. The false-negative rate of fine-needle aspiration cytology for diagnosing thyroid carcinoma in thyroid nodules. Langenbecks Arch Surg 2010;395:127–32.
25. Mehanna R, Murphy M, McCarthy J, et al. False negatives in thyroid cytology: impact of large nodule size and follicular variant of papillary carcinoma. Laryngoscope 2013;123:1305–9.
26. Raj MD, Grodski S, Woodruff S, et al. Diagnostic lobectomy is not routinely required to exclude malignancy in thyroid nodules greater than four centimetres. ANZ J Surg 2012;82:73–7.
27. Rosario PW, Salles DS, Bessa B, et al. Low false-negative rate of cytology in thyroid nodules >or= 4 cm. Arq Bras Endocrinol Metabol 2009;53(9):1143–5.
28. Shrestha M, Crothers BA, Burch HB. The impact of thyroid nodule size on the risk of malignancy and accuracy of fine-needle aspiration: a 10-year study from a single institution. Thyroid 2012;22(12):1251–6.
29. Yoon JH, Kwak JY, Moon HJ, et al. The diagnostic accuracy of ultrasound-guided fine-needle aspiration biopsy and the sonographic differences between benign and malignant thyroid nodules 3 cm or larger. Thyroid 2011;21(9):993–1000.
30. Wharry LI, McCoy KL, Stang MT, et al. Thyroid nodules (>4 cm): can ultrasound and cytology reliably exclude cancer? World J Surg 2014;38:614–21.
31. Carrillo JF, Frias-Mendivil M, Ochoa-Carrillo FJ, et al. Accuracy of fine-needle aspiration biopsy of the thyroid combined with an evaluation of clinical and radiologic factors. Otolaryngol Head Neck Surg 2000;122:917–21.
32. McCoy KL, Jabbour N, Ogilvie JB, et al. The incidence of cancer and rate of false-negative cytology in thyroid nodules greater than or equal to 4 cm in size. Surgery 2007;142:837–44.
33. Meko JB, Norton JA. Large cystic/solid thyroid nodules: a potential false-negative fine-needle aspiration. Surgery 1995;118:996–1003.
34. Pinchot SN, Al-Wagih H, Schaefer S, et al. Accuracy of fine-needle aspiration biopsy for predicting neoplasm or carcinoma in thyroid nodules 4 cm or larger. Arch Surg 2009;144(7):649–55.
35. McHenry CR, Huh ES, Machekano RN. Is nodule size an independent predictor of thyroid malignancy? Surgery 2008;144:1062–9.
36. Shin JJ, Caragacianu D, Randolph GW. Impact of thyroid nodule size on prevalence and post-test probability of malignancy: a systematic review. Laryngoscope 2015;125:263–72.

37. Proietti A, Borrelli N, Giannini R, et al. Molecular characterization of 54 cases of false-negative fine-needle aspiration among 1347 papillary thyroid carcinomas. Cancer Cytopathol 2014;122:751–9.

38. Steward DL, Carty SE, Sippel RS, et al. Performance of a multigene genomic classifier in thyroid nodules with indeterminate cytology: a prospective blinded multicenter study. JAMA Oncol 2019;5(2):204–12 [Erratum in: JAMA Oncol. 2019;5(2):271].

39. Lupo MA, Walts AE, Sistrunk JW, et al. Multiplatform molecular test performance in indeterminate thyroid nodules. Diagn Cytopathol 2020;48(12):1254–64.

40. Wells SA Jr, Asa SL, Dralle H, et al. Revised American Thyroid Association guidelines for the management of medullary thyroid carcinoma. Thyroid 2015;25(6):567–610.

41. Meltzer C, Klau M, Gurushanthaiah D, et al. Surgeon volume in thyroid surgery: surgical efficiency, outcomes, and utilization. Laryngoscope 2016;126(11):2630–9.

42. Kim HI, Kim TH, Choe JH, et al. Surgeon volume and prognosis of patients with advanced papillary thyroid cancer and lateral nodal metastasis. Br J Surg 2018;105(3):270–8.

43. Dwarakanathan AA, Staren ED, D'Amore MJ, et al. Importance of repeat fine-needle biopsy in the management of thyroid nodules. Am J Surg 1993;166:350–2.

44. Flanagan MB, Ohori NP, Carty SE, et al. Repeat thyroid nodule fine-needle aspiration in patients with initial benign cytologic results. Am J Clin Pathol 2006;125:698–702.

45. Durante C, Costante G, Lucisano G, et al. The natural history of benign thyroid nodules. JAMA 2015;313(9):926–35.

46. Papini E, Petrucci L, Guglielmi R, et al. Long-term changes in nodular goiter: a 5-year prospective randomized trial of levothyroxine suppressive therapy for benign cold thyroid nodules. J Clin Endocrinol Metab 1998;83(3):780–3.

47. Erdogan MF, Gursoy A, Erdogan G. Natural course of benign thyroid nodules in a moderately iodine-deficient area. Clin Endocrinol (Oxf) 2006;65:767–71.

48. Furlan JC, Bedard YC, Rosen IB. Single versus sequential fine-needle aspiration biopsy in the management of thyroid nodular disease. Can J Surg 2005;48(1):12–8.

49. Illouz F, Rodien P, Saint-André JP, et al. Usefulness of repeated fine-needle cytology in the follow-up of non-operated thyroid nodules. Eur J Endocrinol 2007;156:303–8.

50. Nou E, Kwong N, Alexander LK, et al. Determination of the optimal time interval for repeat evaluation after a benign thyroid nodule aspiration. J Clin Endocrinol Metab 2014;99(2):510–6.

51. Oertel YC, Miyahara-Felipe L, Mendoza MG, et al. Value of repeated fine needle aspirations of the thyroid: an analysis of over ten thousand FNAs. Thyroid 2007;17(11):1061–6.

52. Orlandi A, Puscar A, Capriata E, et al. Repeated fine-needle aspiration of the thyroid in benign nodular thyroid disease: critical evaluation of long-term follow-up. Thyroid 2005;15(3):274–8.

53. Rosário PW, Purisch S. Ultrasonographic characteristics as a criterion for repeat cytology in benign thyroid nodules. Arq Bras Endocrinol Metabol 2010;54(1):52–5.

54. Erdogan MF, Kamel N, Aras D, et al. Value of re-aspirations in benign nodular thyroid disease. Thyroid 1998;8(12):1087–90.

55. Alexander EK, Hurwitz S, Heering JP, et al. Natural history of benign solid and cystic thyroid nodules. Ann Intern Med 2003;138:315–8.
56. Albuja-Cruz MB, Goldfarb M, Gondek SS, et al. Reliability of fine-needle aspiration for thyroid nodules greater than or equal to 4 cm. J Surg Res 2013;181:6–10.
57. Porterfield JR, Grant CS, Dean DS, et al. Reliability of benign fine needle aspiration cytology of large thyroid nodules. Surgery 2008;144:963–9.

Decision Making in Subclinical Thyroid Disease

Josh M. Evron, MD[a], Maria Papaleontiou, MD[b],*

KEYWORDS

- Subclinical hypothyroidism • Subclinical hyperthyroidism • Decision making

KEY POINTS

- Subclinical thyroid disease is defined by a serum thyroid-stimulating hormone (TSH) level either greater than or less than the reference range with normal thyroxine (T_4) concentrations.
- Subclinical hypothyroidism may be associated with increased cardiovascular events and death, particularly when TSH level is greater than 10 mIU/L.
- Although recommendations for treatment vary, there is limited evidence that treatment of subclinical hypothyroidism reduces the risk of cardiovascular events and no evidence that it improves quality of life or cognitive function.
- Subclinical hyperthyroidism has been associated with increased risk of atrial fibrillation and osteoporosis in multiple studies.
- Treatment of subclinical hyperthyroidism is generally recommended when the TSH is suppressed (<0.1 mIU/L) with variable recommendations when the TSH is between 0.1 mIU/L and the lower limit of normal.

INTRODUCTION

Despite variable recommendations from professional societies, thyroid function testing has become ubiquitous in modern medicine.[1,2] As a consequence, subtle abnormalities in serum thyroid-stimulating hormone (TSH) levels have become a commonly encountered clinical scenario. Overt thyroid dysfunction is defined by thyroid hormone levels (thyroxine [T4] and triiodothyronine [T3]) greater than or less than the reference range in addition to an abnormal serum TSH level. A significantly more common finding is a TSH level outside of the reference range with thyroid hormone levels within the reference range (**Fig. 1**).[3,4] Although purely a biochemical diagnosis,

[a] Division of Endocrinology and Metabolism, Department of Internal Medicine, University of North Carolina, Burnett-Womack, CB 7172, Chapel Hill, NC 27599, USA; [b] Division of Metabolism, Endocrinology and Diabetes, Department of Internal Medicine, University of Michigan, North Campus Research Complex, 2800 Plymouth Road, Bldg. 16, Rm 453S, Ann Arbor, MI 48109, USA
* Corresponding author.
E-mail address: mpapaleo@med.umich.edu

Med Clin N Am 105 (2021) 1033–1045
https://doi.org/10.1016/j.mcna.2021.05.014
0025-7125/21/© 2021 Elsevier Inc. All rights reserved.

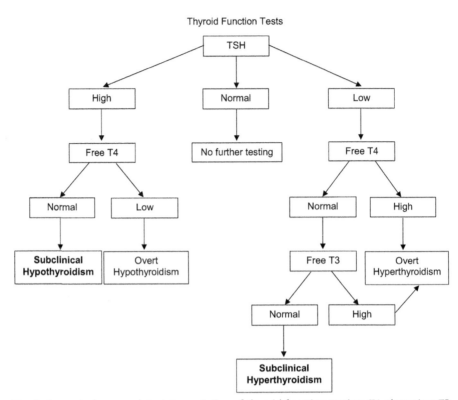

Fig. 1. Suggested approach to interpretation of thyroid function testing. T4, thyroxine; T3, triiodothyronine; TSH, thyroid-stimulating hormone.

these thyroid function test abnormalities are collectively classified as subclinical thyroid disease.

Prior epidemiologic studies suggest that the prevalence of subclinical hypothyroidism and subclinical hyperthyroidism in the general US population are between 4.0% and 9.0% and 1.8% and 2.1%, respectively, with higher rates in women and older adults.[5,6] Although it is widely accepted that overt hypothyroidism and hyperthyroidism should be treated, significant uncertainty remains regarding the management of subclinical thyroid disease. Complementary to previous expert reviews[7–12] we summarize the available evidence on the implications of subclinical thyroid disease and provide a practical guide for clinical decision making and management.

DISCUSSION
Overview

Physiology of subclinical thyroid disease
Thyroid hormone production and secretion are tightly regulated by an endocrine feedback loop in which hypothalamic thyroid-releasing hormone (TRH) stimulates anterior pituitary production and release of TSH, which in turn acts directly on thyroidal TSH receptors.[13] Prior work has demonstrated that intraindividual variations in T4 concentrations are much smaller than interindividual variations, such that an individual's normal range is generally narrower than the reference range for a population.[14] This finding may explain the prevalence of subclinical disease.[7,15]

Changes in thyroid function with age

There has been considerable debate regarding the most appropriate reference range for serum TSH.[3,16] In general, a reference range is determined based on the values found in healthy, disease-free individuals in a population and encompasses two standard deviations on either side of the mean value. With modern immunometric assays, the upper limit of the range for TSH in most laboratories is considered to be between 4.0 and 5.0 mIU/L. Notably, TSH does not follow a normal distribution, and levels vary diurnally by up to approximately 50% of mean values.[2,17] According to National Health and Nutrition Examination Survey (NHANES) III, in a reference population defined as being disease free without pregnancy, taking estrogen or androgen, without detectable thyroid antibodies, and without laboratory evidence of hypothyroidism or hyperthyroidism, the range is narrower, with the upper limit of normal of serum TSH level being 4.12 mIU/L.[5]

In addition, a shift to higher TSH values has been demonstrated with increasing age, such that more than 14% of healthy individuals older than 80 years may have a TSH level greater than 4.5 mIU/L.[18,19] Indeed, the 97.5% confidence interval for serum TSH level in healthy persons older than 80 years increases to 7.5 mIU/L[19]; this is particularly notable given prior studies suggesting that any increased cardiovascular risk associated with mild subclinical hypothyroidism may be attenuated in those older than 80 years[20,21] and that there may be an association with improved survival in those older than 85 years with TSH values greater than the reference range.[22] Taken together, these findings have prompted some experts to recommend age-specific TSH reference ranges.[16,23]

Subclinical Hypothyroidism

Evaluation

The causes of subclinical hypothyroidism and overt hypothyroidism are the same. The most common cause in the United States is autoimmune or lymphocytic thyroiditis, although the differential is extensive.[7,15] Many investigators have, arbitrarily, classified subclinical hypothyroidism as grade 1, or mild, if the initial TSH level is less than 10 mIU/L and grade 2, or severe, if the initial TSH is 10 mIU/L or more.[8,11,15,24] Prior work suggests that in the vast majority of cases of subclinical hypothyroidism, the initial abnormal TSH level is less than 10 mIU/L.[25]

The natural history seems to depend on the degree of initial TSH level elevation. In a study by Somwaru and colleagues,[25] among adults aged 65 years and older with an initial TSH level 4.5 to 7 mIU/L, 46% had normalization of TSH level and only 1% showed progression to overt hypothyroidism over 2 years. Conversely, when initial TSH was greater than 10 mIU/L, only 7% demonstrated normalization, whereas 10% progressed to overt hypothyroidism over 2 years. Therefore, the finding of an abnormal TSH level should lead to measurement of free thyroxine (free T_4). If this value is within the normal range, repeat testing should be performed after an interval of 1 to 3 months, erring toward a shorter interval for those with grade 2 subclinical hypothyroidism.[8,15] It is unclear whether detection of thyroid peroxidase antibodies (TPOAb) changes management; however, several studies demonstrated that progression to overt hypothyroidism is more likely when TPOAb are detected, and their presence provides confirmation of an autoimmune cause (ie, Hashimoto disease).[25–27]

Implications

Cardiovascular disease. Several prior studies evaluated the relationship between subclinical hypothyroidism and cardiovascular disease. Although there are limitations, older studies suggest that subclinical hypothyroidism may be associated with worsening of various measures of cardiac performance, including impaired left ventricular systolic and diastolic function.[28,29] Also, whereas the relationship between overt hypothyroidism and hyperlipidemia is well established, the impact of subclinical hypothyroidism on lipid metabolism is less certain.[3,30] Some cross-sectional studies have suggested increases in levels of total cholesterol and low-density lipoprotein,[6,31] whereas others, including NHANES III, have not shown an association.[32,33]

Perhaps more clinically relevant is the potential increased risk of major cardiovascular events, heart failure, and death.

Several large cohort studies have found no association between subclinical hypothyroidism and cardiovascular disease.[34,35] In the Cardiovascular Health Study, a cohort of adults aged 65 years and older followed longitudinally, there was no association between subclinical hypothyroidism and increased risk of coronary heart disease (CHD) events (hazard ratio [HR], 1.04; 95% confidence interval [CI], 0.86–1.26), heart failure (HR, 0.95; 95% CI, 0.78–1.15), or CHD mortality (HR, 1.06; 95% CI, 0.86–1.30), even for those with TSH level greater than 10 mIU/L.[34] In a separate cohort of adults older than 85 years, despite combining subclinical and overt hypothyroidism, no association was found with cardiovascular or all-cause mortality.[20] A recent cohort study of 9020 adults used NHANES data to evaluate the association between subclinical hypothyroidism and overall mortality. In multivariable analysis, after adjusting for age, sex, race/ethnicity, education status, smoking cancer history, and estimated glomerular filtration rate, subclinical hypothyroidism was associated with an increased risk of all-cause mortality (HR, 1.90; 95% CI, 1.14–3.19). In mediation analyses, it was estimated that cardiovascular disease was responsible for 14.3% of the association between subclinical hypothyroidism and all-cause mortality.[36] Even though this latter study yielded compelling results, risk of bias due to unmeasured confounders, such as obesity and diabetes, cannot be ruled out.

Furthermore, a meta-analysis evaluated the association between subclinical hypothyroidism and cardiovascular outcomes using individual participant data.[37,38] In age- and sex-adjusted analyses, there was a nonsignificant trend toward increased CHD events, CHD mortality, and total mortality. Notably, when stratified analyses were performed, a TSH level greater than 10 mIU/L was associated with significantly increased risk of heart failure (HR, 1.86; 95% CI, 1.27–2.72), CHD events (HR, 1.89; 95% CI, 1.28–2.80), and CHD mortality (HR, 1.58; 95% CI, 1.10–2.27). In addition, a TSH level of 7 to 9.9 mIU/L was associated with significantly increased risk of CHD mortality (HR, 1.42; 95% CI, 1.03–1.95). Age did not impact these findings.[37,38] These findings suggest that grade 2 subclinical hypothyroidism may potentially be associated with increased risk of cardiovascular disease and even mortality.

Osteoporosis and fractures. Multiple studies have evaluated the potential relationship between subclinical hypothyroidism and osteoporosis and fractures. Wirth and colleagues[39] conducted a meta-analysis of high-quality studies and found no relationship between subclinical hypothyroidism and hip (HR, 1.12; 95% CI, 0.76–1.42) or non-spine (HR, 1.04; 95% CI, 0.76–1.42) fractures. An additional meta-analysis using individual participant data found no association between subclinical hypothyroidism and hip fractures (HR, 0.96; 95% CI, 0.83–1.10) or vertebral fractures (HR, 0.96; 95% CI, 0.59–1.55).[40]

Cognitive decline and dementia. The association between subclinical hypothyroidism and cognitive decline is controversial. A recent prospective cohort study evaluated adults aged 70 to 79 years over a median of 9 years using data from the Health, Aging, and Body Composition study. This study found no association between subclinical hypothyroidism and increased risk of dementia (HR, 0.91; 95% CI, 0.70–1.19).[41] Several meta-analyses have also been performed and generally have found no association with increased risk of dementia.[42,43] However, in stratified analysis from one such study, a significantly increased risk was seen in adults younger than 75 years (odds ratio, 1.81; 95% CI, 1.43–2.28).[44] These findings suggest that, at least in adults aged 75 and older, there is a lack of a consistent association between subclinical hypothyroidism and cognitive function.

Treatment of subclinical hypothyroidism: evidence and decision-making. In general, large randomized controlled trials (RCTs) evaluating the effects of treatment of subclinical hypothyroidism on important clinical outcomes are lacking. As a result, it is unknown whether treatment reduces the apparent increased cardiovascular risk associated with subclinical hypothyroidism. A retrospective cohort study in the United Kingdom found that in patients with subclinical hypothyroidism aged 40 to 70 years, treatment with levothyroxine was associated with a lower risk of fatal and nonfatal ischemic heart disease events (HR, 0.61; 95% CI, 0.39–0.95) and all-cause mortality (HR, 0.36; 95% CI, 0.19–0.66), after controlling for age, sex, conventional cardiovascular risk factors, and baseline serum TSH level. There was no association with reduced risk of either outcome in those older than 70 years.[45] These results should be interpreted with caution in view of the retrospective nature of this study and possible unmeasured confounders. Only adequately powered RCTs will be able to demonstrate whether treatment of subclinical hypothyroidism is beneficial in these patients in terms of mitigating cardiovascular risk. Contrary to this study, another retrospective cohort study in Sweden found no association between treatment and risk of myocardial infarction or cardiovascular death, although there was an association with decreased all-cause mortality in those younger than 65 years (incidence rate ratio, 0.63; 95% CI, 0.40–0.99).[46] Although underpowered for cardiovascular outcomes, a large RCT discussed further later in the article found no decreased risk of fatal or nonfatal cardiovascular events in adults 65 years or older (HR, 0.89; 95% CI, 0.47–1.69).[47]

Multiple studies have examined the effect of thyroid hormone treatment on cognitive performance and quality of life measures.[47–50] A small double-blind, randomized, placebo-controlled trial in adults 65 years or older evaluated the effects of thyroid hormone therapy on cognitive function over 12 months and found no significant change in any measure of cognitive performance.[50] Stott and colleagues[47] conducted a larger double-blind, randomized, placebo-controlled trial of low-dose levothyroxine therapy in adults 65 years or older with persistent subclinical hypothyroidism. The primary outcome was change in Thyroid-Related Quality-of-Life Patient-Reported Outcome measure (ThyPRO) Hypothyroid Symptoms score and Tiredness score. Over 12 months, compared with placebo, there was no significant difference in either measure. An additional analysis combined data from this trial with a second similar RCT of adults aged 80 years or older. There was no improvement in either hypothyroid symptoms or fatigue scores.[49] Also, a meta-analysis of RCTs found that treatment with thyroid hormone was not associated with improvement in general quality of life, thyroid-specific symptoms, depressive symptoms, fatigue, strength, or body mass index.[48]

Given a general lack of evidence that treatment of subclinical hypothyroidism ameliorates possible cardiovascular risk or improves quality of life, recommendations for treatment are based primarily on expert opinion. Most guidelines and expert reviews agree that treatment should be initiated in those younger than 65 to 70 years when the TSH level is greater than 10 mIU/L[2,7,11,24]; however, recommendations are more variable for older individuals and when the TSH level is between the upper limit of normal and 10 mIU/L. When the TSH level is between the upper limit of normal and 10 mIU/L, the American Thyroid Association recommends consideration of treatment in those who are symptomatic (eg, with symptoms of fatigue, lack of energy, constipation), at high risk for progression (positive TPOAb), or at high cardiovascular risk.[2] The European Thyroid Association guidelines are similar, although they recommend against treatment in those older than 70 years.[24] Some investigators more strongly recommend treatment in those with TSH values between 7 and 9.9 mIU/L, particularly when younger than 65 years based on observational evidence of increased risk of CHD mortality.[8,51] Notably, a clinical practice guideline published in response to the meta-analysis by Bekkering and colleagues[52] recommends against treatment of subclinical hypothyroidism in most adults with the exception of those with TSH level greater than 20 mIU/L and women pursuing pregnancy.

If the decision is made to initiate treatment, levothyroxine (LT_4) should be used.[2,7,53] As subclinical hypothyroidism is a state of subtotal thyroid hormone deficiency, many patients may not require a full, weight-based replacement dose (1.6 μg/kg/d for the average adult), and starting with doses of 25 to 75 μg/d should be considered, particularly in those older than 65 years or with risk factors for cardiovascular disease.[2,53] Dose adjustment is made every 6 to 8 weeks based on serum TSH values, and the goal is a TSH level within the reference range.[24,53] However, it should be acknowledged that normal serum TSH ranges may be higher in the older adult population, and it is reasonable to consider a target TSH level of 4 to 6 mIU/L in those older than 70 to 80 years.[53] Examples of subclinical hypothyroidism scenarios and decision-making considerations in management are shown in **Table 1**.

Table 1
Examples of subclinical hypothyroidism scenarios and decision-making considerations

Case Scenario	Decision-Making Considerations
Case 1: A healthy 85-year-old man was screened for thyroid dysfunction. He is asymptomatic. Laboratory test results show TSH level 6.1 mIU/L, normal free T_4	The TSH reference range shifts higher with aging, and this result is within the age-adjusted reference range. Treatment is not recommended. Thyroid function tests should be repeated in 1–3 mo
Case 2: A 50-year-old woman with a history of type 1 diabetes underwent screening for thyroid dysfunction. Her TSH level has increased from 4.5 to 7.5 to 10 mIU/L over the last year but free T_4 level remains normal. TPOAb are positive. She feels well	This patient most likely has underlying lymphocytic thyroiditis. She has progressive subclinical hypothyroidism and has an increased risk of progressing to overt hypothyroidism due to the presence of TPOAb. Although data demonstrating that treatment reduces cardiovascular risk are lacking, treatment with levothyroxine should be strongly considered given her age, underlying disease, and degree of TSH elevation
Case 3: A 55-year-old woman with a history of hypertension, on lisinopril, was found to have a TSH level of 7.5 mIU/L with repeat value of 7.8 mIU/L 2 months later. Free T_4 level is normal. She has worsening fatigue	This is a relatively young individual with TSH values greater than the reference range, but less than 10 mIU/L. She has symptoms that could relate to thyroid dysfunction, but are nonspecific. Although there is no evidence that treatment will improve her symptoms or cardiovascular risk, a trial of treatment is reasonable with reassessment of symptoms once TSH level is normalized. An alternative approach is observation.

SUBCLINICAL HYPERTHYROIDISM
Evaluation

As outlined in prior reviews, several clinical conditions and medications can lead to a low TSH level and should be considered before making a diagnosis of subclinical hyperthyroidism.[8,11] In a similar manner to subclinical hypothyroidism, patients are stratified by TSH level into grade 1 (TSH level 0.1–0.4 mIU/L) and grade 2 (TSH level <0.1 mIU/L) subclinical hyperthyroidism. Initial TSH level is the best predictor of the clinical course; although overall rates of progression to overt hyperthyroidism vary by study, the risk is greater in those with initial TSH level less than 0.1 mIU/L when compared with TSH level 0.1 to 0.4 mIU/L.[54–56] Repeat biochemical testing at an interval of 1 to 3 months is recommended to document persistence with a shorter interval favored for those with initial TSH level less than 0.1 mIU/L.[8,57] The most likely cause depends on the patient's age and iodine status; Graves disease is the most likely diagnosis in young individuals and in iodine-replete areas, whereas toxic multinodular goiter and toxic adenomas become more common in older adults and in areas of iodine deficiency.[10,11] Evaluation depends on the clinical scenario. In a patient with classic signs of Graves disease, including a smooth, diffusely enlarged thyroid, thyroid bruit, and/or orbitopathy, no additional workup may be needed. Otherwise, measurement of thyrotropin receptor antibodies or thyroid-stimulating immunoglobulin provides high sensitivity and specificity for Graves disease. If negative, 24-h radioactive iodine uptake provides quantification of iodine uptake and thyroid scintigraphy allows visualization of the uptake pattern; this is particularly helpful in differentiating between hyperfunctioning nodules and Graves disease and can additionally identify subacute thyroiditis, which demonstrates very low iodine uptake.[57] Thyroid ultrasonography is primarily useful when thyroid scan suggests hyperfunctioning nodules to further define the size and extent of nodular disease and for "cold nodules" to evaluate for biopsy.

Implications

Cardiovascular disease
Both population-based studies and a meta-analysis have demonstrated an association between subclinical hyperthyroidism and increased risk of incident atrial fibrillation.[58–62] It is uncertain whether this risk applies generally to those with subclinical hyperthyroidism or only to those with grade 2 subclinical hyperthyroidism. The largest population-based study to date, conducted in Denmark, found that the risk of atrial fibrillation progressively increased with decreasing TSH level, although there was a statistically significant increased risk only for those subjects with TSH level less than 0.1 mIU/L (HR, 1.41; 95% CI, 1.25–1.59).[61] On the other hand, Cappola and colleagues[58] found that in a population-based cohort of subjects older than 65 years, the increased risk remained in stratified analyses of those with TSH level 0.1 to 0.44 mIU/L (HR, 1.85; 95% CI, 1.14–3.00).

Studies on the association between subclinical hyperthyroidism and cardiovascular disease are more heterogeneous. The Cardiovascular Health Study found no increased risk of cardiovascular events or death,[58] whereas other population-based studies have demonstrated an association with increased risk of nonfatal cardiovascular events[35,62] and cardiovascular mortality.[63] A meta-analysis using individual participant data found that when adjusting for age and sex, subclinical hyperthyroidism was associated with an increased risk of CHD mortality (HR, 1.29; 95% CI, 1.02–1.62). In stratified analyses, however, this increased risk was seen only in those with TSH level less than 0.1 mIU/L.[59] Notably, when controlling for additional cardiovascular risk factors, in multivariable analyses, the association with increased cardiovascular death was no longer present.[59] A meta-analysis using individual partic- ipant data found that subclinical hyperthyroidism was associated with significantly increased risk of heart failure events in those with TSH level less than 0.1 mIU/L (HR, 1.94; 95% CI, 1.01–3.72).[37] Last, a recent meta-analysis found no relationship with increased risk of stroke.[64]

Osteoporosis and fractures
Owing to effects of thyroid hormone on bone turnover, there has been significant concern about the possibility of increased risk of osteoporosis and fractures in pa- tients with subclinical hyperthyroidism. Wirth and colleagues[39] evaluated this relation- ship in a meta-analysis of prospective population-based studies. Although limited by study heterogeneity, there was a trend toward increased risk of hip and nonspine frac- tures; however, this did not reach statistical significance. A follow-up meta-analysis published in 2015 used individual participant data and found that compared with euthyroid controls, subclinical hyperthyroidism was associated with an increased risk of hip fracture (HR, 1.36; 95% CI, 1.13–1.64), increased risk of any fracture (HR, 1.28; 95% CI, 1.06–1.53), and a trend toward increased risk of clinical vertebral frac- ture (HR, 1.51; 95% CI, 0.93–2.45). In stratified analyses, there was a significant trend toward increased hip fracture and any fracture with decreasing TSH level.[40]

Cognitive decline and dementia
Two recent studies evaluated the possible association between subclinical hyperthy- roidism and cognitive decline and dementia. Rieban and colleagues[43] conducted a meta-analysis of prospective studies and found a positive association (relative risk, 1.67; 95% CI, 1.04–2.69). Subsequently, the results of the Health, Aging, and Body Composition Study were published in 2017,[41] which was a prospective cohort study of adults aged 70 to 89 years followed for 10 years. This study demonstrated a signif- icantly increased risk of dementia in those with suppressed TSH levels (<0.1 mIU/L) (HR, 2.38; 95% CI, 1.13–5.04) but no association in those with mildly decreased TSH levels (0.10–0.44 mIU/L) (HR, 0.79; 95% CI, 0.45–1.38).

Treatment of subclinical hyperthyroidism: evidence and decision making
Ideally, decisions for initiating treatment in patients with subclinical hyperthyroidism should be based on high-quality evidence demonstrating reduced risk of one or more of the outcomes discussed earlier. Unfortunately, these data are generally lacking.

In their absence, recommendations are based predominantly on expert opinion.

With subtle differences, recommendations for treatment of subclinical hyperthyroid- ism are generally consistent.[8,11,57,65] The main considerations are the degree of TSH suppression and the age and risk factors of the patient. When the TSH level is persis- tently less than 0.1 mIU/L, treatment is strongly recommended for those older than 65 years and for those with or at high risk for complications including osteoporosis, arrhythmia, and heart disease. Owing to lack of robust data, for patients younger than age 65 years without risk factors or symptoms and a persistent TSH level less than 0.1 mIU/L, guidelines recommend that treatment can be considered at the phy- sician's discretion given possible improvement in symptoms and risk of progression. When TSH level is persistently between 0.1 mIU/L and the lower limit of normal, treat- ment is generally favored for those older than 65 years and for those with risk factors. On the other hand, for asymptomatic individuals younger than 65 years and a TSH level between 0.1 mIU/L and the lower limit of normal, observation is generally appro- priate. The specific treatment chosen (antithyroid medications, radioactive iodine, or surgery) depends on the underlying cause and patient preferences. Toxic multinodular

Table 2	
Examples of subclinical hyperthyroidism scenarios and decision-making considerations	
Case Scenario	**Decision-Making Considerations**
Case 1: A healthy 39-year-old woman has had TSH values between 0.3 and 0.4 mIU/L over the last year. Free T_4 and free T_3 levels are normal. TRAb are negative, and she has a normal 24-h iodine uptake and scan. She is asymptomatic	This is a young patient with a TSH level slightly less than the reference range (grade 1 subclinical hyperthyroidism) without an identified cause. There is no evidence that treatment will be beneficial and observation is appropriate
Case 2: A 75-year-old woman with a history of coronary artery disease, hypertension, and hyperlipidemia is found to have a TSH level of 0.05 mIU/L. Repeat TSH a month later is 0.08 mIU/L. Free T_4 and free T_3 levels remain normal. She has palpable thyroid nodules, and thyroid scintigraphy demonstrates toxic multinodular goiter	This is an older, postmenopausal woman with known coronary artery disease. She has grade 2 subclinical hyperthyroidism. Given her age and risk factors, treatment is appropriate. Radioactive iodine is generally the preferred treatment, which would lead to hypothyroidism and the need for lifelong thyroid hormone replacement therapy. Antithyroid drugs can be used, but likely need to be continued indefinitely. Significant comorbidity (cardiovascular disease) weighs against the choice of surgery in this patient
Case 3: A 59-year-old woman with osteopenia is found to have TSH values between 0.2 and 0.3 mIU/L over the last 6 mo. Free T_4 and free T_3 levels remain normal. TRAb is elevated	This is a middle-aged woman with asymptomatic grade 1 subclinical hyperthyroidism. The cause is likely Graves disease. Because she is postmenopausal and has low bone density, treatment should be considered, although observation with close monitoring for progression is reasonable

Abbreviation: TRAb, thyrotropin receptor antibodies.

goiter does not spontaneously remit and therefore many experts favor treatment with radioactive iodine or surgery,[57,65] although it should be noted that thionamides can be used effectively. For those with Graves disease, a trial of thionamides is often appropriate, particularly in young patients. With this treatment, remission may occur in up to 40% to 50% of patients after 12 to 18 months.[66] Alternative options for definitive management include radioactive iodine and thyroidectomy.[57,66] Examples of subclinical hyperthyroidism scenarios and decision-making considerations in management are shown in **Table 2**.

SUMMARY

Subclinical thyroid disease is a frequently encountered clinical problem. Although uncertainty remains, subclinical hypothyroidism seems to be associated with an increased risk of cardiovascular disease and death, particularly when TSH is >10 mIU/L. Subclinical hyperthyroidism has been shown to be associated with an increased risk of atrial fibrillation and osteoporosis. In addition, there may be an increased risk of cardiovascular disease in those with TSH level less than 0.1 mIU/L.

There is a lack of large, adequately powered randomized controlled trials evaluating the effects of treatment of subclinical thyroid disease on meaningful clinical outcomes. Treatment of subclinical hypothyroidism should generally be considered when TSH level is greater than 10 mIU/L and possibly in younger individuals with TSH levels between the upper limit of normal and 10 mIU/L with convincing symptoms, positive TPOAb, or at high risk for cardiovascular disease. In subclinical hyperthyroidism, treatment decisions should be based on patient age, risk factors for cardiovascular disease and osteoporosis, and the degree of TSH suppression. Treatment is more strongly favored for those 65 years and older and for those with or at high risk for cardiovascular disease or osteoporosis. Future studies, including randomized prospective controlled trials, aimed at better understanding the potential benefits of treatment of subclinical thyroid disease would greatly add to our current understanding of this topic and improve our ability to make evidence-based recommendations to our patients.

CLINICS CARE POINTS

- Many factors affect thyroid function testing, and a review of these should be undertaken when abnormal results are encountered.
- Subclinical thyroid disease is defined by TSH values persistently outside the reference range with normal levels of serum free T_4.
- The TSH reference range shifts higher with advancing age, and this should be considered when interpreting results in older individuals.
- Treatment decisions in subclinical thyroid disease should take into account the age and comorbidities of the individual, as well as the degree of the derangement in TSH.

DISCLOSURE

The authors have nothing to disclose. Dr Papaleontiou is funded by K08 AG049684 from the National Institute on Aging of the National Institutes of Health.

REFERENCES

1. LeFevre ML. Screening for thyroid dysfunction: U.S. Preventive Services Task Force recommendation statement. Ann Intern Med 2015;162(9):641–50.
2. Garber JR, Cobin RH, Gharib H, et al. Clinical practice guidelines for hypothyroidism in adults: cosponsored by the American Association of Clinical Endocrinologists and the American Thyroid Association. Thyroid 2012;22(12):1200–35.
3. Biondi B, Cooper DS. The clinical significance of subclinical thyroid dysfunction. Endocr Rev 2008;29(1):76–131.
4. Surks MI, Ortiz E, Daniels GH, et al. Subclinical thyroid disease: scientific review and guidelines for diagnosis and management. JAMA 2004;291(2):228–38.
5. Hollowell JG, Staehling NW, Flanders WD, et al. Serum TSH, T(4), and thyroid antibodies in the United States population (1988 to 1994): National Health and Nutrition Examination Survey (NHANES III). J Clin Endocrinol Metab 2002;87(2):489–99.
6. Canaris GJ, Manowitz NR, Mayor G, et al. The colorado thyroid disease prevalence study. Arch Intern Med 2000;160(4):526–34.
7. Biondi B, Cappola AR, Cooper DS. Subclinical hypothyroidism: a review. JAMA 2019;322(2):153–60.
8. Biondi B, Cooper DS. Subclinical hyperthyroidism. N Engl J Med 2018;378(25):2411–9.
9. Peeters RP. Subclinical hypothyroidism. N Engl J Med 2017;377(14):1404.

10. Carlé A, Andersen SL, Boelaert K, et al. Management of endocrine disease: subclinical thyrotoxicosis: prevalence, causes and choice of therapy. Eur J Endocrinol 2017;176(6):R325.

11. Cooper DS, Biondi B. Subclinical thyroid disease. Lancet 2012;379(9821): 1142–54.

12. Sue LY, Leung AM. Levothyroxine for the treatment of subclinical hypothyroidism and cardiovascular disease. Front Endocrinol 2020;11(824):591588.

13. Jameson JL, Mandel SJ, Weetman AP. Thyroid gland physiology and testing. In: Jameson JL, Fauci AS, Kasper DL, et al, editors. Harrison's principles of internal medicine, 20e. New York, NY: McGraw-Hill Education; 2018. p. 2692–7.

14. Andersen S, Pedersen KM, Bruun NH, et al. Narrow individual variations in serum T4 and T3 in normal subjects: a clue to the understanding of subclinical thyroid disease. J Clin Endocrinol Metab 2002;87(3):1068–72.

15. Peeters RP. Subclinical hypothyroidism. N Engl J Med 2017;376(26):2556–65.

16. Cappola AR. The thyrotropin reference range should be changed in older patients. JAMA 2019;322(20):1961–2.

17. Caron PJ, Nieman LK, Rose SR, et al. Deficient nocturnal surge of thyrotropin in central hypothyroidism. J Clin Endocrinol Metab 1986;62(5):960–4.

18. Bremner AP, Feddema P, Leedman PJ, et al. Age-related changes in thyroid function: a longitudinal study of a community-based cohort. J Clin Endocrinol Metab 2012;97(5):1554–62.

19. Surks MI, Hollowell JG. Age-specific distribution of serum thyrotropin and antithyroid antibodies in the US population: implications for the prevalence of subclinical hypothyroidism. J Clin Endocrinol Metab 2007;92(12):4575–82.

20. Pearce SH, Razvi S, Yadegarfar ME, et al. Serum thyroid function, mortality and disability in advanced old age: the newcastle 85+ study. J Clin Endocrinol Metab 2016;101(11):4385–94.

21. Waring AC, Arnold AM, Newman AB, et al. Longitudinal changes in thyroid function in the oldest old and survival: the cardiovascular health study all-stars study. J Clin Endocrinol Metab 2012;97(11):3944–50.

22. Gussekloo J, van Exel E, de Craen AJ, et al. Thyroid status, disability and cognitive function, and survival in old age. JAMA 2004;292(21):2591–9.

23. Baloch Z, Carayon P, Conte-Devolx B, et al. Laboratory medicine practice guidelines. Laboratory support for the diagnosis and monitoring of thyroid disease. Thyroid 2003;13(1):3–126.

24. Pearce SH, Brabant G, Duntas LH, et al. 2013 ETA guideline: management of subclinical hypothyroidism. Eur Thyroid J 2013;2(4):215–28.

25. Somwaru LL, Rariy CM, Arnold AM, et al. The natural history of subclinical hypothyroidism in the elderly: the cardiovascular health study. J Clin Endocrinol Metab 2012;97(6):1962–9.

26. Díez JJ, Iglesias P. Spontaneous subclinical hypothyroidism in patients older than 55 years: an analysis of natural course and risk factors for the development of overt thyroid failure. J Clin Endocrinol Metab 2004;89(10):4890–7.

27. Huber G, Staub JJ, Meier C, et al. Prospective study of the spontaneous course of subclinical hypothyroidism: prognostic value of thyrotropin, thyroid reserve, and thyroid antibodies. J Clin Endocrinol Metab 2002;87(7):3221–6.

28. Biondi B, Palmieri EA, Lombardi G, et al. Subclinical hypothyroidism and cardiac function. Thyroid 2002;12(6):505–10.

29. Biondi B, Palmieri EA, Lombardi G, et al. Effects of subclinical thyroid dysfunction on the heart. Ann Intern Med 2002;137(11):904–14.

30. Pearce EN. Update in lipid alterations in subclinical hypothyroidism. J Clin Endocrinol Metab 2012;97(2):326–33.

31. Kanaya AM, Harris F, Volpato S, et al. Association between thyroid dysfunction and total cholesterol level in an older biracial population: the health, aging and body composition study. Arch Intern Med 2002;162(7):773–9.

32. Hueston WJ, Pearson WS. Subclinical hypothyroidism and the risk of hypercholesterolemia. Ann Fam Med 2004;2(4):351–5.

33. Vierhapper H, Nardi A, Grösser P, et al. Low-density lipoprotein cholesterol in subclinical hypothyroidism. Thyroid 2000;10(11):981–4.

34. Hyland KA, Arnold AM, Lee JS, et al. Persistent subclinical hypothyroidism and cardiovascular risk in the elderly: the cardiovascular health study. J Clin Endocrinol Metab 2013;98(2):533–40.

35. Selmer C, Olesen JB, Hansen ML, et al. Subclinical and overt thyroid dysfunction and risk of all-cause mortality and cardiovascular events: a large population study. J Clin Endocrinol Metab 2014;99(7):2372–82.

36. Inoue K, Ritz B, Brent GA, et al. Association of subclinical hypothyroidism and cardiovascular disease with mortality. JAMA Netw Open 2020;3(2):e1920745.

37. Gencer B, Collet TH, Virgini V, et al. Subclinical thyroid dysfunction and the risk of heart failure events: an individual participant data analysis from 6 prospective cohorts. Circulation 2012;126(9):1040–9.

38. Rodondi N, den Elzen WP, Bauer DC, et al. Subclinical hypothyroidism and the risk of coronary heart disease and mortality. JAMA 2010;304(12):1365–74.

39. Wirth CD, Blum MR, da Costa BR, et al. Subclinical thyroid dysfunction and the risk for fractures: a systematic review and meta-analysis. Ann Intern Med 2014; 161(3):189–99.

40. Blum MR, Bauer DC, Collet TH, et al. Subclinical thyroid dysfunction and fracture risk: a meta-analysis. JAMA 2015;313(20):2055–65.

41. Aubert CE, Bauer DC, da Costa BR, et al. The association between subclinical thyroid dysfunction and dementia: The Health, Aging and Body Composition (Health ABC) study. Clin Endocrinol (Oxf) 2017;87(5):617–26.

42. Akintola AA, Jansen SW, van Bodegom D, et al. Subclinical hypothyroidism and cognitive function in people over 60 years: a systematic review and meta-analysis. Front Aging Neurosci 2015;7:150.

43. Rieben C, Segna D, da Costa BR, et al. Subclinical thyroid dysfunction and the risk of cognitive decline: a meta-analysis of prospective cohort studies. J Clin Endocrinol Metab 2016;101(12):4945–54.

44. Pasqualetti G, Pagano G, Rengo G, et al. Subclinical hypothyroidism and cognitive impairment: systematic review and meta-analysis. J Clin Endocrinol Metab 2015;100(11):4240–8.

45. Razvi S, Weaver JU, Butler TJ, et al. Levothyroxine treatment of subclinical hypothyroidism, fatal and nonfatal cardiovascular events, and mortality. Arch Intern Med 2012;172(10):811–7.

46. Andersen MN, Olsen AM, Madsen JC, et al. Levothyroxine substitution in patients with subclinical hypothyroidism and the risk of myocardial infarction and mortality. PLoS One 2015;10(6):e0129793.

47. Stott DJ, Rodondi N, Kearney PM, et al. Thyroid hormone therapy for older adults with subclinical hypothyroidism. N Engl J Med 2017;376(26):2534–44.

48. Feller M, Snel M, Moutzouri E, et al. Association of thyroid hormone therapy with quality of life and thyroid-related symptoms in patients with subclinical hypothyroidism: a systematic review and meta-analysis. JAMA 2018;320(13):1349–59.

49. Mooijaart SP, Du Puy RS, Stott DJ, et al. Association between levothyroxine treatment and thyroid-related symptoms among adults aged 80 years and older with subclinical hypothyroidism. JAMA 2019;322(20):1–11.

50. Parle J, Roberts L, Wilson S, et al. A randomized controlled trial of the effect of thyroxine replacement on cognitive function in community-living elderly subjects with subclinical hypothyroidism: the Birmingham Elderly Thyroid study. J Clin Endocrinol Metab 2010;95(8):3623–32.

51. Ross DS. Subclinical hypothyroidism in nonpregnant adults. Waltham, MA: UpToDate; 2020.

52. Bekkering GE, Agoritsas T, Lytvyn L, et al. Thyroid hormones treatment for subclinical hypothyroidism: a clinical practice guideline. BMJ 2019;365:l2006.

53. Jonklaas J, Bianco AC, Bauer AJ, et al. Guidelines for the treatment of hypothyroidism: prepared by the american thyroid association task force on thyroid hormone replacement. Thyroid 2014;24(12):1670–751.

54. Das G, Ojewuyi TA, Baglioni P, et al. Serum thyrotrophin at baseline predicts the natural course of subclinical hyperthyroidism. Clin Endocrinol (Oxf) 2012;77(1):146–51.

55. Vadiveloo T, Donnan PT, Cochrane L, et al. The Thyroid Epidemiology, Audit, and Research Study (TEARS): the natural history of endogenous subclinical hyperthyroidism. J Clin Endocrinol Metab 2011;96(1):E1–8.

56. Díez JJ, Iglesias P. An analysis of the natural course of subclinical hyperthyroidism. Am J Med Sci 2009;337(4):225–32.

57. Ross DS, Burch HB, Cooper DS, et al. 2016 American Thyroid Association guidelines for diagnosis and management of hyperthyroidism and other causes of thyrotoxicosis. Thyroid 2016;26(10):1343–421.

58. Cappola AR, Fried LP, Arnold AM, et al. Thyroid status, cardiovascular risk, and mortality in older adults. JAMA 2006;295(9):1033–41.

59. Collet TH, Gussekloo J, Bauer DC, et al. Subclinical hyperthyroidism and the risk of coronary heart disease and mortality. Arch Intern Med 2012;172(10):799–809.

60. Gammage MD, Parle JV, Holder RL, et al. Association between serum free thyroxine concentration and atrial fibrillation. Arch Intern Med 2007;167(9):928–34.

61. Selmer C, Olesen JB, Hansen ML, et al. The spectrum of thyroid disease and risk of new onset atrial fibrillation: a large population cohort study. BMJ 2012;345:e7895.

62. Vadiveloo T, Donnan PT, Cochrane L, et al. The Thyroid Epidemiology, Audit, and Research Study (TEARS): morbidity in patients with endogenous subclinical hyperthyroidism. J Clin Endocrinol Metab 2011;96(5):1344–51.

63. Sgarbi JA, Matsumura LK, Kasamatsu TS, et al. Subclinical thyroid dysfunctions are independent risk factors for mortality in a 7.5-year follow-up: the Japanese–Brazilian thyroid study. Eur J Endocrinol 2010;162(3):569.

64. Chaker L, Baumgartner C, Ikram MA, et al. Subclinical thyroid dysfunction and the risk of stroke: a systematic review and meta-analysis. Eur J Epidemiol 2014;29(11):791–800.

65. Biondi B, Bartalena L, Cooper DS, et al. The 2015 European Thyroid Association guidelines on diagnosis and treatment of endogenous subclinical hyperthyroidism. Eur Thyroid J 2015;4(3):149–63.

66. Burch HB, Cooper DS. Management of graves disease: a review. JAMA 2015;314(23):2544–54.

Approach to the Patient with an Incidental Adrenal Mass

Xin He, MD, MBA[a], Patricia R. Peter, MD[b], Richard J. Auchus, MD, PhD[a,c,d],*

KEYWORDS

- Adrenal • Aldosterone • Hypertension • Cortisol • Pheochromocytoma • Adenoma

KEY POINTS

- Clinical evaluation, biochemical testing, and imaging characteristics aid in identifying the incidental adrenal lesions that are hormone-producing and/or concerning for malignancy, and therefore require further intervention. Any positive biochemical screening tests or concerning features on imaging should prompt specialist referral for guidance as to appropriate next steps in evaluation and management.
- Cortisol-producing adenomas are the most common functional adrenal lesion, so this should be investigated in all cases with the 1 mg dexamethasone suppression test.
- Aldosterone-producing lesions are common in the hypertensive population. Rather than relying on the aldosterone/renin ratio, interpreting these levels separately enables the assessment of these values in a clinical context. Medication withdrawal before screening is generally unnecessary in the initial evaluation, although mineralocorticoid-receptor antagonists are the most likely drugs to cause false-negative results by raising plasma renin activity.
- Screening for pheochromocytomas is essential, given the profound hemodynamic consequences of a missed diagnosis. Measurement of plasma and urine metanephrines can identify these lesions, but false-positive results can frequently occur, so further testing often needs to be directed by a specialist.
- On imaging, smaller adrenal lesion size, homogenous appearance, lower Hounsfield units on computed tomography, and higher loss of signal intensity between in- and out-of-phase images on MRI, are reassuring features suggestive of benign etiology.

Sources of Funding: X. He is supported by grant T32DK07245 from the National Institutes of Diabetes and Digestive and Kidney Diseases.

[a] Division of Metabolism, Endocrinology, and Diabetes, Department of Internal Medicine, University of Michigan, 1500 East Medical Center Drive, Ann Arbor, MI 48109, USA; [b] Section of Endocrinology, Department of Internal Medicine, Yale School of Medicine, 333 Cedar Street, FMP 110, PO Box 208020, New Haven, CT 06520, USA; [c] Department of Pharmacology, University of Michigan, Ann Arbor, MI, USA; [d] Ann Arbor Veterans Affairs Medical Center, Ann Arbor, MI, USA

* Corresponding author. Division of Metabolism, Endocrinology and Diabetes, University of Michigan, 1150 West Medical Center Drive, MSRB II, 5560A, Ann Arbor, MI 48109.

E-mail address: rauchus@med.umich.edu

Med Clin N Am 105 (2021) 1047–1063
https://doi.org/10.1016/j.mcna.2021.06.009
0025-7125/21/© 2021 Elsevier Inc. All rights reserved.

medical.theclinics.com

INTRODUCTION

The frequent use of cross-sectional imaging in routine clinical practice, including computed tomography (CT) and MRI, has been both a blessing and a curse. The high-resolution images with functional correlates speed the evaluation of symptoms and follow-up of disease, but often the studies identify abnormalities for which the ordering physicians were not searching. The adrenal glands, ~15 g endocrine organs situated superior to the kidneys, are a common locus of such incidental findings. Like the thyroid and pituitary glands, the adrenals are prone to developing benign tumors with age, but as internal organs unlike the thyroid, adrenals are not palpable. Like the pituitary, the adrenal is composed of several cell types. The outer cortex produces steroids, whereas the chromaffin cells of the medulla produce catecholamines, primarily epinephrine. The cortex itself is divided into 3 zones: The outer zona glomerulosa, which synthesizes the mineralocorticoid aldosterone, primarily under the control of angiotensin II and elevated plasma potassium; the zona fasciculata, which synthesizes cortisol, primarily under the control of corticotropin (ACTH); and the zona reticularis, which synthesizes the androgen precursor dehydroepiandrosterone (DHEA) and its sulfate (DHEAS), also under ACTH stimulation.

Tumors might arise from any of these zones or from neoplastic cells that do not precisely mimic a particular zone of origin. Tumors of the medulla are called pheochromocytomas, and the catecholamine excess can cause hypertension and paroxysms of sweating, palpitations, and acute blood pressure elevations. These tumors are rarely malignant, and catecholamine production is typically proportionate to size. However, most incidentally discovered pheochromocytomas are small and thus minimally symptomatic.[1] Cortical adenomas can produce aldosterone, cortisol, a mixture of these two hormones, and rarely DHEAS. Adrenocortical carcinoma (ACC) represents less than 0.1% of adrenal tumors but are highly malignant and often secrete multiple steroids and steroid hormone precursors such as 11-deoxycortisol and pregnenolone.[2] Cortical adenomas that primarily produce aldosterone (aldosterone-producing adenoma, APA) often cause hypertension that is poorly responsive to conventional treatments and cause hypokalemia in a minority of cases. Most cortisol-producing adenomas (CPAs) are difficult to ascertain clinically, but even mild hypercortisolemia can also cause hypertension as well as glucose intolerance and bone loss. When severe, CPAs result in overt ACTH-independent Cushing syndrome and warrant treatment. A variation on the CPA is macronodular adrenocortical hyperplasia, a "goiter of the adrenals," in which both adrenals are enlarged and nodular. Similar to the CPA, these tumors are relatively inefficient cortisol producers and are typically large before ascertained. Lastly, the differential for adrenal masses also includes less common and non–hormone-producing pathologies such as myelolipomas, cysts, lymphomas, hematomas, hemangiomas, and infiltrative diseases, as well as tumors arising from adjacent tissues that grow against the adrenals, such as ganglioneuromas, renal cell carcinomas, and sarcomas of the retroperitoneum.

To summarize, most incidentally discovered adrenal masses are cortical adenomas that are poorly functional. Most commonly, these tumors make variable amounts of cortisol proportionate to their size, and a central part of the evaluation is to gauge how much cortisol is produced and how significant this ACTH-independent synthesis is above the normal, regulated production to the patient's physiology. APAs of any size, in contrast, can cause hypertension and should be strongly considered in any patient with hypertension and an adrenal mass. Pheochromocytomas and ACCs are rare and often large, with distinct imaging characteristics compared with cortical adenomas. Other primary adrenal masses and metastases or para-adrenal tumors complete the differential diagnosis. Most patients in whom an adrenal mass is incidentally discovered will have initial laboratory screening tests and one follow-up imaging study in a year, after which no directed testing is necessary. The purpose of the evaluation, therefore, is primarily to identify the minority of patients with tumors of greater significance due to hormone production or biological activity and to focus attention on these patients in greater detail.

APPROACH TO THE PATIENT

The assessment of the patient with an incidentally identified adrenal mass can be operationally divided into 3 parts. First, the review of the imaging study should be at a level of detail that might not be found in the report. Size is a very important factor, not only in raising concern for malignancy or an uncommon tumor but also as a predictor of hormone (specifically cortisol) production. Imaging characteristics are likewise important, as discussed in the following sections. One must also visualize the contralateral adrenal gland and determine whether it is normal, atrophic, or also nodular—to narrow the differential diagnosis and tailor the approach. Second, the history and physical examination are very important in guiding the direction and intensity of the evaluation. The presence of hypertension might suggest pheochromocytoma, but primary aldosteronism is roughly 100 times more common and should be considered first. Cushingoid features and symptoms should be vigorously probed. Recent changes in weight and control of blood pressure, lipids, or glucose are tip-offs to tumor function, and medication increases are another variable to assess. Third, standard biochemical testing follows, and higher-risk individuals might have additional testing. The screening tests used for adrenal hyperfunction are designed to have high sensitivity, but at the cost of significant false-positive rates. Consequently, the pretest probability of a patient having the disease is critical to the interpretation (positive predictive value) of the screening tests.

Biochemical Evaluation

Why is biochemical evaluation of hormone secretion needed in the assessment of adrenal nodules? Which hormones are assessed? Which adrenal nodules should be screened?
Although the vast majority of incidentally identified adrenal nodules are nonfunctional (produce negligible amounts of hormones), around 10% to 15% are hormonally active,[3] leading to clinically significant consequences. Adrenal nodules can be evaluated for cortisol, aldosterone, and catecholamine secretion, with assessments guided by clinical findings and imaging characteristics, while taking into account relative prevalence and the potential consequences of a missed diagnosis.

Approximately 6% of adrenal nodules secrete excess cortisol,[3] so given this relatively high prevalence, ACTH-independent cortisol production should be investigated in all nodules.[4–6] The degree of glucocorticoid secretion can range from profound, presenting with overt signs of classic Cushing syndrome such as facial plethora, violaceous striae, and proximal muscle weakness, to mild ACTH-independent cortisol secretion. Although physical manifestations of hypercortisolism may be absent, mild ACTH-independent cortisol excess is associated with a higher prevalence of conditions such as hypertension, diabetes, obesity, or osteoporosis, as well as higher cardiovascular and all-cause mortality.[7] On imaging, cortisol hypersecretion is more often found in those with large (>2.5 cm) lipid-rich adrenal lesions or in bilateral disease.[7,8]

Primary aldosteronism (see Chapter "Primary Hyperaldosteronism: Approach to Diagnosis and Management") is the most common cause of secondary hypertension with a prevalence ranging from 4% in the hypertensive primary care population to around 10% to 20% in those with resistant hypertension.[9–12] Although hypokalemia is frequently described as a classic manifestation of primary aldosteronism, most of the patients actually present with normokalemia, so current guidelines recommend screening for this condition in all hypertensive patients presenting with an adrenal nodule.[13,14] On imaging, primary aldosteronism can present as a unilateral and small (typically <2 cm in size) adenoma, as well as bilateral hyperplasia, or with completely normal adrenal imaging.[10,15]

Pheochromocytomas, adrenal tumors that produce catecholamines, comprise approximately 3% of adrenal nodules.[3] Classically, patients present with hypertension and paroxysms of headaches, palpitations, and sweating, but up to 20% might be normotensive.[16] Given the absence of symptoms in some patients and the potentially devastating cardiovascular consequences of missing this diagnosis, many have advocated for screening all adrenal incidentalomas for excess catecholamine secretion.[4,17] However, more recent data have emphasized the importance of imaging characteristics in guiding this decision, finding that lesions with an unenhanced attenuation of less than 10 Hounsfield units (HU) on CT scan are only very rarely associated with a true pheochromocytoma.[18,19] Thus, given the not insignificant risk of false-positive results that arise in biochemical testing for this condition, some experts now advocate biochemical pheochromocytoma screening only for adrenal lesions with unenhanced attenuation of greater than 10 HU.[20] In addition, pheochromocytoma should always be ruled out before adrenal biopsy or any planned surgical intervention given the risk of hypertensive crisis that can occur with manipulation of a catecholamine-producing lesion.[4]

What are the best screening tests to identify abnormal biochemical activity in an adrenal nodule? What is considered a "positive" result?

There are several tests that can be used to screen for excess cortisol production by an adrenal nodule, each one investigating a different potential pathophysiologic defect. Typically, the diagnosis of ACTH-independent cortisol secretion is only made if more than one test is abnormal. The preferred initial test is the low-dose dexamethasone suppression test, which identifies inappropriate cortisol secretion in the absence of ACTH stimulation. In this test, the patient is instructed to take 1 mg dexamethasone at 11 PM to midnight and obtain serum cortisol measurement at 8 to 9 AM the next morning. Various cut-offs have been proposed to identify abnormal cortisol secretion, ranging from 1.8 μg/dL (50 nmol/L) to 5 μg/dL (138 nmol/L) with sensitivities and specificities of this test differing based on the cut-off used. A value of 1.8 μg/dL essentially excludes clinically meaningful hypercortisolemia but is subject to a 20% false-positive rate,[6,21] whereas a higher cut-off of 5 μg/dL is highly specific at the expense of missing some clinically important cases of ACTH-independent cortisol secretion.[4,21] Thus, as an initial screening test, several guidelines recommend using the more sensitive 1.8 μg/dL cut-off as an indication that ACTH-independent cortisol secretion is possible, and therefore, an additional workup is indicated (**Fig. 1**).[5,6] A simultaneous dexamethasone level ensures that the medication has reached the target range for suppression. Other commonly used screening tests, late-night salivary cortisol and 24-h urine-free cortisol, are insensitive for detecting mild forms of hypercortisolemia.[4,6] Rather than additional testing of cortisol production per se, indirect testing for attenuation of the hypothalamic-pituitary-adrenal axis are more useful to support the diagnosis of ACTH-independent hypercortisolemia in a patient with an adrenal mass and an abnormal dexamethasone suppression test. These tests include measurement of plasma ACTH and serum DHEAS, both expected to be near or below the lower end of the normal range but not necessarily suppressed or undetectable.

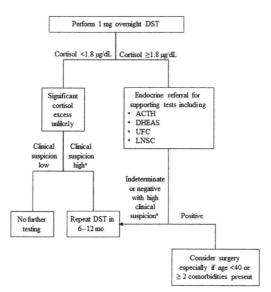

Fig. 1. Biochemical screening for hypercortisolemia. [a]Based on the patient's clinical features and/or if adrenal lesion greater than 2.5 cm. ACTH, adrenocorticotropic hormone; DHEAS, dehydroepiandrosterone sulfate; DST, dexamethasone suppression test; LNSC, late-night salivary cortisol; UFC, 24-h urine free cortisol.

The plasma ACTH must be drawn in the early morning when values are normally the highest, and an ACTH less than 15 pg/mL (<3.3 pmol/L) is suspicious of adrenal hypercortisolemia.[4,22,23] Because DHEAS production from the normal adrenal gland, like cortisol, is ACTH-dependent, chronic dampening of ACTH release due to the heightened negative feedback from a CPA will lower circulating DHEAS concentrations. A very good metric for diagnosing ACTH-independent hypercortisolemia is a significant fall in serial DHEAS measurements over time. Given the multitude of options for cortisol testing, controversy regarding cut-offs and potential pitfalls of each test, any abnormal result should prompt a referral to endocrinology for further evaluation.

Screening for primary aldosteronism consists of measuring serum aldosterone and plasma renin (**Fig. 2**). Although many antihypertensives influence the renin-angiotensin-aldosterone axis, medication withdrawal is generally unnecessary. A positive case-detection test includes a suppressed plasma renin activity less than 1 ng/mL/h or direct renin less than 10 pg/mL and a serum aldosterone ≥10 ng/dL (277 pmol/L).[24,25] These tests should be drawn simultaneously in the morning after the patient has been ambulatory for about 2 hours. Rather than using aldosterone-to-renin ratios, we advocate for interpreting the plasma renin and serum aldosterone levels in a clinical context, which includes consideration of their antihypertensive regimen and serum potassium level. Resistant hypertension and hypokalemia raise the pretest probability of primary aldosteronism; however, hypokalemia attenuates aldosterone production even from tumors and can cause false-negative screens, so hypokalemia should be corrected before testing. Elevation of plasma renin because of antihypertensives (such as calcium channel blockers, angiotensin-converting enzyme inhibitors, angiotensin receptor blockers, other vasodilators) or diuretics, particularly mineralocorticoid receptor antagonists (spironolactone and eplerenone), is a second major cause of false-negative screens, but simultaneously elevated aldosterone is a

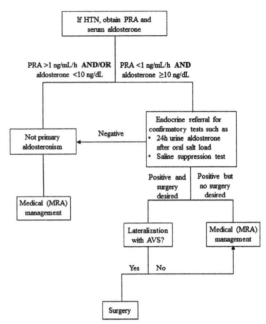

Fig. 2. Biochemical screening for primary aldosteronism. AVS, adrenal vein sampling; MRA, mineralocorticoid receptor antagonist; PRA, plasma renin activity, or direct renin—PRA of 1 ng/mL/h ∼ direct renin of 10 pg/mL.

clue to a medication effect, which warrants repeat screening after medication withdrawal. False-positive tests, in contrast, are rare when the aldosterone and renin are interpreted sequentially and not only assessed together as the aldosterone-to-renin ratio. As with other cases of potential hormonal hypersecretion, a positive screening test warrants referral to an endocrinologist for confirmatory testing.

Patients with pheochromocytomas reliably demonstrate elevated levels of metanephrines in a 24-h urine specimen or in the plasma (**Fig. 3**). Plasma metanephrines are perhaps simpler to obtain in the primary care setting but are not usually drawn in the ideal way (supine after an indwelling catheter has been in place for 30 minutes) and so are often plagued by false-positive results.[17] In particular, the stress of a venipuncture frequently results in activation of the sympathetic nervous system and slight elevations of plasma normetanephrine, up to twice the upper limit of normal. As a result, approximately 3 out of 4 patients with an incidentaloma who have positive plasma metanephrines do not end up having a true pheochromocytoma.[26] In addition, the normal range of normetanephrines observed in individuals with essential hypertension are higher than those without the condition. Despite these limitations, elevations of either plasma normetanephrines or metanephrines >3 to 4 times the upper limit of normal[4,17] or any elevation of both metanephrines and normetanephrines[17] increases suspicion of a true catecholamine-producing tumor. Although antihypertensive agents do not need to be held, psychiatric drugs that block catecholamine reuptake (most commonly tricyclic antidepressants and selective serotonin or norepinephrine reuptake inhibitors) and high doses of adrenergic agonists will interfere with these assays and so should be tapered and discontinued at least 2 weeks before testing.[17] If pheochromocytoma cannot be excluded from initial screening, an endocrinologist should complete the evaluation with additional testing on an individualized basis according

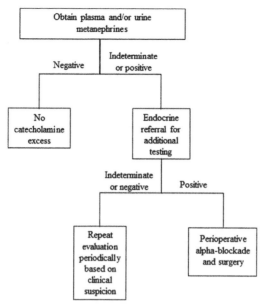

Fig. 3. Biochemical screening for pheochromocytoma. Recommend screening all adrenal nodules for pheochromocytoma, although future guidelines might only recommend screening if the nodule density is >10 HU.

to the degree of clinical suspicion. Options for additional testing that specialists may pursue include repeating the biochemical testing (immediately or a few months later), obtaining a supine plasma sample or a 24-h urine collection (if not obtained previously), checking for elevated chromogranin A, performing a clonidine suppression test, or obtaining additional imaging.[17] To avoid false-positive results in patients with a low index of suspicion, 24-h urine metanephrines can be used as the initial screen when feasible. In addition to the aforementioned medications as well as transient stress, the main causes of false-positive urine metanephrines are sleep apnea and clonidine withdrawal, which can occur within hours even despite consistent dosing schedules.

What are the potential pitfalls of these screening tests?
There are potential drawbacks to each of the screening tests for ACTH-independent hypercortisolemia, so these factors need to be taken into account when performing these tests (**Table 1**). Various medications can alter dexamethasone metabolism through induction or inhibition of cytochrome P450 3A4, and rapid dexamethasone clearance leads to inadequate suppression of ACTH and ultimately a false-positive result. Measuring dexamethasone levels can help identify those situations and aid in the correct interpretation of the cortisol results; alternatively, a larger dose of dexamethasone (3 mg) to assure ACTH suppression can be used.[27] In addition, the cortisol assay measures total cortisol levels, and about 90% of cortisol is protein-bound and biologically inactive. Alterations in corticosteroid-binding globulin and albumin may lead to artificially higher (ie, in women taking estrogen-containing contraception pills) or lower levels (ie, in those with nephrotic syndrome or hypoalbuminemia). Measurement of free cortisol in the saliva avoids this problem but may not be interpretable in a shift worker whose circadian rhythm is altered. Last, urine-free cortisol levels can be

Table 1
Potential sources of error in biochemical testing

Test	Causes of False Positives	Causes of False Negatives

Dexamethasone suppression test	Drugs that increase dexamethasone metabolism
	  Antiepileptics
	  Pioglitazone
	  Rifampin
	Increased CBG
	  Estrogen (ie, OCPs, pregnancy)
		Drugs that impair dexamethasone metabolism
		  Aprepitant
		  Cimetidine
		  Diltiazem
		  Fluoxetine
		  Itraconazole
		  Ritonavir
		Decreased CBG
		  Nephrotic syndrome
		  Critical illness
		  Malnutrition
		  Liver disease

Salivary cortisol	Contamination by topical steroids Licorice ingestion Shift workers Tobacco use	
Urine free cortisol	>5 L/d fluid intake	CrCl <60 mL/min Cyclic CS Mild forms of hypercortisolism

Metanephrines	Drugs
	  Amphetamines
	  Buspirone
	  Decongestants
	  Ethanol
	  Levodopa
	  Prochlorperazine
	  SNRIs
	  TCAs
	  Withdrawal from clonidine
	Acute illness and/or hospitalization
	Autonomic dysfunction
	Hemodialysis (plasma)
		Reduced renal filtration (urine)

Plasma Renin Activity	Direct renin inhibitors	ACEi/ARB Diuretics Mineralocorticoid receptor antagonists Pregnancy Sodium restriction
Aldosterone	Hyperkalemia	Hypokalemia

Abbreviations: ACEi, angiotensin-converting enzyme inhibitor; ARB, angiotensin II receptor blocker; CBG, cortisol-binding globulin; CrCl, creatinine clearance; CS, Cushing's syndrome; OCP, oral contraceptives; TCA, tricyclic antidepressants.
Sources[6,25,63]

elevated in cases of high fluid intake (>5 L/d) or depressed if renal impairment is present.

Although the testing for primary aldosteronism can be influenced by many classes of antihypertensive agents, initial screening can usually be attempted without making changes to a patient's medical regimen. The mechanism of most antihypertensives is either volume depletion or vasodilation, which raises plasma renin and subsequently aldosterone. In contrast, beta-blockers lower renin, but also lower aldosterone. Consequently, screening results are always interpretable as long as the plasma renin is suppressed.[28] This principle is true even for patients taking mineralocorticoids receptor antagonists such as spironolactone and eplerenone.[29] However, if plasma renin is not suppressed, potentially interfering medications should be held for 2 to 4 weeks, hypokalemia corrected and salt intake liberalized.[30] Alternative antihypertensives that do not impact aldosterone and renin levels include alpha-antagonists, calcium channel blockers, and hydralazine, so these agents can be used to control blood pressures while other agents are withheld.[14] (See Chapter "Primary Hyperaldosteronism: Approach to Diagnosis and Management" for more information on the evaluation of hyperaldosteronism.)

As alluded to previously, while antihypertensive agents can and should be continued, certain psychoactive medications and stimulants will impact the measurement of plasma and urine metanephrines, so these should be tapered and discontinued a few weeks before testing (see **Table 1**).

Once a patient screens positive for hormone secretion, what are the next steps in diagnosis and management?

Although surgery is the standard of care treatment of overt Cushing syndrome, management of mild ACTH-independent cortisol secretion, often referred to as "subclinical Cushing's" is less straightforward. Several recent studies found increased morbidity and mortality in patients with mild ACTH-independent cortisol secretion, presumably due to hypertension, glucose intolerance, and dyslipidemia. Although several small studies have shown improvements in glycemia, blood pressure, and dyslipidemia after surgical resection of a CPA, clear evidence of a mortality benefit from treatment has not been demonstrated.[31–37] Thus, given the relatively low-quality evidence available thus far, current guidelines do not unequivocally favor surgical management for all patients with mild ACTH-independent hypercortisolemia. Instead, it is best to take an individualized approach to management with more serious consideration of surgery in those likely to derive the most benefit such as younger patients (<40 years) or those with multiple cortisol-mediated comorbidities, especially if any are progressive or uncontrolled.[5] If surgery is pursued, glucocorticoid replacement might be necessary perioperatively given the risk of contralateral adrenal suppression and transient postoperative adrenal insufficiency.[38] Patients with postoperative adrenal insufficiency are difficult to identify from preoperative laboratory testing but might be ascertained from a cosyntropin stimulation test on the first postoperative day.[39] If there is clinical equipoise regarding the diagnosis, continued biochemical monitoring can be pursued annually for up to 5 years, because while hypercortisolism can manifest over time, it does not typically progress to overt Cushing syndrome.[4,40,41] Medical management of hypertension with spironolactone is generally successful, and a variety of glucose-lowering agents can be used to control diabetes. However, the other consequences of hypercortisolemia, including the catabolic features, require additional targeted therapies that carry either high cost or significant risks.[42]

Once a patient screens positive for primary aldosteronism, endocrinologists will often confirm the diagnosis by demonstrating lack of normal aldosterone suppression after salt loading (see Chapter "Primary Hyperaldosteronism: Approach to Diagnosis and Management"). Most commonly this is done by collecting a 24-h urine sample after 3 days of oral salt loading, but some centers administer 2 L saline intravenously over 4 hours and measure serum aldosterone instead. Spontaneous hypokalemia coupled with a completely suppressed plasma renin and an aldosterone level greater than 20 ng/dL is diagnostic of this condition and so does not require additional confirmatory testing.[14] The most common forms of primary aldosteronism are a unilateral APA, which is surgically curable, or bilateral hyperaldosteronism, which is medically managed.[43,44] Thus, if a patient is an appropriate and willing surgical candidate, adrenal vein sampling is recommended to determine whether this is unilateral or bilateral disease, as adrenal imaging is unreliable in making this distinction and determining lateralization.[45] Furthermore, an imaged adenoma in a patient with primary aldosteronism might not be the source of aldosterone, even when adrenal vein sampling lateralizes to the adrenal with the tumor.[46] Given the technical challenges associated with this procedure, this should be done in a tertiary care center by an experienced interventional radiologist.[47] If the patient is not a surgical candidate, all forms of primary aldosteronism can be managed medically with spironolactone titrated every 4 to 8 weeks until blood pressure and serum potassium normalize and the plasma renin is no longer suppressed.[25] Eplerenone can be used instead if adverse effects such as menstrual irregularity or gynecomastia develop with spironolactone.

If an adrenal mass is consistent with pheochromocytoma based on biochemical and imaging findings, surgical resection is indicated. To avoid intraoperative hemodynamic instability and crisis, patients need to be prepared for surgery a few weeks before with a combination of alpha-adrenergic blockers such as phenoxybenzamine or doxazosin, followed by beta-blockade until blood pressures and heart rates normalize. To offset the orthostasis often induced by medical therapy, patients are encouraged to liberalize their sodium (>5 g/d) and fluid intake (>2.5 L/d) as well.[20]

Imaging Evaluation

What are typical imaging modalities used to evaluate adrenal nodules? What imaging characteristics are concerning?

CT and MRI are the most common cross-sectional imaging modalities that identify incidental adrenal lesions and can also further characterize adrenal masses. Several features on CT and MRI have been identified that help distinguish between benign and malignant lesions (**Table 2**). In general, benign tumors are smaller, homogenous, have lower HU on precontrast CT images and loss of signal intensity between in- and out-of-phase images on MRI.

Nodule size is important, with larger or growing lesions more concerning for malignancy[48] and more likely to show hyperfunction. Specifically, lesions larger than 4 cm in patients without prior history of cancer are associated with a higher probability of ACC.[49] Several society guidelines recommend surgical resection for masses greater than 4 cm, with or without other concerning radiologic features.[4,5,50] Some exceptions to this size limit include myelolipomas, which are benign tumors identified by the presence of macroscopic fat in the tumor, and tumors that have not enlarged over many months of careful surveillance—an approach often chosen for patients at high risk for surgical complications. Meanwhile, lesions smaller than 4 cm with benign features can often be monitored with follow-up imaging, unless significant hormone production is found. Size stability over 6 to 12 months makes malignancy unlikely.

The preferred imaging scan to characterize an otherwise identified adrenal tumor is a triphasic CT scan without and with contrast, plus a washout scan. The CT images

Table 2		
Imaging characteristics of benign versus suspicious or indeterminate adrenal tumors		
Imaging Feature	Benign Lesions	Suspicious or Indeterminate Lesions
Size	<4 cm	>4 cm
	Size stability over time	Size increase over time
CT	Homogeneous	Heterogeneous
	Regular margins	Irregular margins
	Presence of macroscopic fat	Presence of necrosis or hemorrhage
	Hounsfield units $\leq$10	Hounsfield units >10
	Relative washout $\geq$40%	Relative washout <40%
	Absolute washout $\geq$60%	Absolute washout <60%
MRI	Homogeneous, regular margins	Heterogeneous, irregular margins
	Loss of intensity	No loss of intensity
	between in-phase	between in-phase
	and out-of-phase imaging	and out-of-phase imaging
PET	Low ratio of adrenal	High ratio of adrenal
	SUV_{max} to liver SUV_{max}	SUV_{max} to liver SUV_{max}
	or SUV_{mean}	or SUV_{mean}

Absolute washout is calculated as follows: $(HU_{postcontrast} - HU_{washout})/(HU_{postcontrast} - HU_{precontrast})$.
Relative washout is calculated as follows: $(HU_{postcontrast} - HU_{washout})/(HU_{postcontrast})$.

without contrast assess the density of tissues in the body compared to water, which is allocated the tissue attenuation value of 0 measured in HU. HU are only meaningful in homogenous lesions, as heterogeneous lesions by definition have various attenuations in different regions of the tumor. Of note, noncontrast CT images are required for interpretation of HU; HU of adrenal lesions incidentally found on contrast-enhanced scans alone cannot be interpreted. Most benign adrenal adenomas are lipid-rich, have homogenous appearance, regular borders, and low Hounsfield units on CT. The conventional cut-off of $\leq$10 HU is 71% sensitive and 98% specific for benign lipid-rich adenomas.[51] In fact, some guidelines state that tumors less than 4 cm in size, homogenous, and have HU $\leq$10 are benign, and no further imaging is required.[5]

Upon administration of contrast, the HU of the lesion are measured at 2 time points: about 5 minutes, corresponding to peak enhancement, and 15 minutes during washout. These values are used to calculate the relative and absolute contrast enhancement washout percentages. Benign tumors have faster washout compared with malignant tumors. A relative washout of $\geq$40% and an absolute washout $\geq$60% are associated with benign tumors.[52,53] The converse, however, is not always true; benign pheochromocytomas and some cortical adenomas can demonstrate delayed contrast washout.

The MRI technique of chemical shift imaging has also been used, which relies on the differences in resonance frequencies of proton nuclei for water and lipid molecules in a magnetic field, because of their distinct chemical environments. When the signal intensity is compared with the in-phase images, lipid-rich adenomas have loss of signal intensity on the out-of-phase images, whereas malignant tumors or pheochromocytomas do not.[54,55] Owing to the lack of standardization in MRI techniques and measurements, this imaging modality is generally less preferred but avoids ionizing radiation.

When should I monitor adrenal nodules with repeat imaging versus refer to a specialist?

The European Society of Endocrinology clinical practice guidelines recommend that for nonfunctioning adrenal nodules that are less than 4 cm in size, homogenous, and have a density of ≤10 HU on noncontrast CT, no further evaluation or follow-up imaging is needed.[5] Nevertheless, most endocrinologists conservatively perform a single follow-up (generally noncontrasted) scan for most tumors, particularly those between 2 and 4 cm, in 6 to 12 months after the initial study based on size. As discussed earlier, the probability of hypercortisolemia increases with size, and repeat screening should be considered for tumors greater than 2 cm unless unequivocally normal on initial testing. For example, a 50-year-old patient with a 3 cm cortical adenoma has a dexamethasone-suppressed cortisol of 1.5 µg/dL, ACTH of 18 pg/mL, and DHEAS of 80 µg/dL (low-normal). Given the marginally normal results in a patient with a fairly large mass, repeat testing for hypercortisolemia is warranted in 6 to 12 months, independent of the decision to repeat imaging. If imaging and biochemical stability is observed after 6 to 12 months, no further evaluation is generally warranted, although subsequent rescreening is prudent if the clinical status changes. Lesions with concerning features, such as those greater than 4 cm, heterogeneous appearance, or greater than 10 HU, can be referred to an endocrinologist or endocrine surgeon independent of hormone production.

What other imaging should a primary care provider order?

We recommend deferring the decision for additional imaging to specialists. Under most circumstances, CT or MRI will both provide specialists with adequate information to determine the most appropriate management. Approximately 12% of the time, adrenal tumors may be indeterminate on CT or MRI.[56] For large or hormone-producing masses, specialists might recommend further evaluation with fluorodeoxyglucose positron-emission tomography ([18F]-FDG-PET/CT) or meta-iodobenzguanine ([123I]-MIBG) scans. [18F]-FDG-PET/CT can be useful to rule out malignancy, particularly in patients with known or suspected cancer.[57–60] [123I]-MIBG scan uses an iodine-labeled norepinephrine analog that is transported via the catecholamine reuptake system, which is specifically accumulated in pheochromocytomas but not cortical tumors.[61,62]

How does imaging impact clinical management?

Several features of imaging can impact clinical management. Small, lipid-rich adenomas that are nonfunctional on hormonal testing generally require no intervention. Lesions that are larger, heterogeneous, or have higher HU may warrant further diagnostic imaging, biopsy, or surgery. For lesions that warrant surgery, surgeons may prefer open over laparoscopic surgery for large tumors with concern for malignancy or pheochromocytoma, because spillage of tumor cells can spread disease and thwart a curative operation.[4,5]

SUMMARY

Most incidentally discovered adrenal masses are benign and poorly functional adrenal tumors. Nevertheless, these tumors do require further investigation. Physicians should remain alert for concerning imaging findings and features of hormone excess. Screening biochemical studies in conjunction with history, physical examination, and review of the images are used to triage patients to specialists, determine if follow-up imaging is necessary, and recommend therapies for comorbidities.

CLINICS CARE POINTS

Pearls
- Primary aldosteronism is far more common than pheochromocytoma.
- Antihypertensive medication withdrawal is generally unnecessary before screening for primary aldosteronism with a plasma renin and serum aldosterone.
- ACTH-independent hypercortisolemia is uncommon for adrenal cortex adenomas less than 2 cm and becomes proportionately more common as the size increases greater than 2.5 cm.
- Imaging features of adrenal masses that warrant concern for malignancy include large size (>4 cm), heterogenous appearance such as hemorrhage, irregular borders, density greater than 10 Hounsfield units on computed tomography (CT), and no signal loss between in- and out-of-phase images on MRI.

Pitfalls
- Hormone testing results should be interpreted in the clinical context and pretest probability of disease.
- Most slightly elevated plasma metanephrines in asymptomatic patients with an adrenal mass are false-positive results.
- Urine-free cortisol and late-night saliva cortisol are insensitive tests for ACTH-independent hypercortisolemia; the 1 mg overnight dexamethasone suppression test is preferred.
- MRI is typically not necessary to characterize masses already visualized on CT, which provides superior resolution and adequate initial imaging assessment.

DISCLOSURE

The authors have nothing to disclose.

REFERENCES

1. Gruber LM, Hartman RP, Thompson GB, et al. Pheochromocytoma characteristics and behavior differ depending on method of discovery. J Clin Endocrinol Metab 2019;104(5):1386–93.
2. Arlt W, Biehl M, Taylor AE, et al. Urine steroid metabolomics as a biomarker tool for detecting malignancy in adrenal tumors. J Clin Endocrinol Metab 2011;96(12): 3775–84.
3. Cawood TJ, Hunt PJ, O'Shea D, et al. Recommended evaluation of adrenal incidentalomas is costly, has high false-positive rates and confers a risk of fatal cancer that is similar to the risk of the adrenal lesion becoming malignant; time for a rethink? Eur J Endocrinol 2009;161(4):513–27.
4. Zeiger M, Thompson G, Duh Q-Y, et al. American Association of Clinical Endocrinologists and American Association of Endocrine Surgeons Medical Guidelines for the Management of Adrenal Incidentalomas. Endocr Pract 2009; 15(Supplement 1):1–20.
5. Fassnacht M, Arlt W, Bancos I, et al. Management of adrenal incidentalomas: European Society of Endocrinology Clinical Practice Guideline in collaboration with the European Network for the Study of Adrenal Tumors. Eur J Endocrinol 2016; 175(2):G1–34.
6. Nieman LK, Biller BMK, Findling JW, et al. The diagnosis of Cushing's syndrome: an Endocrine Society Clinical Practice Guideline. J Clin Endocrinol Metab 2008; 93(5):1526–40.
7. Nieman LK. Update on subclinical Cushing's syndrome. Curr Opin Endocrinol Diabetes Obes 2015;22(3):180–4.

8. Vassilatou E, Vryonidou A, Ioannidis D, et al. Bilateral adrenal incidentalomas differ from unilateral adrenal incidentalomas in subclinical cortisol hypersecretion but not in potential clinical implications. Eur J Endocrinol 2014;171(1):37–45.

9. Hannemann A, Wallaschofski H. Prevalence of primary aldosteronism in patient's cohorts and in population-based studies–a review of the current literature. Horm Metab Res 2012;44(3):157–62.

10. Monticone S, Burrello J, Tizzani D, et al. Prevalence and clinical manifestations of primary aldosteronism encountered in primary care practice. J Am Coll Cardiol 2017;69(14):1811–20.

11. Douma S, Petidis K, Doumas M, et al. Prevalence of primary hyperaldosteronism in resistant hypertension: a retrospective observational study. Lancet 2008; 371(9628):1921–6.

12. Calhoun DA, Nishizaka MK, Zaman MA, et al. Hyperaldosteronism among black and white subjects with resistant hypertension. Hypertension 2002;40(6):892–6.

13. Mulatero P, Stowasser M, Loh K-C, et al. Increased diagnosis of primary aldosteronism, including surgically correctable forms, in centers from five continents. J Clin Endocrinol Metab 2004;89(3):1045–50.

14. Funder JW, Carey RM, Mantero F, et al. The Management of Primary Aldosteronism: Case Detection, Diagnosis, and Treatment: An Endocrine Society Clinical Practice Guideline. J Clin Endocrinol Metab 2016;101(5):1889–916.

15. White ML, Gauger PG, Doherty GM, et al. The role of radiologic studies in the evaluation and management of primary hyperaldosteronism. Surgery 2008; 144(6):926–33 [discussion: 933].

16. Lenders JWM, Eisenhofer G, Mannelli M, et al. Phaeochromocytoma. Lancet 2005;366(9486):665–75.

17. Lenders JWM, Duh Q-Y, Eisenhofer G, et al. Pheochromocytoma and paraganglioma: an endocrine society clinical practice guideline. J Clin Endocrinol Metab 2014;99(6):1915–42.

18. Canu L, Van Hemert JAW, Kerstens MN, et al. CT Characteristics of Pheochromocytoma: Relevance for the Evaluation of Adrenal Incidentaloma. J Clin Endocrinol Metab 2019;104(2):312–8.

19. Buitenwerf E, Berends AMA, van Asselt ADI, et al. Diagnostic Accuracy of Computed Tomography to Exclude Pheochromocytoma: A Systematic Review, Meta-analysis, and Cost Analysis. Mayo Clin Proc 2019;94(10):2040–52.

20. Neumann HPH, Young WF, Eng C. Pheochromocytoma and Paraganglioma. N Engl J Med 2019;381(6):552–65.

21. Stewart PM. Is subclinical Cushing's syndrome an entity or a statistical fallout from diagnostic testing? Consensus surrounding the diagnosis is required before optimal treatment can be defined. J Clin Endocrinol Metab 2010;95(6):2618–20.

22. Yener S, Yilmaz H, Demir T, et al. DHEAS for the prediction of subclinical Cushing's syndrome: perplexing or advantageous? Endocrine 2015;48(2):669–76.

23. Dennedy MC, Annamalai AK, Prankerd-Smith O, et al. Low DHEAS: A Sensitive and Specific Test for the Detection of Subclinical Hypercortisolism in Adrenal Incidentalomas. J Clin Endocrinol Metab 2017;102(3):786–92.

24. Auchus RJ. Primary aldosteronism and a Texas two-step. Rev Endocr Metab Disord 2011;12(1):37–42.

25. Byrd JB, Turcu AF, Auchus RJ. Primary Aldosteronism: Practical Approach to Diagnosis and Management. Circulation 2018;138(8):823–35.

26. Sawka AM, Prebtani AP, Thabane L, et al. A systematic review of the literature examining the diagnostic efficacy of measurement of fractionated plasma free

metanephrines in the biochemical diagnosis of pheochromocytoma. BMC Endocr Disord 2004;4(1):2.

27. Reincke M. Subclinical Cushing's syndrome. Endocrinol Metab Clin North Am 2000;29(1):43–56.

28. Rye P, Chin A, Pasieka J, et al. Unadjusted Plasma Renin Activity as a "First-Look" Test to Decide Upon Further Investigations for Primary Aldosteronism. J Clin Hypertens Greenwich Conn 2015;17(7):541–6.

29. Haase M, Riester A, Kröpil P, et al. Outcome of adrenal vein sampling performed during concurrent mineralocorticoid receptor antagonist therapy. J Clin Endocrinol Metab 2014;99(12):4397–402.

30. Baudrand R, Guarda FJ, Torrey J, et al. Dietary Sodium Restriction Increases the Risk of Misinterpreting Mild Cases of Primary Aldosteronism. J Clin Endocrinol Metab 2016;101(11):3989–96.

31. Di Dalmazi G, Vicennati V, Garelli S, et al. Cardiovascular events and mortality in patients with adrenal incidentalomas that are either non-secreting or associated with intermediate phenotype or subclinical Cushing's syndrome: a 15-year retrospective study. Lancet Diabetes Endocrinol 2014;2(5):396–405.

32. Morelli V, Reimondo G, Giordano R, et al. Long-term follow-up in adrenal incidentalomas: an Italian multicenter study. J Clin Endocrinol Metab 2014;99(3):827–34.

33. Debono M, Bradburn M, Bull M, et al. Cortisol as a marker for increased mortality in patients with incidental adrenocortical adenomas. J Clin Endocrinol Metab 2014;99(12):4462–70.

34. Chiodini I, Morelli V, Salcuni AS, et al. Beneficial metabolic effects of prompt surgical treatment in patients with an adrenal incidentaloma causing biochemical hypercortisolism. J Clin Endocrinol Metab 2010;95(6):2736–45.

35. Toniato A, Merante-Boschin I, Opocher G, et al. Surgical versus conservative management for subclinical Cushing syndrome in adrenal incidentalomas: a prospective randomized study. Ann Surg 2009;249(3):388–91.

36. Tsuiki M, Tanabe A, Takagi S, et al. Cardiovascular risks and their long-term clinical outcome in patients with subclinical Cushing's syndrome. Endocr J 2008; 55(4):737–45.

37. Iacobone M, Citton M, Viel G, et al. Adrenalectomy may improve cardiovascular and metabolic impairment and ameliorate quality of life in patients with adrenal incidentalomas and subclinical Cushing's syndrome. Surgery 2012;152(6):991–7.

38. Eller-Vainicher C, Morelli V, Salcuni AS, et al. Post-surgical hypocortisolism after removal of an adrenal incidentaloma: is it predictable by an accurate endocrinological work-up before surgery? Eur J Endocrinol 2010;162(1):91–9.

39. Ortiz DI, Findling JW, Carroll TB, et al. Cosyntropin stimulation testing on postoperative day 1 allows for selective glucocorticoid replacement therapy after adrenalectomy for hypercortisolism: Results of a novel, multidisciplinary institutional protocol. Surgery 2016;159(1):259–65.

40. Libè R, Dall'Asta C, Barbetta L, et al. Long-term follow-up study of patients with adrenal incidentalomas. Eur J Endocrinol 2002;147(4):489–94.

41. Giordano R, Marinazzo E, Berardelli R, et al. Long-term morphological, hormonal, and clinical follow-up in a single unit on 118 patients with adrenal incidentalomas. Eur J Endocrinol 2010;162(4):779–85.

42. Hinojosa-Amaya JM, Cuevas-Ramos D, Fleseriu M. Medical Management of Cushing's Syndrome: Current and Emerging Treatments. Drugs 2019;79(9): 935–56.

43. Williams TA, Lenders JWM, Mulatero P, et al. Outcomes after adrenalectomy for unilateral primary aldosteronism: an international consensus on outcome

measures and analysis of remission rates in an international cohort. Lancet Diabetes Endocrinol 2017;5(9):689–99.

44. Sukor N, Gordon RD, Ku YK, et al. Role of unilateral adrenalectomy in bilateral primary aldosteronism: a 22-year single center experience. J Clin Endocrinol Metab 2009;94(7):2437–45.

45. Kempers MJE, Lenders JWM, van Outheusden L, et al. Systematic review: diagnostic procedures to differentiate unilateral from bilateral adrenal abnormality in primary aldosteronism. Ann Intern Med 2009;151(5):329–37.

46. Nanba AT, Nanba K, Byrd JB, et al. Discordance between imaging and immunohistochemistry in unilateral primary aldosteronism. Clin Endocrinol (Oxf) 2017; 87(6):665–72.

47. Rossi GP, Auchus RJ, Brown M, et al. An expert consensus statement on use of adrenal vein sampling for the subtyping of primary aldosteronism. Hypertension 2014;63(1):151–60.

48. Pantalone KM, Gopan T, Remer EM, et al. Change in adrenal mass size as a predictor of a malignant tumor. Endocr Pract 2010;16(4):577–87.

49. Sturgeon C, Shen WT, Clark OH, et al. Risk assessment in 457 adrenal cortical carcinomas: how much does tumor size predict the likelihood of malignancy? J Am Coll Surg 2006;202(3):423–30.

50. Mayo-Smith WW, Song JH, Boland GL, et al. Management of Incidental Adrenal Masses: A White Paper of the ACR Incidental Findings Committee. J Am Coll Radiol 2017;14(8):1038–44.

51. Boland GW, Lee MJ, Gazelle GS, et al. Characterization of adrenal masses using unenhanced CT: an analysis of the CT literature. Am J Roentgenol 1998;171(1): 201–4.

52. Peña CS, Boland GWL, Hahn PF, et al. Characterization of Indeterminate (Lipid-poor) Adrenal Masses: Use of Washout Characteristics at Contrast-enhanced CT. Radiology 2000;217(3):798–802.

53. Szolar DH, Kammerhuber FH. Adrenal adenomas and nonadenomas: assessment of washout at delayed contrast-enhanced CT. Radiology 1998;207(2): 369–75.

54. Korobkin M, Giordano TJ, Brodeur FJ, et al. Adrenal adenomas: relationship between histologic lipid and CT and MR findings. Radiology 1996;200(3):743–7.

55. Haider MA, Ghai S, Jhaveri K, et al. Chemical Shift MR Imaging of Hyperattenuating (>10 HU) Adrenal Masses: Does It Still Have a Role? Radiology 2004; 231(3):711–6.

56. Song JH, Chaudhry FS, Mayo-Smith WW. The incidental adrenal mass on CT: prevalence of adrenal disease in 1,049 consecutive adrenal masses in patients with no known malignancy. AJR Am J Roentgenol 2008;190(5):1163–8.

57. Brady MJ, Thomas J, Wong TZ, et al. Adrenal Nodules at FDG PET/CT in Patients Known to Have or Suspected of Having Lung Cancer: A Proposal for an Efficient Diagnostic Algorithm. Radiology 2009;250(2):523–30.

58. Caoili EM, Korobkin M, Brown RKJ, et al. Differentiating Adrenal Adenomas From Nonadenomas Using ^{18}F-FDG PET/CT: Quantitative and Qualitative Evaluation. Acad Radiol 2007;14(4):468–75.

59. Metser U, Miller E, Lerman H, et al. ^{18}F-FDG PET/CT in the Evaluation of Adrenal Masses. J Nucl Med 2006;47(1):32–7.

60. Delivanis DA, Bancos I, Atwell TD, et al. Diagnostic performance of unenhanced computed tomography and ^{18}F-fluorodeoxyglucose positron emission tomography in indeterminate adrenal tumours. Clin Endocrinol (Oxf) 2018;88(1):30–6.

61. Bhatia KSS, Ismail MM, Sahdev A, et al. [^{123}I]-metaiodobenzylguanidine (MIBG) scintigraphy for the detection of adrenal and extra-adrenal phaeochromocytomas: CT and MRI correlation. Clin Endocrinol (Oxf) 2008;69(2):181–8.

62. van der Harst E, de Herder WW, Bruining HA, et al. [^{123}I]metaiodobenzylguanidine and [^{111}In]octreotide uptake in begnign and malignant pheochromocytomas. J Clin Endocrinol Metab 2001;86(2):685–93.

63. Young WF. Clinical presentation and diagnosis of pheochromocytoma - UpToDate. UpToDate. 2020. Available at: https://www.uptodate.com/contents/clinical-presentation-and-diagnosis-of-pheochromocytoma. Accessed November 30, 2020.

Primary Hyperaldosteronism

Approach to Diagnosis and Management

Nadine El-Asmar, MD[a,b], Aman Rajpal, MD[b,c],
Baha M. Arafah, MD[a,b],*

KEYWORDS

- Hyperaldosteronism • Aldosterone • Plasma renin activity • Secondary hypertension

KEY POINTS

- Hyperaldosteronism is more common than previously appreciated and the diagnosis should be suspected in patients with difficult to control hypertension, those with unprovoked hypokalemia, and those with hypertension and incidental adrenal masses.
- Initial screening tests (plasma renin activity and serum aldosterone levels) can be followed in most patients by salt loading to confirm the diagnosis. Although adrenal computed tomography/magnetic resonance imaging scans often can define a disease's subtype, adrenal vein sampling might be necessary in some patients who are surgical candidates.
- Medical therapy using selective mineralocorticoid receptor antagonists can be effective in most patients.
- The long-term outcome of patients treated with either surgical or optimal medical therapy appears to be similar.

INTRODUCTION

Hypertension is a common disorder that is associated with increased morbidity and mortality related to its impact on the cardiovascular and renal systems. Although a majority of patients with this disorder have essential hypertension, many have other diseases or conditions that can increase blood pressure (BP). Such conditions, known as secondary causes of hypertension, account for up to 10% of all cases. The secondary causes of hypertension include but are not limited to diseases of the kidney (renovascular and parenchymal), vascular abnormalities, certain medications or drugs, states of high cardiac output, and endocrine disorders. It is estimated that endocrine disorders account for up to 5% of all cases of hypertension.[1–3] Although the focus of this review is on hyperaldosteronism, many other disorders of the adrenal cortex can cause hypertension, as shown in **Table 1**.

---

[a] Division of Clinical and Molecular Endocrinology, University Hospitals Cleveland Medical Center, 11100 Euclid Avenue, Cleveland, OH 44106, USA; [b] Case Western Reserve University, Cleveland, OH, USA; [c] Louis Stokes VA Medical Center, 10701 East Blvd, Cleveland OH 44106, USA
* Corresponding author.
E-mail address: baha.arafah@case.edu

Med Clin N Am 105 (2021) 1065–1080
https://doi.org/10.1016/j.mcna.2021.06.007
medical.theclinics.com
0025-7125/21/© 2021 Elsevier Inc. All rights reserved.

Table 1 Adrenocortical causes of hypertension	
Primary hyperaldosteronism	Excess mineralocorticoid syndromes other than aldosterone
Aldosterone-secreting adenoma	Congenital adrenal hyperplasia (11β-hydroxylase deficiency or 17α-hydroxylase deficiency)
Bilateral hyperplasia	Cushing syndrome (excess cortisol)
Aldosterone-producing adrenocortical carcinoma	Deoxycorticosterone-producing tumor
FH (glucocorticoid-remediable hyperaldosteronism type I, FH type II, FH type III, and FH type IV)	AME (11β-HSD2 deficiency)

Hyperaldosteronism represents the most common endocrine disorder causing secondary hypertension. Older studies suggested that the prevalence of primary hyperaldosteronism among the hypertensive population to be nearly 1%. Recent studies, however, indicate that the prevalence may be as high as 5% of the hypertensive population seen by primary care physicians.[1–3] This article provides an overview of aldosterone secretion in healthy individuals, the impact of commonly used antihypertensive medications on its secretion, and the parameters used to diagnose states of excessive aldosterone production. This review discusses clinical and biochemical alterations that should raise concern for hyperaldosteronism and address potential diagnostic and therapeutic management approaches related to this disease.

THE PHYSIOLOGY OF THE RENIN-ANGIOTENSIN-ALDOSTERONE SYSTEM

The adrenal cortex is composed of 3 distinct regions, each of which has specific set of enzymes that regulate the synthesis and secretion of 3 classes of steroid hormones. The outermost layer, the zona glomerulosa, secretes aldosterone; the middle region, the zona fasciculata, is where cortisol is synthesized; and the innermost one, the zona reticularis, is where adrenal androgens are secreted. Aldosterone secretion (100–150 μg/d) from the zona glomerulosa is regulated by angiotensin II (**Fig. 1**) acting on several key enzymes, the most specific being the CYP11B2 (aldosterone synthase). Potassium and to a lesser extent adrenocorticotropic hormone (ACTH), also are known to stimulate the release of aldosterone.[4] Angiotensin II and potassium increase the transcription of CYP11B2 through common intracellular signaling pathways, leading to the production of aldosterone from the adrenal cortex. Angiotensin II binds to the surface AT1 receptor present in the adrenal gland, vessels, kidneys, heart, and brain. In addition to aldosterone production, angiotensin II exerts its effects on different tissues and results in constriction of vascular smooth muscle and release of norepinephrine and epinephrine. The effect of ACTH on aldosterone secretion is rather modest and is more pronounced in the acute setting after a bolus of ACTH, mainly through stimulating the early steroidogenic pathways. Chronic and sustained ACTH stimulation has either no effect or an actual inhibitory effect on aldosterone production. Other factors, such as somatostatin, heparin, atrial natriuretic factor, and dopamine, can inhibit aldosterone synthesis partially.

Renin is an enzyme produced in the juxtaglomerular cells of the kidney and stored in granules. Renin is cleaved from its precursor prorenin into the active enzyme. Renin

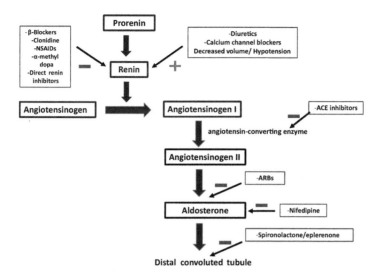

Fig. 1. Overview of the parameters modulating the renin-angitensin-aldosterone system (RAAS). The graph illustrates the physiologic regulators of the system as well as the impact of medications (positive and negative) of administered medications on components of the system. +, stimulatory effect; −, inhibitory effect; ARBs, Angiotensin receptor blockers..

release in the circulation is the rate-limiting step in the renin-angiotensin-aldosterone system (RAAS). There are multiple factors that control renin release.[5] These include the following:

1. The juxtaglomerular cells in the kidneys, which act as pressure transducers that sense the stretch of the afferent arteriolar wall and thus renal perfusion pressure
2. The macula densa, which is a group of distal convoluted tubular cells that function as chemoreceptors for monitoring the sodium and the chloride present in the distal tubule
3. The sympathetic nervous system in response to upright posture
4. Circulating factors, including potassium, angiotensin II, and atrial natriuretic peptides[5]

Renin in turn breaks down angiotensinogen, a protein synthesized in the liver, into angiotensin I. The latter peptide, angiotensin I, does not appear to have any biological activity but rather is cleaved by the angiotensin-converting enzyme (ACE) into angiotensin II, which is the main biologically active angiotensin (see **Fig. 1**). ACE is located in the cell membranes of the lung and certain tissues that produce angiotensin II. Physiologic functions of angiotensin II include not only the promotion of aldosterone production from the adrenal cortex but also multiple additional effects, including constricting vascular smooth muscle, increasing BP, increasing release of norepinephrine and epinephrine from the adrenal medulla, enhancing the activity of the sympathetic nervous system, and increasing release of vasopressin.[6]

ALDOSTERONE FUNCTION AND METABOLISM

Although 60% to 70% of aldosterone in the circulation is protein-bound (albumin and cortisol-binding globulin [CBG]), approximately 30% to 40% is unbound or free. Thus, alterations in plasma binding proteins can have an impact on measurements because current assay systems for aldosterone determine the total (bound + free) serum concentration. Aldosterone is inactivated in the liver to tetrahydroaldosterone. Free aldosterone binds to the mineralocorticoid receptor located in the cytosol of epithelial cells in the kidney. Aldosterone regulates extracellular volume and renal arterial pressure through enhancing sodium retention and also controls potassium homeostasis. Its action results in increased sodium ion transport across the cell membranes in the kidney and tubular secretion of potassium along with loss of hydrogen ions resulting in hypokalemia and metabolic alkalosis. Endogenous glucocorticoids and mineralocorticoids both bind to the mineralocorticoid receptor in peripheral tissues. The specificity of cortisol binding to the mineralocorticoid receptor is controlled mainly by the 11β–hydroxysteroid dehydrogenase type 2 (11β-HSD2) enzyme activity, which converts cortisol to cortisone and mitigates the action of cortisol as a mineralocorticoid. This mechanism becomes pathophysiologically relevant in conditions of apparent mineralocorticoid excess (AME) (discussed later). Aldosterone has additional nonclassic effects that include increasing the expression of genes controlling tissue growth factors and genes mediating inflammation. The resultant actions lead to microangiopathy, necrosis, and fibrosis in various tissues, such as the heart, the vasculature, and the kidney, which can be seen in patients with primary hyperaldosteronism where aldosterone secretion is dysregulated.[7]

PRIMARY VERSUS SECONDARY HYPERALDOSTERONISM

In individuals with intact adrenal mineralocorticoid production, multiple factors influence the RAAS system, as discussed previously, including volume status, changes to arterial pressure, and salt intake (**Table 2**). It is important to distinguish between primary and secondary hyperaldosteronism because the latter condition occurs when the elevated aldosterone levels result from increased renin activity. In contrast, primary hyperaldosteronism is a condition where aldosterone secretion is independent of renin stimulation. For example, individuals with heart failure or liver cirrhosis sustain an activation of the RAAS in the form of secondary hyperaldosteronism due to relative intravascular volume depletion. Other causes of secondary hyperaldosteronism include renal artery stenosis or, rarely, renin-secreting tumors.

There are rare genetic syndromes that can result in secondary hyperaldosteronism without hypertension. Bartter and Gitelman syndromes occur as a result of an impairment in 1 of the transporters involved in sodium chloride reabsorption in the loop of Henle or the distal tubule, respectively. Consequently, there is impaired sodium

Table 2 Alterations in plasma renin activity and serum aldosterone levels during various clinical settings				
Condition	Plasma Renin Activity	Angiotensin II	Aldosterone	Blood Pressure
Volume depletion/hypotension	↑	↑	↑	↓
Renal artery stenosis	↑	↑	↑	↑
Renin-secreting tumor	↑	↑	↑	↑
High-salt diet	↓	↓	↓	↑ or normal
Low-salt diet	↑	↑	↑	↓ or normal
Heart failure/liver cirrhosis	↑	↑	↑	Variable

reabsorption, volume depletion, and subsequent activation of the RAAS, resulting in hyperreninemia and secondary hyperaldosteronism which, in turn, lead to hypokalemia and metabolic alkalosis but in the absence of hypertension. These syndromes are autosomal recessive in transmission.[8]

PRIMARY HYPERALDOSTERONISM

Primary hyperaldosteronism is an autonomous production of aldosterone, which results in renin suppression. It almost always causes hypertension and commonly hypokalemia. The most common causes[9] include

a. Aldosterone-producing adenoma (APA) in approximately 30% of cases
b. Idiopathic bilateral adrenal hyperplasia in approximately 60% of cases
c. Adrenocortical carcinoma
d. Familial hyperaldosteronism (FH)

FAMILIAL HYPERALDOSTERONISM

These disorders typically are diagnosed when primary hyperaldosteronism is discovered at age less than 20 or when there are multiple family members with hyperaldosteronism. Currently, there are 4 types of FH recognized, with a germline gene mutation specific to each type.

1. FH type I, also known as glucocorticoid-remediable aldosteronism: in this variant of FH, the causative agent is the CYP11B1/CYP11B2 chimeric gene, whereby ACTH rather than angiotensin II becomes the main regulator of aldosterone secretion. In this condition, hypersecretion of aldosterone can be controlled by administering exogenous glucocorticoids, thereby lowering ACTH secretion, hence the name, glucocorticoid remediable hyperaldosteronism. There also is increased production of 18-hydroxycortisol and 18-oxocortisol, which can be measured in the urine or plasma. Genetic testing typically confirms the diagnosis.
2. FH type II is caused by a germline CLCN2 chloride channel mutation and is autosomal dominant. Here, the hyperaldosteronism does not suppress with exogenous glucocorticoids.
3. FH type III is caused by germline KCNJ5 mutations. Patients typically have refractory hypertension before age 7 and have bilateral massive hyperplasia, often requiring bilateral adrenalectomy.
4. FH type IV is caused by germline CACNA1H gene mutations, which is inherited in an autosomal dominant pattern.[9]

OTHER CAUSES OF MINERALOCORTICOID EXCESS

Other mineralocorticoids secreted by the adrenal cortex include corticosterone and deoxycorticosterone. Conditions that cause excess production of these mineralocorticoids result in hypertension, such as congenital adrenal hyperplasia and certain adrenal tumors (see **Table 1**).

AME syndrome occurs when cortisol acts as a mineralocorticoid in the setting of impaired conversion of cortisol to cortisone by the enzyme 11β-HSD2. Normally, cortisol and mineralocorticoids bind receptors in the kidneys with similar affinity. The concentration of cortisol is 100 times more than that of aldosterone; however, due to the function of 11β-HSD2, activation of these receptors by cortisol is limited due the conversion of cortisol to cortisone.[10] In the genetic form of AME, there is a mutation in the kidney isoform of 11β-HSD2, which prevents the conversion of cortisol into cortisone. This leads to markedly increased cortisol activity at the mineralocorticoid receptor, resulting in hypertension and hypokalemia. Acquired AME occurs after licorice ingestion, a product that contains glycyrrhetinic acid that inhibits 11β-HSD2 activity.[10] Clinically, all conditions of mineralocorticoid excess are characterized by hypertension and hypokalemia, along with low renin and aldosterone levels.

NON–MINERALOCORTICOID-RELATED HYPERTENSION AND HYPOKALEMIA

In the rare autosomal dominant Liddle syndrome, gain-of-function pathogenic variants of the amiloride-sensitive collecting tubule sodium channel, results in increased sodium reabsorption, potassium wasting, hypertension, and hypokalemia. Importantly, patients with Liddle syndrome have suppressed plasma renin activity (PRA) and low serum aldosterone levels. Definitive diagnosis of Liddle syndrome requires genetic testing.[11]

DIAGNOSIS OF PRIMARY ALDOSTERONISM

Unless suspected, primary hyperaldosteronism often is missed. When diagnosed, patients typically are in the third to sixth decades of life. Marked hypokalemia due to excess aldosterone may result in muscle cramps and weakness, in addition to polyuria due to the development of hypokalemia-induced nephrogenic diabetes insipidus. Hypokalemia is an important finding but has low sensitivity and specificity for the diagnosis and often is confounded by the use of diuretics. It is estimated that unprovoked hypokalemia is evident in only 30% to 35% of patients with primary hyperaldosteronism and, therefore, a majority of patients with this disorder have normal potassium levels.

WHO SHOULD BE TESTED FOR HYPERALDOSTERONISM?

The following patient populations and others with certain biochemical features should be tested for primary hyperaldosteronism:

1. Hypertension diagnosed at a young age less than 40
2. Severe hypertension at any age
3. Uncontrolled hypertension on 3 or more medications
4. Hypertension with hypokalemia
5. Hypertension with adrenal incidentaloma
6. All hypertensive first-degree relatives of patients with primary hyperaldosteronism
7. Hypertension and family history of early-onset hypertension or cerebrovascular accident at age less than 40

INITIAL SCREENING TESTS FOR PRIMARY HYPERALDOSTERONISM

There are few symptoms or physical signs specific to this diagnosis, and often a diagnosis is made biochemically after the measurement of low PRA and elevated serum aldosterone levels. When primary aldosteronism is suspected, PRA and aldosterone levels should be measured in a random ambulatory blood sample. Due to the dynamic variation of renin and aldosterone, the measurement must be done on the same sample at the same point in time. Serum electrolytes must be measured concomitantly as well. The evaluating physician also must be aware of the patient's volume status and medications to aid in interpreting laboratory values. Urine sodium evaluation can prove helpful as a reflection of sodium balance. It also is important to replete potassium prior to measuring serum aldosterone because hypokalemia can reduce the secretion of aldosterone even in patients with autonomous aldosterone production. Urinary potassium excretion should be assessed in patients who present with spontaneous or unprovoked hypokalemia before potassium repletion because this can offer clues to the cause of hypokalemia. The demonstration of potassium loss (urinary potassium of >30 meq/L) in someone with unexplained hypokalemia indicates inappropriate kaliuresis, a feature that is expected in patients with the diagnosis of hyperaldosteronism.

Most patients being evaluated for aldosterone over-production already are on anti-hypertensive medications that, in themselves, have varying effects on renin and aldo-sterone levels (**Fig. 2**; **Table 3**). β-Blockers are known to have a significant impact on renin production, resulting in falsely low renin values.[12] Other drugs that suppress renin production include clonidine, α-methyldopa, and nonsteroidal anti-inflammatory drugs (NSAIDs). Direct renin inhibitors lower PRA but increase direct renin concentration. In contrast, diuretics, including spironolactone, dihydropyridine calcium channel blockers, ACE inhibitors, and angiotensin receptor blockers (ARBs) increase PRA (see **Fig. 2**). In addition, nifedipine, which is a dihydropyridine calcium channel blocker, has been shown in some in vitro and in vivo studies to inhibit aldoste-rone synthesis.[13]

Hypertensive patients who do not have hyperaldosteronism and are being treated with ACE inhibitors or ARBs typically have low serum aldosterone levels and elevated PRA. Thus, the finding of a suppressed PRA and high serum aldosterone levels in in-dividuals treated with the latter medications should raise concern for the diagnosis of hyperaldosteronism.

It is not necessary to hold these or most other hypertension medications when eval-uating for primary hyperaldosteronism. The exception is mineralocorticoid receptor blockers, such as spironolactone and eplerenone, which block the aldosterone recep-tor and result in an elevation in renin, which may lead to false-negative results. There-fore, both spironolactone and eplerenone should be held approximately 4 weeks to 6 weeks prior to measuring renin and aldosterone levels. As discussed previously,

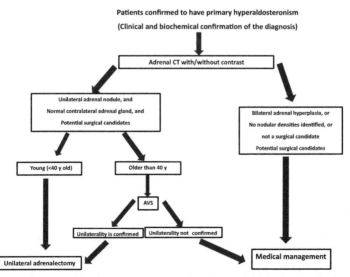

Fig. 2. Suggested protocol in the management of patients with biochemically documented hyperaldosteronism.

Table 3
The influence of various medications on parameters of the renin-angiotensin-adlosterone system

	Plasma Renin Activity	Plasma Angiotensin II	Serum Aldosterone
β-Blockers	↓	↓	↓
Clonidine	↓	↓	↓
NSAIDs	↓	↓	↓
α-Methyldopa	↓	↓	↓
Direct renin inhibitors	↓	↓	↓
Diuretics	↑	↑	↑
Dihydropyridine calcium channel blockers (amlodipine)	↑	↑	↑
ACE inhibitors	↑	↓	↓
Angiotensin receptor blockers	↑	↑	↓
Spironolactone/eplerenone	↑	↑	↑

the finding of suppressed PRA (<1 ng/mL/h) in patients on an ACE inhibitor or an ARB, actually is highly suggestive of primary hyperaldosteronism.

Primary hyperaldosteronism should be suspected when the PRA is suppressed (<1 ng/mL/h) and the plasma aldosterone concentration is greater than 10 ng/dL. These measurements are done only as initial testing for case detection and often more confirmatory tests are needed,[14] as discussed later.

LABORATORY ASSAY CONSIDERATIONS

Different laboratory assays have variable PRA cutoffs as well as assay detectability limits and, therefore, relying solely on using the well-known approach of calculating the aldosterone/renin ratio might be misleading. Another important aspect when obtaining renin and aldosterone measurements is distinguishing between renin concentration and PRA. PRA is a more reliable method of assessing renin function. Starting with the premise that renin exerts its effects on peripheral tissue via angiotensin, PRA measures angiotensin I generated per unit of time through the activity of renin. This is important in individuals on estrogen replacement therapy because this gonadal steroid is known to stimulate the production of renin substrate, that is, angiotensinogen. This creates a falsely elevated aldosterone/renin ratio if the measurement relies on renin concentration rather than activity.[15]

During the luteal phase of the menstrual cycle, it commonly is reported that aldosterone/renin ratios are falsely elevated if direct renin concentration is measured.[16] Endogenous or exogenous progestins can have varying effects on the RAAS; for examples, progestins, such as drospirenone with anti-mineralocorticoid receptor activity, can stimulate production of both renin and aldosterone.[17]

Other caveats to keep in mind when interpreting serum aldosterone levels include falsely elevated levels due to elevated CBG. As discussed previously, aldosterone is partially bound to CBG and, therefore, any condition that may elevate CBG values results in a falsely higher aldosterone concentration. A common cause of elevated CBG is the use of oral contraceptives or estrogen replacement therapy in women observed in women. Aldosterone levels can be 10 times the normal range during pregnancy.[17]

Other causes include conditions, such as chronic hepatitis C. Conversely, in patients with hypoalbuminemia, serum aldosterone may be lower and may cause a falsely low aldosterone/renin ratio.

CONFIRMATORY TESTS OF PRIMARY HYPERALDOSTERONISM

Patients whose preliminary data are suggestive of primary hyperaldosteronism often require additional confirmatory testing to establish a diagnosis. Specifically, confirmatory tests are needed in individuals who have only modest elevation in serum aldosterone levels (<20 ng/dL) and a low but measurable PRA (<1 ng/mL/h). Such testing is not necessary, however, in other patients who have a classic clinical presentation and strong biochemical data consistent with hyperaldosteronism, including a serum aldosterone of greater than 20 ng/dL and a suppressed PRA (<1 ng/mL/h). The need for confirmatory testing is less compelling the lower the PRA and the higher the serum aldosterone level. A retrospective Japanese study, including 327 patients with hypertension and suppressed PRA (<1 ng/mL/h), found that patients who had typical features of primary hyperaldosteronism, such as serum aldosterone greater than 30 ng/dL, and others who have levels between 20 and 30 along with spontaneous hypokalemia (<3.5 mEq/L) potentially can be spared from confirmatory testing.[18] Suppressed PRA (<1 ng/mL/h) in patients receiving mineralocorticoid receptor antagonist (MRA) should be a strong indicator that these patients have primary hyperaldosteronism and may not need confirmatory testing. Therefore, confirmatory testing should be reserved for patients with less clear indication of primary hyperaldosteronism on initial testing.

If confirmatory testing is needed, oral salt loading in the outpatient setting is the test of choice. The idea is that during volume expansion in normal individuals as well as in patients with essential hypertension, PRA decreases and, consequently, aldosterone secretion falls (see **Table 2**), whereas in patients with primary hyperaldosteronism, due to autonomous nature of aldosterone production, additional volume expansion does not decrease aldosterone levels to the same extent as in normal subjects or patients with essential hypertension. Salt loading testing can be done either via oral salt loading or saline infusion.

Oral Salt Loading Test

Patients are given 2-g oral sodium chloride tablets, 3 times daily, and are advised to monitor their BP. Serum potassium should be corrected before the test because sodium loading can lead to increased kaliuresis and hypokalemia. On the third day of the high-sodium diet, serum electrolytes and aldosterone as well as PRA are measured along with a 24-hour urine specimen collected for measurement of aldosterone, sodium, potassium, and creatinine. The 24-hour urine sodium excretion should exceed 200 mEq to document adequate salt loading. Urine aldosterone excretion greater than 12 μg/24 h in this setting is consistent with hyperaldosteronism.[19] Also, prior studies have shown that serum aldosterone levels are suppressed to approximately 4 ng/dL in normal subjects after high salt diet.[20] Therefore, the authors suggest that serum aldosterone level of greater than 5 ng/dL with undetectable PRA after salt loading remains highly suggestive of primary hyperaldosteronism.

Saline Infusion Test

The test is performed by the intravenous administration of 2 L of isotonic saline over 4 hours, ideally while the patient is seated.[21] As discussed previously, serum aldosterone levels are expected to be less than 5 ng/dL in normal individuals after salt loading; therefore, a level above 5 ng/dL is consistent with primary hyperaldosteronism.[22]

Although the test can provide useful data, the authors minimize its use because this amount of volume potentially precipitates hypertensive urgency and heart failure in some tenuous patients with primary hyperaldosteronism.

Other confirmatory tests are available but are not used routinely. These include fludrocortisone suppression test and the captopril challenge test. To conduct the former test, 0.2 mg of fludrocortisone are administered daily for 3 days, and urinary aldosterone excretion is measured on the third day of its administration. Urine aldosterone excretion greater than 10 ug/24 h confirms primary hyperaldosteronism.[23] Given the many adverse effects encountered with the administration of this large dose of fludrocortisone, such as severe hypokalemia, however, worsening of hypertension and heart failure, this test is not recommended routinely. To perform the captopril challenge test, patients are given 50 mg of captopril orally in the morning and blood samples subsequently are drawn for measurement of serum aldosterone levels and PRA at time zero and 2 hours after the challenge. The administration of an ACE inhibitor, such as captopril, results in an increase in PRA and a decrease in serum aldosterone levels (see **Fig. 1** and **Table 3**). Different studies have recommended examining different parameters, such as absolute or percentage change in aldosterone levels (before and after Captopril administration), a change in PRA, and/or a change in their ratios. One study suggests that a serum aldosterone level of greater than 13 ng/dL after captopril indicates probable hyperaldosteronism whereas a level less than 8 ng/dL makes the diagnosis unlikely.[24] Even though the Captopril challenge test is easy to conduct and does not risk cardiac decompensation, the large number of hypertensive patients already treated with an ACE inhibitor as well as high frequency of false-negative or equivocal results makes the test less desirable to use for confirmation of hyperaldosteronism.

The authors recommend using oral salt loading as the preferred test for confirmation of diagnosis of primary hyperaldosteronism, when necessary. Once a diagnosis of primary hyperaldosteronism is confirmed, the next step is to localize the source of hyperaldosteronism.

LOCALIZATION/SUBTYPE CLASSIFICATION

Adrenal computed tomography (CT) scan is the first test of choice to differentiate between unilateral APA from bilateral adrenal hyperplasia and to eliminate other possibilities, such as adrenal carcinoma. Alternatively, magnetic resonance imaging (MRI) can be used. Lingam and colleagues[25] showed that the sensitivity and specificity for detecting APA was similar for both CT and MRI. Additional detailed attempts at localization are not needed in all patients with primary hyperaldosteronism, especially those who are not surgical candidates. Other patients with primary hyperaldosteronism should undergo further testing for subtype classification.

In addition to variations in expertise in interpreting adrenal imaging studies, one of the difficulties commonly encountered in the work up of patients with hyperaldosteronism is the presence of an incidental nonfunctional adrenal nodule or tumor. These are more likely to be encountered with increasing age (>40 years), because the prevalence of incidental and usually nonfunctional adrenal adenomas can reach 10% in older individuals.[26] Thus, older patients with biochemical features of hyperaldosteronism require further localizing tests if they are surgical candidates. In contrast, young patients (<40 y old) have very low incidence of adrenal incidentalomas; therefore, it commonly is accepted that the presence of a solitary, hypodense, unilateral nodule with normal contralateral adrenal gland imaging, in this age group with biochemically confirmed primary hyperaldosteronism, suggests a diagnosis of aldosteronoma, and unilateral adrenalectomy is a reasonable therapeutic option.[27] Alternatively, patients with bilateral adrenal hyperplasia on CT scan can be treated directly with MRA rather than further testing.[28] A graphic representation of the authors' management decision protocol is shown in **Fig. 2**. For older patients who are surgical candidates and who have adrenal nodules on CT scanning, the main additional localizing or confirmatory study is adrenal vein sampling (AVS), as discussed later.

ADRENAL VEIN SAMPLING

AVS has been billed as the gold standard by the 2016 Endocrine Society Guidelines, to distinguish between unilateral and bilateral aldosterone overproduction and, therefore, to safely refer patients with primary hyperaldosteronism to surgery.[29] These recommendations are based on observational and retrospective studies, with not well-defined selection criteria for AVS and treatment based only on that procedure.[30] Also, AVS remains a costly and challenging procedure and is not needed routinely in most cases of primary hyperaldosteronism. The Adrenal venous sampling-guided adrenalectomy rates in primary aldosteronism: results of an international Cohort (AVSTAT) study evaluated 200 patients with primary hyperaldosteronism and found that treatment based on CT or AVS did not show significant differences in intensity of antihypertensive medication or clinical benefits for patients after 1 year of follow-up.[31] Similarly, Dekkers and colleagues[32] conducted a randomized controlled trial aimed at comparing 2 groups of CT-based and AVS-based management in patients with confirmed primary hyperaldosteronism. They evaluated 184 patients with primary hyperaldosteronism (92 received CT-based treatment and 92 AVS-based treatment) and found no difference between the 2 groups in the intensity of drug treatment required to obtain a target BP, biochemical cure rate, health-related quality of life, and adverse events.[32] Recently, a multicenter retrospective study analyzed data on 125 patients with confirmed primary hyperaldosteronism (45 cross-sectional imaging with AVS and 80 imaging only) who underwent adrenalectomy.[33] The AVSTAT investigation found no difference in complete biochemical success (defined as normokalemia and normalization of aldosterone levels) or complete clinical success (defined as normal BP without aid of any antihypertensive medications) postsurgery based on whether or not AVS was performed preoperatively.[33] These findings suggest that AVS may not be necessary in all patients but could be considered in certain patients with confirmed primary hyperaldosteronism, who are eligible surgical candidates and who have no obvious adrenal nodules identified on CT/MRI or others who have more than one adrenal nodule. The procedure technically is difficult and should be performed by an experienced interventional radiologist with proper coordination of sample collection and labeling.

Methodology and Interpretation of Adrenal Vein Sampling

Most centers conduct AVS with continuous cosyntropin infusion (50 μg/h) started approximately 30 minutes prior to sequential sampling of the adrenal veins and continued throughout the procedure. Continuous cosyntropin infusion helps minimize stress-induced fluctuations in aldosterone secretion and maximizes the gradient in cortisol from adrenal vein to inferior vena cava (IVC), thus confirming successful sampling of the adrenal veins.[29] Aldosterone and cortisol concentrations are measured sequentially from 3 sites (right adrenal vein, left adrenal vein, and IVC).

Confirming catheterization was successful is an important initial step in evaluating AVS data. This can be done by measuring the cortisol levels from the adrenal veins and IVC. With continuous cosyntropin infusion, the adrenal vein–to–IVC cortisol ratio greater than 10:1 confirms successful cannulation on that side. After confirming accurate catheter localization in both adrenal veins, the cortisol-corrected serum aldosterone levels should be calculated by dividing the right and left adrenal vein aldosterone levels by their respective cortisol levels. The latter calculation corrects for the dilutional effect of the inferior phrenic vein flow into the left adrenal vein. Most patients with a unilateral source of aldosterone have cortisol-corrected aldosterone lateralization ratios greater than 4.[29]

AVS has certain limitations, especially the inability to obtain good samples, because the right adrenal vein is small and difficult to locate and success rates are dependent on experience of the interventional radiologist conducting the procedure and, to some degree, the patient's anatomy. Failure to cannulate the right adrenal vein can lead to an incorrect diagnosis of unilateral disease when both glands are affected. AVS can have large variability because the success is dependent on procedure expertise and coordinated sample handling. The most common complications are groin hematoma, adrenal hemorrhage, and adrenal vein dissection.[34]

MANAGEMENT

Multiple studies have shown increased cardiovascular risk associated with primary hyperaldosteronism. Milliez and colleagues[35] conducted a retrospective study in 124 patients with confirmed primary hyperaldosteronism and compared them to 465 control patients with essential hypertension. Despite a similar BP control, patients with primary hyperaldosteronism were significantly more likely to have stroke, myocardial infarction, and atrial fibrillation.[35] Similarly, another study conducted by Reincke and colleagues[36] using a German registry of Conn syndrome patients who had been treated medically or surgically found that patients with primary hyperaldosteronism were significantly more likely to have died from cardiovascular complications than the control patients. These studies suggest that patients with hyperaldosteronism clearly have increased morbidity and would benefit from optimal therapy.

The goals of treatment of patients with primary hyperaldosteronism include maintaining normal or physiologic aldosterone levels, prevention of adverse cardiovascular effects of hyperaldosteronism, normalization of the serum potassium levels, and finally normalization of BP. Such goals can be achieved in some patients following surgical and/or medical therapy.

Surgical Management

In patients with hyperaldosteronism who have an adrenal adenoma, unilateral laparoscopic adrenalectomy is the treatment of choice. Given that some patients have underlying essential hypertension along with primary hyperaldosteronism, it is possible that surgery may not lead to BP normalization. Therefore, these patients often require continued use of antihypertensive medications, albeit less than what they were using preoperatively. Furthermore, eliminating hyperaldosteronism leads to lowering of future cardiovascular risk.[37]

Medical Management

Treatment with MRA is the appropriate approach in patients with hyperaldosteronism who either have bilateral adrenal hyperplasia or adrenal adenoma who are not surgical candidates. The primary goal of these drugs is to adequately block the aldosterone effects. The 2 MRAs that are widely available are spironolactone and eplerenone. Spironolactone is more potent MRA and usually is started at a dose of 50 mg daily, typically increased every 4 weeks to 8 weeks with a goal of normalizing serum potassium without supplementation. Dose of spironolactone can be as high as 200 mg/d to 400 mg/d in certain patients. On the other hand, eplerenone is a more selective MRA agent but is only half as potent as spironolactone. It usually is started at a dose of 50 mg daily but in some cases has been used in higher doses around 100 mg/d to 200 mg/d. Common side effects are hyperkalemia and renal failure; therefore, renal function panel should be monitored routinely in these patients. Also, because spironolactone binds and bocks the androgen receptor, its use can lead to the development of some antiandrogen effects, with gynecomastia a common side effect in men. In patients using these drugs, avoiding the use of other drugs that have potential interaction, such as NSAIDs, is needed, because this also can lead to decreased glomerular filtration rate and hyperkalemia. Patients should be counseled adequately about cautious use of these drugs because many are available over the counter. Most patients with primary hyperaldosteronism have been on several antihypertensive drugs at the time of diagnosis and before MRA therapy is initiated. With the introduction of MRA therapy, other antihypertensive medications need to be tapered gradually as the dose of MRA drugs is increased. This often requires close monitoring of patients' BP and renal function. Measurements of PRA are helpful in determining optimal suppression of the increased mineralocorticoid function, with the goal of greater than 1 ng/mL/h.

Monitoring while using medical treatment
1. Renal function panel: because hyperkalemia and renal failure are known side effects of the MRA agents, renal function panel should be monitored routinely in these patients.
2. PRA: as discussed previously, the primary goal of these drugs is to adequately block the aldosterone effect. Thus, one way to indirectly measure the amount of drug needed is to titrate the MRA dose to raise PRA greater than 1 ng/mL/h.

Cardiovascular Outcome

In line with studies showing higher rates of cardiovascular disease in patients with primary hyperaldosteronism, there are data suggesting improvement in cardiovascular outcomes in patients who are treated with either surgical adrenalectomy and/or MRA agents. Recently, there have been some studies comparing the efficacy of surgical adrenalectomy and MRA on cardiovascular outcomes in patients with primary hyperaldosteronism. All have been observational, with the potential for channeling bias, that is, poorer surgical candidates may be more likely to be treated medically, whereas more severe disease may be more likely to be dealt with surgically.

Wu and colleagues[38] conducted a longitudinal analysis of 3362 patients with primary hyperaldosteronism with an average follow-up of 5.75 years using a Taiwan National Health Insurance database. Consistent with earlier findings, the investigators showed that patients with primary hyperaldosteronism were more likely to have major cardiovascular events. The study by Wu and colleagues also demonstrated that adrenalectomy was associated with greater reductions in all-cause mortality compared with treatment with MRAs alone.[38] Similarly, Rossi and colleagues[39] evaluated 107 patients with primary hyperaldosteronism for a median follow-up of 11.8 years, out of whom 41 underwent adrenalectomy and remaining 66 patients were treated medically. The latter study also showed that patients with primary hyperaldosteronism who were treated medically trended to have a higher rate of incident atrial fibrillation compared with surgically treated patients.[39] A recent study by Hundemer and colleagues[40] evaluated 602 patients with primary hyperaldosteronism treated medically found that the adverse cardiovascular outcomes are mitigated if the MRA dose is titrated to raise PRA to greater than 1 ng/mL/h. Therefore, if the MRAs are used in appropriate dosing to block the aldosterone effects, they likely reduce the cardiovascular events in patients with primary hyperaldosteronism. The study by Hundemer and colleagues suggests that PRA should be monitored in medically treated patients with hyperaldosteronism with the goal being an increase in that activity to greater than 1 ng/mL/h.

CLINICS CARE POINTS

Pearls
- Consider the diagnosis of hyperaldosteronism in hypertensive patients on multiple drugs, those with unprovoked hypokalemia, and others with adrenal nodule(s).
- Initial screening for the diagnosis includes measurements of PRA and serum aldosterone levels.
- Confirmatory testing of the diagnosis using salt loading often is needed.
- AVS can be performed after a diagnosis is confirmed in older patients with adrenal nodule (s) who are surgical candidates.
- Optimal medical therapy using MRAs often leads to a rise in PRA.

Pitfalls
- PRA should not be confused with direct-measure renin level or concentrations.
- Many drugs may influence PRA and aldosterone levels independently.
- Assays for PRA have different sensitivities and detectability levels.
- Serum aldosterone level can be influenced by variation in binding proteins (albumin and CBG).
- The prevalence of incidental adrenal nodules/masses increases with age.

ACKNOWLEDGEMENTS

Funding source was received from Local/ departmental support.

DISCLOSURE

Nothing to disclose by all authors.

REFERENCES

1. Hannemann A, Wallaschofski H. Prevalence of primary aldosteronism in patient's cohorts and in population-based studies–a review of the current literature. Horm Metab Res 2012;44(3):157–62.
2. Monticone S, Burrello J, Tizzani D, et al. Prevalence and clinical manifestations of primary aldosteronism encountered in primary care practice. J Am Coll Cardiol 2017;69(14):1811–20.
3. Brown JM, Siddiqui M, Calhoun DA, et al. The unrecognized prevalence of primary aldosteronism: a cross-sectional study. Ann Intern Med 2020;173(1):10–20.
4. Rainey WE. Adrenal zonation: clues from 11beta-hydroxylase and aldosterone synthase. Mol Cell Endocrinol 1999;151(1–2):151–60.
5. Skøtt O, Jensen BL. Cellular and intrarenal control of renin secretion. Clin Sci (Lond) 1993;84(1):1–10.
6. Corvol P, Jeunemaitre X. Molecular genetics of human hypertension: role of angiotensinogen. Endocr Rev 1997;18(5):662–77.
7. Funder JW. The nongenomic actions of aldosterone. Endocr Rev 2005;26(3):313–21.

8. Kurtz I. Molecular pathogenesis of Bartter's and Gitelman's syndromes. Kidney Int 1998;54(4):1396–410.

9. Funder JW. Primary aldosteronism. Hypertension 2019;74(3):458–66.

10. Quinkler M, Stewart PM. Hypertension and the cortisol-cortisone shuttle. J Clin Endocrinol Metab 2003;88(6):2384–92.

11. Cui Y, Tong A, Jiang J, et al. Liddle syndrome: clinical and genetic profiles. J Clin Hypertens (Greenwich) 2017;19(5):524–9.

12. Seifarth C, Trenkel S, Schobel H, et al. Influence of antihypertensive medication on aldosterone and renin concentration in the differential diagnosis of essential hypertension and primary aldosteronism. Clin Endocrinol (Oxf) 2002;57(4): 457–65.

13. Fiad TM, Cunningham SK, Hayes FJ, et al. Effects of nifedipine treatment on the renin-angiotensin-aldosterone axis*. J Clin Endocrinol Metab 1997;82(2):457–60.

14. Blumenfeld JD, Sealey JE, Schlussel Y, et al. Diagnosis and treatment of primary hyperaldosteronism. Ann Intern Med 1994;121(11):877–85.

15. Ahmed AH, Gordon RD, Taylor PJ, et al. Effect of contraceptives on aldosterone/ renin ratio may vary according to the components of contraceptive, renin assay method, and possibly route of administration. J Clin Endocrinol Metab 2011; 96(6):1797–804.

16. Ahmed AH, Gordon RD, Taylor PJ, et al. Are women more at risk of false-positive primary aldosteronism screening and unnecessary suppression testing than men? J Clin Endocrinol Metab 2011;96(2):E340–6.

17. Oelkers WK. Effects of estrogens and progestogens on the renin-aldosterone system and blood pressure. Steroids 1996;61(4):166–71.

18. Umakoshi H, Sakamoto R, Matsuda Y, et al. Role of aldosterone and potassium levels in sparing confirmatory tests in primary aldosteronism. J Clin Endocrinol Metab 2019;105(4):1284–9.

19. Young WFJ. Primary aldosteronism: update on diagnosis and treatment. Endocrinologist 1997;7(4):213–21.

20. Arafah BM, Gordon NH, Salazar R, et al. Modulation of tissue responsiveness to angiotensin-II in hyperprolactinemic subjects*. J Clin Endocrinol Metab 1990; 71(1):60–6.

21. Stowasser M, Ahmed AH, Cowley D, et al. Comparison of seated with recumbent saline suppression testing for the diagnosis of primary aldosteronism. J Clin Endocrinol Metab 2018;103(11):4113–24.

22. Holland OB, Brown H, Kuhnert L, et al. Further evaluation of saline infusion for the diagnosis of primary aldosteronism. Hypertension 1984;6(5):717–23.

23. Westerdahl C, Bergenfelz A, Larsson J, et al. Re-evaluation of the fludrocortisone test: duration, NaCl supplementation and cut-off limits for aldosterone. Scand J Clin Lab Invest 2009;69(2):234–41.

24. Song Y, Yang S, He W, et al. Confirmatory tests for the diagnosis of primary aldosteronism: a prospective diagnostic accuracy study. Hypertension 2018;71(1): 118–24.

25. Lingam RK, Sohaib SA, Rockall AG, et al. Diagnostic performance of CT versus MR in detecting aldosterone-producing adenoma in primary hyperaldosteronism (Conn's syndrome). Eur Radiol 2004;14(10):1787–92.

26. Bovio S, Cataldi A, Reimondo G, et al. Prevalence of adrenal incidentaloma in a contemporary computerized tomography series. J Endocrinol Invest 2006;29(4): 298–302.

27. Lim V, Guo Q, Grant CS, et al. Accuracy of adrenal imaging and adrenal venous sampling in predicting surgical cure of primary aldosteronism. J Clin Endocrinol Metab 2014;99(8):2712–9.

28. Mulatero P, Bertello C, Rossato D, et al. Roles of clinical criteria, computed tomography scan, and adrenal vein sampling in differential diagnosis of primary aldosteronism subtypes. J Clin Endocrinol Metab 2008;93(4):1366–71.

29. Young WF, Stanson AW, Thompson GB, et al. Role for adrenal venous sampling in primary aldosteronism. Surgery 2004;136(6):1227–35.

30. Nwariaku FE, Miller BS, Auchus R, et al. Primary hyperaldosteronism: effect of adrenal vein sampling on surgical outcome. Arch Surg 2006;141(5):497–502 [discussion: 502–3].

31. Ohno Y, Naruse M, Beuschlein F, et al. Adrenal venous sampling–guided adrenalectomy rates in primary aldosteronism: results of an international cohort (AV-STAT). J Clin Endocrinol Metab 2021;106:1400–7.

32. Dekkers T, Prejbisz A, Kool LJS, et al. Adrenal vein sampling versus CT scan to determine treatment in primary aldosteronism: an outcome-based randomised diagnostic trial. Lancet Diabetes Endocrinol 2016;4(9):739–46.

33. Thiesmeyer JW, Ullmann TM, Stamatiou AT, et al. Association of adrenal venous sampling with outcomes in primary aldosteronism for unilateral adenomas. JAMA Surg 2021;156:165–71.

34. Monticone S, Satoh F, Dietz AS, et al. Clinical management and outcomes of adrenal hemorrhage following adrenal vein sampling in primary aldosteronism. Hypertension 2016;67(1):146–52.

35. Milliez P, Girerd X, Plouin P-F, et al. Evidence for an increased rate of cardiovascular events in patients with primary aldosteronism. J Am Coll Cardiol 2005;45(8):1243–8.

36. Reincke M, Fischer E, Gerum S, et al. Observational study mortality in treated primary aldosteronism. Hypertension 2012;60(3):618–24.

37. Vorselaars W, Nell S, Postma EL, et al. Clinical outcomes after unilateral adrenalectomy for primary aldosteronism. JAMA Surg 2019;154(4):e185842.

38. Wu VC, Wang SM, Chang CH, et al. Long term outcome of aldosteronism after target treatments. Sci Rep 2016;6:32103.

39. Rossi GP, Maiolino G, Flego A, et al. Adrenalectomy lowers incident atrial fibrillation in primary aldosteronism patients at long term. Hypertension 2018;71(4):585–91.

40. Hundemer GL, Curhan GC, Yozamp N, et al. Incidence of atrial fibrillation and mineralocorticoid receptor activity in patients with medically and surgically treated primary aldosteronism. JAMA Cardiol 2018;3(8):768–74.

What to Do with Incidentally Discovered Pituitary Abnormalities?

Fabienne Langlois, MD[a], Maria Fleseriu, MD[b],*

KEYWORDS

- Incidentaloma • Macroadenoma • Magnetic resonance imaging • Microadenoma
- Pituitary adenoma • Prolactinomas • Rathke cleft cyst

KEY POINTS

- As evidenced by MRI, small pituitary lesions are found in approximately 1 in 5 individuals.
- Lesions less than 6 mm are most often not clinically significant.
- A complete history, physical examination, and hormonal workup are indicated in all cases.
- Contrast-enhanced pituitary MRI is the imaging modality of choice to characterize lesions.
- Individualized patient follow-up is tailored to lesion size and nature.

INTRODUCTION

Incidentalomas in endocrinology patients are frequent, with thyroid and adrenal incidentalomas being the most common.[1,2] By definition, a pituitary incidentaloma is a sellar lesion typically discovered by imaging ordered to investigate an unrelated condition. Approximately 1 in 5 individuals will harbor a pituitary lesion of at least a few millimeters.[3] Incidental diagnosis does not preclude clinical impact and hormonal abnormalities or mass effects that may occur. Diagnosis of pituitary dysfunction can be challenging, and this further complicates pituitary tumor management; one cannot rely on the presence of a lesion to conclude a pituitary cause of hormonal dysfunction. This review will assess the challenges associated with pituitary incidentaloma management.

[a] Division of Endocrinology, Department of Medicine, Centre intégré universitaire de santé et de services sociaux de l'Estrie - Centre Hospitalier Universitaire de Sherbrooke, Sherbrooke, Quebec, Canada; [b] Departments of Medicine (Division of Endocrinology, Diabetes and Clinical Nutrition), and Neurological Surgery, and Pituitary Center, Oregon Health & Science University, CH8N 3303 South Bond Avenue, Portland, OR, USA
* Corresponding author.
E-mail address: fleseriu@ohsu.edu

Med Clin N Am 105 (2021) 1081–1098
https://doi.org/10.1016/j.mcna.2021.05.015   medical.theclinics.com
0025-7125/21/Crown Copyright © 2021 Published by Elsevier Inc. All rights reserved.

CASE PRESENTATION

A 60-year-old woman underwent brain MRI for investigation of chronic, severe daily headaches. A 1 cm pituitary mass was discovered; the radiology report concludes that the mass is a cystic adenoma or Rathke cleft cyst (RCC).

QUESTIONS

Is this an incidentaloma?
 What initial clinical evaluation is warranted, and what follow-up is indicated?

EPIDEMIOLOGY

The epidemiology of pituitary lesions is uncertain because of the intrinsic nature of clinically silent abnormalities. In 1936, Russel T. Costello published a series of over 1000 pituitary postmortem cases and found 225 adenomas—so-called subclinical pituitary adenomas.[3] In 2008, Mark E. Molitch published a combined autopsy series of close to 19,000 pituitary cases and reported a pituitary lesion prevalence of 10.7%.[4] These lesions were almost exclusively under 1 cm in size and affected all ages and sex.

 Brain imaging also reveals a high prevalence of abnormalities; 4% to 20% of pituitary lesions can be seen on brain CT compared with 10% to 40% by MRI.[5–9] Overall, depending on cyst inclusion/exclusion, technique sensitivity, and the population studied, lesions are discovered in approximately 1 in 5 individuals. Therefore, a pituitary MRI should not be ordered unless there is high clinical suspicion of pituitary dysfunction and a confirmed biochemical diagnosis.

 As with all pituitary lesions, incidentalomas are classified by size as macro if $\geq$1 cm and micro if <1 cm. In terms of clinical significance, adenomas that are less than 6 mm are probably inconsequential.[10–13] However, the prevalence of clinically significant lesions (either by size or hyperfunctioning status) is high, affecting approximately 1 in 1000 individuals.[14–19]

PITUITARY ANATOMY AND NORMAL PHYSIOLOGY

The pituitary gland sits in sella turcica, a cavity in the sphenoid bone located at the skull base. Cavernous sinuses containing important neurovascular structures, such as the internal carotid artery and cranial nerves III, IV, V1, V2, and VI, are lateral to the sella (**Fig. 1**[20]). Anterior pituitary cells receive direct hormonal input from the hypothalamus through vascular channels. Various cells with the anterior gland then secrete hormonal products into the bloodstream targeting a peripheral gland (**Fig. 2**[21]). Antidiuretic hormone and oxytocin are produced in the hypothalamus and then neuronally transported and secreted by the posterior pituitary.

NORMAL PITUITARY IMAGING

Pituitary incidentalomas are discovered by imaging, that is typically ordered for neurologic complaints such as headaches, cerebrovascular events, vertigo, dizziness, or visual changes.[22,23]

 MRI is the modality of choice in diagnosing pituitary lesions. Pituitary MRI is superior to CT; it provides higher definition and soft-tissue contrast. T1-weighted and T2-weighted images and various acquisition sequences provide complementary data on lesion nature and content. For example, cerebrospinal fluid (CSF) appears hypointense (dark) on T1 and hyperintense (white) on T2. High-resolution MR images are

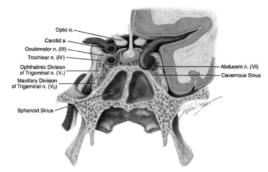

Fig. 1. Normal pituitary and sellar/parasellar anatomy. From Christina Jackson, Jordina Rincon-Torroella, Alfredo Quiñones-Hinojosa. Parasellar Tumors, Video Atlas of Neurosurgery, 2016, 33; 221 to 228 (*with permission*).[20]

usually acquired with 1.5, 3, or 5 MRI tesla scanners. A higher tesla number relates to magnetic field strength and magnetic flux density, providing greater imaging detail.

A specific pituitary MRI protocol is essential and typically includes thin cuts (usually 2 mm) of the pituitary sellar region and images that are pregadolinium and postgadolinium (if renal function allows; glomerular filtration rate (GFR) >30 cc/min). Contrast agents and dynamic images allow for better definition of adenomas that appear hypoenhanced compared with normal pituitary tissue.[24]

DIFFERENTIAL DIAGNOSIS

A pituitary incidentaloma etiologic diagnosis is similar to that of other sellar masses; however, it also includes technical artifacts, pituitary hyperplasia, and variants of normal anatomy (**Table 1**).

Visualizing an abnormal density often envisioned on only 1 cut can be a technical artifact of either the lateral/posterior pituitary or a portion of the dorsum sellae. Additional, thinner cuts may resolve this.[25] Furthermore, image noise leading to gland heterogeneity may be due to adjacent bony structures, sinus air content, or carotid arteries.[26]

Pituitary hyperplasia is a globally enlarged pituitary, likely due to physiologic cell hyperplasia related to somatotroph hyperplasia (adolescence), lactotroph hyperplasia (pregnancy), thyrotroph hyperplasia (severe untreated primary hypothyroidism), corticotroph hyperplasia (Addison's disease), or gonadotroph hyperplasia (perimenopause). Upon resolution of the underlying condition, the pituitary returns to a normal concave form.[27] In the pediatric population, pituitary hyperplasia is the most common type of pituitary incidentaloma.[28]

Variants of normal anatomy include the normal hypersignal of neurohypophysis (may be ectopic in congenital forms of hypopituitarism), thicker bony components such as dorsum sellae, or a smaller sella resulting in the appearance of an enlarged pituitary.[25]

Generally, more than 90% of pituitary incidentalomas are either pituitary adenomas or RCCs.[23,26] Clinical characteristics can lead to a diagnosis, but a definitive diagnosis can only be made by histopathology determinants.

Pituitary adenomas are monoclonal cell tumors arising from various lineages.[29,30] Hormones may be secreted but may have reduced or absent biological activity. Thus, pituitary adenomas are often classified as functioning or not functioning

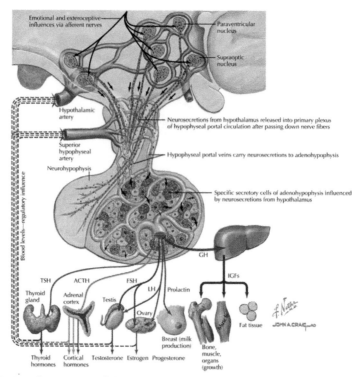

Fig. 2. Pituitary hormones and their target glands. Overview of anterior pituitary function. The anterior pituitary gland is controlled by releasing and inhibitory hormones secreted into the hypophyseal portal circulation; these hormones reach the anterior pituitary directly through this portal circulation without entering the general circulation. Under control of these factors, specific secretory cell types of the anterior pituitary secrete 6 major tropic hormones (TSH, ACTH, FSH, LH, prolactin, and GH), that act on distal endocrine glands. Tropic hormones and the target gland hormones have feedback effects on these endocrine systems designed to regulate blood levels of the target gland hormone. (*Arrows*) color dotted line = inhibiting action; full line =stimulating action.ACTH, adrenocorticotropic hormone; FSH, follicle-stimulating hormone; GH, growth hormone; IGF, insulin-like growth factor; LH, luteinizing hormone; TSH, thyroid-stimulating hormone. From Susan E. Mulroney PhD, Adam K. Myers PhD. *General Principles of Endocrinology and Pituitary and Hypothalamic Hormones*, Netter's Essential Physiology, 2016, Chapter 27; 314 to 327 (*with permission*).[21]

(silent).[31] Prolactinomas cause hyperprolactinemia, oligomenorrhea in females, and hypogonadism in males, and galactorrhea.[19,32] In general, prolactinomas are the most prevalent pituitary adenoma subtype, followed by nonfunctioning pituitary adenomas (NFPAs). In the context of pituitary incidentalomas, silent adenomas and NFPAs make up approximately 50% to 70%, and prolactinomas approximately 15%.[11–13,33,34] Histologically, approximately two-thirds of silent adenomas are gonadotroph tumors.[35] Monomorphous somatotroph adenomas and mixed growth hormone–prolactin combined, account for another 10%.[35] Corticotroph adenomas are the least prevalent and may cause Cushing disease (CD). These corticotroph adenomas are most often microadenomas, whereas silent macroadenomas are more invasive.[36] Thyrotropinomas are very rare and are most often diagnosed in the context of clinical hyperthyroidism with normal or elevated thyroid-stimulating hormone (TSH).

Table 1
Sellar mass etiologies

Anterior pituitary lesions		Vascular

• Pituitary
  ○ Adenoma[a]
  ○ Hyperplasia
  ○ Carcinoma
		• Intracavernous carotid aneurysm
		• Arteriovenous malformation
		• Apoplexy

Cysts		**Inflammatory**

• Rathke cleft cysts[a]
• Dermoid cysts
• Epidermoid cysts
	• Arachnoid cysts
	• Empty sella
		• Hypophysitis
		  ○ Lymphocytic
		  ○ Immunotherapy related
		  ○ IgG4-related
		• Lymphocytic neuro-infundibulitis

Other		**Infiltrative**

• Craniopharyngioma
• Meningiomas
• Metastases
  ○ Breast
  ○ Lung
  ○ Prostate
	• Central nervous system
	  lymphomas
	• Plasmacytoma
	• Chondrosarcoma
	• Germinoma
	• Hypothalamic glioma
	• Pituicytoma
		• Sarcoidosis
		• Amyloidosis
		• Hemochromatosis
		• Langerhans cell histiocytosis
		• Eosinophilic granuloma
		• Wegener's granulomatosis

Other		**Infectious**
• Technical artifact • Normal anatomy variant		• Bacterial abscess • Fungal infection • Tuberculosis • Syphilis

[a] Most frequent; 90% of pituitary incidentalomas.

RCCs are the second most commonly encountered pituitary incidentalomas.[10–13] RCCs consist of fluid accumulation within the Rathke cleft. Remnants are located in the pars intermedia between the anterior and posterior lobes. In a few cases, RCCs can be large enough to cause endocrine hypofunction or headaches.[37] Adrenal insufficiency (AI) is relatively frequent and is probably related to inflammation around the cyst due to fluid microleakage.[38] Imaging characteristics vary depending on cyst contents and can appear as either hypointense or hyperintense. Other types of cysts, such as dermoid (fat content), epidermoid (keratin content), or arachnoid (cerebrospinal fluid;CSF), are possible. Craniopharyngiomas are tumors that arise from Rathke pouch epithelium and have an aggressive course; they most often cause headaches, visual defects, and hypothalamic–pituitary dysfunction.[39] Empty sella is defined as an invasion of the sella dura mater causing a local accumulation, either partial or complete, of CSF in sella turcica. Causes may include resorption of a sellar space-occupying lesion (such as hypophysitis, pituitary adenoma infarction/apoplexy), pseudotumor cerebri, or other causes of increased intracranial pressure. Alternatively, the cause may be idiopathic. If this is the case, an impact on pituitary function is rare.[40]

EVALUATION

Clinical evaluation must include a patient's history (age, sex, comorbidities, and medication), hormonal function, signs and symptoms of mass effect, risk of malignancy, and imaging characteristics. A tabulation of large pituitary incidentaloma series with key evaluation features are summarized in **Table 2**.[11–14,22,33,34,41–44]

Table 2
Large pituitary incidentaloma series[11–14,22,33,34,41–44]

Author (Year)	Patients (n)	Macroadenoma (%)	Tumor Subtype; (%)	Hypopituitarism (%)	Surgery (%)	Visual Defect (%)	Tumor Growth or Recurrence (%)
Vaninetti,[12] 2011	222	70	NFPA; 50 RCC; 18 PRLoma;14	31	36	30	4.9 over 5 y
Sanno et al,[11] 2003	506	n/a mean tumor size 1.3 cm	NFPA; 64 RCC; 27 (PRL >100 ng/mL excluded)	0 excluded	51	excluded	13.3 over 3.75 y
Anagnostis,[33] 2018	61	78	NFPA; 77 PRLoma; 18 RCC; 2	12	48	45	observation; 11 surgery; 48
Day,[60] 2016	46	63	PRLoma; 15	41	37	35	n/a
Reincke et al,[44] 1990	18	61	n/a	17	22	11	17 over 2 y
Karavitaki et al,[42] 2007	41 (including 15 incidentalomas)	60	NFPA; 100	27, or higher	2.5	12	35 over 3.5 y
Donovan & Corenblum,[41] 1995	31	52	PRLoma; 0	0	3.2	0	13 over 6.4 y
Feldkamp et al,[43] 1999	67	37	PRLoma; 12	15	n/a	4.5	27 over 2.7 y
Freda et al,[22] 2020	131	85	hyperPRL; 15	27	34	5.9	n/a
Esteves et al,[34] 2015	71	63	Pit adenoma; 70 RCC; 13 PRLoma; 7	15	29	5.6	n/a
Imran et al,[13] 2016	328	71	NFPA; 55 RCC; 14 PRLoma; 11	36	32	excluded	observation only; 12 postsurgical; 22 over 3 y

Abbreviations: NFPA, nonfunctioning pituitary adenoma; PRLoma, prolactinoma; RCCs, Rathke cleft cysts.

HORMONAL WORKUP

A complete pituitary function test should be ordered at baseline. Testing includes insulin-like growth factor-1 (IGF-1) as a marker of growth hormone secretion, luteinizing hormone (LH), and follicle-stimulating hormone (FSH) with either testosterone in male or estradiol in selected premenopausal women, TSH and free T4, morning (8 AM or 9 AM) cortisol, and prolactin.[45] Of note, there is no need to measure estradiol levels in women with normal menses or taking birth control pills. Serum sodium and serum and urine osmolarity may be added if polyuria and polydipsia are present. A dexamethasone suppression test, urinary free cortisol, or late-night salivary cortisol can be ordered if there is clinical suspicion of hypercortisolemia. Furthermore, normal IGF-1 does not exclude a diagnosis of GH deficiency (**Table 3**).

One or more pituitary axes dysfunction (hypopituitarism) is found in 15% to 30% of pituitary incidentalomas, mostly in macroincidentalomas.[10,13,22,33,34] The sequence of affected axes by an enlarged pituitary mass is initially GH and LH-FSH, followed by TSH and adrenocorticotropic hormone.[46] A clinical finding of persistent hypogonadotropic hypogonadism, especially in young adults, should prompt complete pituitary hormone testing and a pituitary MRI, as this can be the first indication of a sellar mass. Diabetes insipidus (DI) may be a clinical manifestation with metastatic tumors to the pituitary (or pituitary stalk) or infiltrative lesions. A combination of anterior pituitary hormone deficits with DI warrants further diagnostic evaluation to rule out malignancy.

As a result of incidental lesion discovery, symptoms of hypersecretion may be mild or absent, and clinicians should be vigilant in evaluating subclinical hypersecretion states. In mild or early acromegaly stages, key symptoms are hyperhidrosis, seborrhea, headaches, and joint pain.[47] Visceromegaly and somatic effects are apparent after many years of disease evolution.[48] Discriminatory signs in CD include skin thinning, easy bruising, facial plethora, proximal myopathy, and the presence of large and violaceous striae.[49] Clinical manifestations of hypopituitarism and other pituitary hypersecretion syndromes are presented in **Table 3**.

A differential diagnosis of mild to moderate hyperprolactinemia is wide-ranging. Medications that can increase prolactin levels include atypical antipsychotics (risperidone > olanzapine > quetiapine), opioids, metoclopramide, domperidone, ranitidine, or verapamil.[50,51] In the presence of a large macroadenoma with mildly elevated prolactin, one must suspect the possibility of a stalk effect or hook effect. Hook effect can occur if an immunoassay is saturated because of markedly elevated prolactin and hence a falsely low result. A serial prolactin dilutional study by the laboratory is needed to unveil the hook effect.[52] Macroprolactin, a nonbioactive prolactin isoform usually composed of a prolactin monomer and an IgG molecule, can interfere with the immunologic assays, leading to a false elevated prolactin level despite normal bioactivity in vivo. This phenomenon is suspected in cases of hyperprolactinemia without symptoms or without a cause. Macroprolactin detection is performed by the laboratory using the polyethylene glycol precipitation method.[52,53]

If there is a personal or familial history of hyperparathyroidism, an assessment of multiple endocrine neoplasias (MEN-1), an autosomal-dominant form, should be undertaken. Family history of pituitary lesions and kidney stones can be revealing. Thirty to forty percent of patients with MEN-1 will have a pituitary tumor, most often a prolactinoma. Pancreatic neuroendocrine tumors, particularly gastrinomas, also affect close to one-third of patients.[54]

Table 3
Disease evaluation and clinical features[31,45,46,95]

| | Hypopituitarism | |
Axis	Clinical Syndrome	Interpretation of Laboratory Results
Growth hormone (GH)	GH deficiency Fatigue, weight gain, decreased productivity and quality of life	Screening low or low-normal IGF-1 Confirmation glucagon or macimorelin GH stimulation test
Luteinizing hormone–follicle-stimulating hormone (LH–FSH)	Hypogonadism Low libido and infertility Women: oligomenorrhea Men: erectile dysfunction, low muscle mass, gynecomastia	Normal or low in postmenopausal women Normal or low in premenopausal women with low estradiol or in men with low testosterone
Thyroid-stimulating hormone (TSH)	Hypothyroidism Fatigue, constipation, weight gain, cold intolerance, hair loss	Normal (low bioactivity) or low TSH with low free T4
Adrenocorticotropic hormone (ACTH)	Adrenal insufficiency Fatigue, orthostatic hypotension, nausea, anorexia, weight loss	Normal-low ACTH with low 8 AM cortisol • 8 AM cortisol <5 μg/dL: adrenal insufficiency • 8 AM cortisol 5–13 μg/dL: need ACTH stimulation test • 8 AM cortisol >13 μg/dL: normal
Prolactin	Prolactin deficiency Inability to lactate	Low prolactin
Antidiuretic hormone	Diabetes insipidus Polyuria, nocturia, polydipsia	Inappropriately low urine osmolarity in the setting of hypernatremia/hyperosmolarity

Pituitary Hypersecretion Syndromes

Axis	Clinical Syndrome	Interpretation of Laboratory Results
Prolactin	Prolactinoma Hypogonadism and galactorrhea	Prolactin <150–250 ng/mL: stalk effect, medication, microprolactinoma, end-stage renal disease, cirrhosis, neurogenic thoracic stimulation Prolactin > 150–250 ng/mL: macroprolactinoma Prolactinoma may co-secrete GH Rule out hook effect or macroprolactinemia (see text)
Growth hormone	Acromegaly Headaches, joint pain, seborrhea, hyperhidrosis, enlargement of hands and feet, macroglossia, teeth spacing, prognathism, visceromegaly, secondary diabetes, hypertension, sleep apnea	Elevated age-sex adjusted IGF-1 GH nadir >0.4 ng/mL at oral glucose tolerance test (OGTT) OGTT suppression test may not be necessary if IGF-1 is clearly elevated in the right clinical context
Adrenocorticotropic hormone	Cushing disease Truncal obesity, weight gain, skin thinning, easy bruising, proximal muscle weakness, secondary diabetes, hypertension, osteoporosis, oligomenorrhea	No adequate suppression of cortisol post-1 mg dexamethasone (>1.8 µg/dL) Elevated 24 h urine free cortisol Elevated late-night salivary cortisol Normal or elevated ACTH (must exclude ectopic Cushing syndrome from nonpituitary ACTH secretion)
Luteinizing hormone-follicle-stimulating hormone	Secondary "hypergonadism" (very rare) Increased libido, hirsutism, menorrhagia, increased muscle mass in men In men, preserved testicular size could be preserved	Normal or elevated LH and FSH with elevated estradiol or testosterone (in the appropriate clinical context)
Thyroid-stimulating hormone	Hyperthyroidism (rare) Tachycardia, weight loss, tremor, heat intolerance, hyperdefecation	Normal or elevated TSH with elevated T3 and free T4 (Must rule out thyroid hormone resistance or laboratory interference)

MASS EFFECTS OF PITUITARY INCIDENTALOMA

Headaches are not necessarily proportional to incidentaloma size and are more prevalent in patients with a personal or familial history of headaches/migraines.[55,56] Pain may be due to stretching the dura mater or inflammation or surrounding invaded tissue[55] unrelated to the pituitary lesion. Indeed, small incidentalomas diagnosed during headache investigation are rarely the cause of the headache, though such a relationship cannot be confirmed preoperatively. As such, a trial of prophylaxis/medical therapy for headaches and a neurology evaluation should be undertaken as a firstline evaluation.[57] If headaches persist or worsen despite therapy, surgery by an experienced neurosurgeon could be considered in selected patients, especially if the tumor is approaching 1 cm in size. In an RCC series, 65% to 90% of patients with cysts greater than 1 cm and refractory headaches had headache improvement after surgery.[38,58,59]

Five to forty percent of pituitary incidentalomas are associated with visual field defects.[22,33,34,43,60] Peripheral visual loss due to optic chiasm compression causes superior quadranopsia progressing to complete temporal hemianopsia. Clinical visual assessment such as finger counting and red color movement recognition comparisons can improve the detection of visual loss.[61] If a lesion is abutting or compressing the optic chiasm, ophthalmologic formal visual field testing is indicated.[10,62] Cavernous sinus invasion may cause cranial nerve (CN) lesions affecting CNs III, IV, VI, and ophthalmic (V1) and maxillary (V2) nerves with diplopia/ophthalmoplegia or facial paresthesia sparing the forehead, as may be observed in cases of pituitary apoplexy.

MALIGNANCY

Malignancy is rarely a concern as pituitary carcinomas are exceedingly rare (0.1%),[63] and pituitary metastases are often spread from a known distant cancer. However, hematological malignancies such as lymphomas and plasmacytomas can present at a primary pituitary site. Metastasis can affect stalk and posterior pituitary, causing central DI with hypopituitarism.[63] A biopsy is usually necessary if there is clinical suspicion.

IMAGING

Lesion size, nature (cystic or solid), location (central or peripheral, intrasellar or suprasellar), distance from the optic chiasm, and the presence of stalk deviation on the radiological report are important data for clinicians.

The optic chiasm is located approximately 6 to 10 mm above the pituitary gland. Thus, an 8 mm lesion located in the suprasellar area could potentially compress the optic chiasm. Coronal postcontrast T1 imaging usually reveals a hypointense pituitary adenoma (**Fig. 3**). Indirect signs for an adenoma are a convex gland with stalk deviation on the opposite side of the lesion. Cystic adenomas and RCCs may prove difficult to distinguish by imaging characteristics alone and will warrant evaluation and follow-up similar to those of pituitary adenomas.

MANAGEMENT
Observation and Follow-Up

In a systematic review and meta-analysis, tumor growth in pituitary incidentalomas was higher in macroadenomas than in microadenomas.[64] Overall, at a mean 4-year follow-up, 10% of microadenomas[65] and 25% to 40% of NFPAs greater than 1 cm

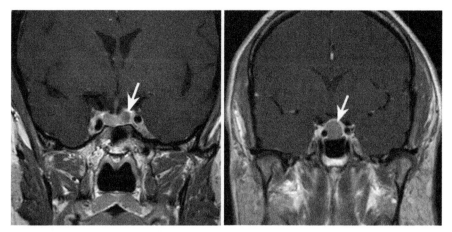

Fig. 3. Coronal T1W MR images—3 mm pituitary microadenoma and 14 mm macroadenoma.

had progressed.[42,65,66] Furthermore, solid lesions tended to grow more than cystic lesions.[64]

In cases of microincidentaloma, follow-up imaging should be planned at 12 months, then yearly for a few years, and then even less frequently if the patient remains stable. If the lesion is >1 cm, follow-up imaging in 6 months, then yearly is judicious.[10] A pituitary incidentaloma management algorithm is provided in **Fig. 4**. Of note, recurrence up to 20 years later has been described; thus, lifelong follow-up is warranted. An imaging plan after initial 5 to 10 years of stability followed by a 5-year interval follow-ups after that has been advocated,[67,68] though more studies are needed to determine the cost-effectiveness of lifelong imaging.

Postoperative surveillance, baseline imaging should be undertaken at 3 months and serially after that, based on the patient's clinical status, tumor pathology, and imaging characteristics.[69] In patients with prolactinomas, repeat imaging after initiation of dopamine agonists should be at 3 to 6 months for macroprolactinomas and 1 year for microprolactinomas. Thereafter, biochemical and structural responses are usually concordant, and serial imaging should be individualized.[70,71]

There is a potential risk in repeating MRIs with evidence of accumulation of gadolinium in the brain and other tissues.[72] A clinical correlation is unknown; however, limiting imaging as much as possible should be envisioned.

Pituitary hormone testing should be tailored based on incidentaloma size. If a lesion is <5 to 6 mm, repeated testing might not be necessary unless clinical symptoms evolve or the adenoma/cyst expands. If a lesion is >6 mm, testing after 1 or 2 years should be planned based on clinical symptoms or imaging results. If a lesion is >1 cm, follow-up in 6 to 12 months and then yearly, followed by every few years, is recommended. The risk of developing hypopituitarism is 2% to 3% per year for macroadenomas and less than 1% for microadenomas.[10]

Pituitary Surgery

Surgical indications include visual field loss, ophthalmoplegia, apoplexy with visual disturbance, and functional tumors (except prolactinomas).[73] Surgery should be considered if a lesion is actively enlarging (especially in the region of the optic chiasm), causing a progression of pituitary hormone loss, in a lesion close to the chiasm in a

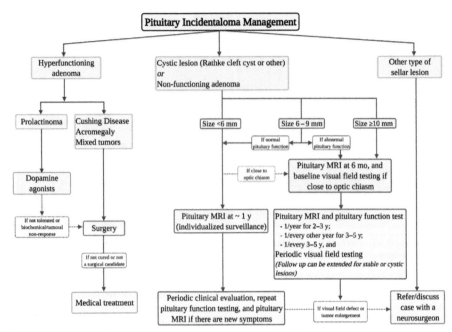

Fig. 4. Pituitary incidentaloma patient-management algorithm.

woman intending pregnancy, in patients with refractory headaches believed to be related to the mass, and indicating the histopathology necessary to establish a diagnosis (ie, if a malignancy or infiltrative disorder is suspected.)[10,74] Tumors abutting the optic chiasm, especially in young patients, are usually resected.[10,62,75] A typical surgical approach is transsphenoidal, and it is highly recommended that an expert neurosurgeon performs the surgery; this increases the likelihood of surgical cure and decreases complication risk.[76] Surgical risks include CSF leak, hemorrhage, infection, pituitary hypofunction, and hyponatremia or hypernatremia.

Medical Treatment

If a prolactinoma is confirmed, DA agonist therapy has been shown to decrease prolactin levels and tumor size in most patients. Bromocriptine (2.5–5 mg daily) and cabergoline (0.25–0.5 mg twice weekly) are mainstays of therapy, the latter being more potent and better tolerated.[50,77–80] Clinicians should be aware that D2-receptor agonists may induce impulse–control disorders such as gambling or deterioration in mood even in patients without histories of mental health issues.[81] Risk of valvular disorders at lower doses (usually used for prolactinomas) is minimal; however, awareness is needed at higher doses (over 2 mg) per week long term. For NFPA, cabergoline at higher doses (1–3 mg per week) has been used occasionally to stabilize tumor size, with variable results (30%–60%).[82]

In patients with acromegaly, somatostatin-receptor ligands (SRLs), such as octreotide or lanreotide, have been shown to achieve disease control in 30% to 40% of patients.[83] Pegvisomant efficacy ranges from 95% in clinical trials to approximately 65% in real-life studies.[84] Pasireotide and cabergoline are other treatment options used as a monotherapy or in combination.[84] In CD, if surgery is unsuccessful or delayed, steroidogenesis inhibitors (osilodrostat, ketoconazole, metyrapone) alone or in combination with pituitary directed therapies (pasireotide or cabergoline) may be used;

mifepristone, a glucocorticoid receptor blocker, has also been approved for the treatment of hyperglycemia or diabetes in patients with hypercortisolism[85,86] Comorbidities or mortalities in patients with acromegaly and CD can return to normal after biochemical remission.[87,88] SRLs have also been used in TSH-omas.

Hypopituitarism physiologic replacement is crucial to improving patient quality of life and survival.[45,89] A brief overview of key axis hormonal replacement is presented in **Table 3**.

Pituitary apoplexy

Overall, the risk of pituitary tumor infarct, necrosis, or bleeding may be as high as 15% to 25%.[90,91] Although only 2% to 5% of patients will present with apoplexy.[43,66] Apoplexy presents as an acute intense headache, often with ophthalmoplegia, due to rapid tumor enlargement and cranial nerve compression. Acute pituitary dysfunction also ensues; AI should be treated promptly. High-dose glucocorticoids could relieve ophthalmic signs and headaches, but surgery is recommended for most patients when there is ophthalmoplegia or visual loss.[92] Apoplexy may be precipitated by surgery, hemodynamic instability, or anticoagulation. Cases due to gonadotropin-releasing hormone agonist initiation have been reported, but its use is not contraindicated in patients with pituitary adenomas.[93,94]

SUMMARY

The pituitary incidentaloma rate as determined by imaging is high—close to 1 in 5 individuals. Most lesions are small or cystic and thus rarely cause a clinical syndrome *per se*. However, approximately one-third will have consequences and warrant management of mass effects or hormone oversecretion. Identifying pituitary incidentalomas is an opportunity for early diagnosis and treatment as well as reduced morbidity and/or mortality.

CLINICS CARE POINTS

- Pituitary incidentalomas will be discovered in 10% to 40% of brain imaging studies.

- Two-thirds of incidentalomas are macroadenomas, and approximately 15% consist of prolactinomas.

- One-third of individuals will undergo surgery, ideally by an expert neurosurgeon in a pituitary center of excellence.

- A small percentage will progress over time, and recurrence may occur and require long-term follow-up.

- In the absence of mass effect, a pituitary MRI should not be ordered without a definite biochemical diagnosis of pituitary dysfunction; the discovery of a pituitary incidentaloma may be unrelated.

ACKNOWLEDGEMENTS

The authors thank Shirley McCartney, PhD, (Oregon Health & Science University) for editorial assistance.

DISCLOSURE

The authors have nothing to disclose.

REFERENCES

1. Jin J, McHenry CR. Thyroid incidentaloma. Best Pract Res Clin Endocrinol Metab 2012;26(1):83–96.
2. Fassnacht M, Arlt W, Bancos I, et al. Management of adrenal incidentalomas: European Society of Endocrinology Clinical Practice Guideline in collaboration with the European Network for the Study of Adrenal Tumors. Eur J Endocrinol 2016; 175(2):G1–34.
3. Costello RT. Subclinical adenoma of the pituitary gland. Am J Pathol 1936;12(2): 205–216.1.
4. Molitch ME. Nonfunctioning pituitary tumors and pituitary incidentalomas. Endocrinol Metab Clin North Am 2008;37(1):151–171,xi.
5. Hall WA, Luciano MG, Doppman JL, et al. Pituitary magnetic resonance imaging in normal human volunteers: occult adenomas in the general population. Ann Intern Med 1994;120(10):817–20.
6. Chambers EF, Turski PA, LaMasters D, et al. Regions of low density in the contrast-enhanced pituitary gland: normal and pathologic processes. Radiology 1982;144(1):109–13.
7. Chong BW, Kucharczyk W, Singer W, et al. Pituitary gland MR: a comparative study of healthy volunteers and patients with microadenomas. AJNR Am J Neuroradiol 1994;15(4):675–9.
8. Carr DH, Sandler LM, Joplin GF. Computed tomography of sellar and parasellar lesions. Clin Radiol 1984;35(4):281–6.
9. Katzman GL, Dagher AP, Patronas NJ. Incidental findings on brain magnetic resonance imaging from 1000 asymptomatic volunteers. JAMA 1999; 282(1):36–9.
10. Freda PU, Beckers AM, Katznelson L, et al. Pituitary incidentaloma: an endocrine society clinical practice guideline. J Clin Endocrinol Metab 2011;96(4):894–904.
11. Sanno N, Oyama K, Tahara S, et al. A survey of pituitary incidentaloma in Japan. Eur J Endocrinol 2003;149(2):123–7.
12. Vaninetti NM, Clarke DB, Zwicker DA, et al. A comparative, population-based analysis of pituitary incidentalomas vs clinically manifesting sellar masses. Endocr Connect 2018;7(5):768–76.
13. Imran SA, Yip CE, Papneja N, et al. Analysis and natural history of pituitary incidentalomas. Eur J Endocrinol 2016;175(1):1–9.
14. Day PF, Loto MG, Glerean M, et al. Incidence and prevalence of clinically relevant pituitary adenomas: retrospective cohort study in a Health Management Organization in Buenos Aires, Argentina. Arch Endocrinol Metab 2016;60(6):554–61.
15. Agustsson TT, Baldvinsdottir T, Jonasson JG, et al. The epidemiology of pituitary adenomas in Iceland, 1955-2012: a nationwide population-based study. Eur J Endocrinol 2015;173(5):655–64.
16. Aldahmani KM, Sreedharan J, Ismail MM, et al. Prevalence and characteristics of sellar masses in the city of Al Ain, United Arab Emirates: 2010 to 2016. Ann Saudi Med 2020;40(2):105–12.
17. Al-Dahmani K, Mohammad S, Imran F, et al. Sellar masses: an epidemiological study. Can J Neurol Sci 2016;43(2):291–7.
18. Daly AF, Rixhon M, Adam C, et al. High prevalence of pituitary adenomas: a cross-sectional study in the province of Liege, Belgium. J Clin Endocrinol Metab 2006;91(12):4769–75.

19. Fernandez A, Karavitaki N, Wass JA. Prevalence of pituitary adenomas: a community-based, cross-sectional study in Banbury (Oxfordshire, UK). Clin Endocrinol (Oxf) 2010;72(3):377–82.
20. Jackson C, Rincon-Torroella J, Quinones-Hinojosa A. Parasellar tumors. In: Quinones-Hinojosa A, editor. Video atlas of neurosirgery: contemporary tumors. New York: Elsevier; 2017. p. 221–8.
21. Mulroney S, Myers A. General principles of endocrinology and pituitary and hypothalamic hormones. In: Mulroney S, Myers A, editors. Netter's essential physiology. Philadelphia, PA: Elsevier; 2016. p. 314–27.
22. Freda PU, Bruce JN, Khandji AG, et al. Presenting features in 269 patients with clinically nonfunctioning pituitary adenomas enrolled in a prospective study. J Endocr Soc 2020;4(4):bvaa021.
23. Famini P, Maya MM, Melmed S. Pituitary magnetic resonance imaging for sellar and parasellar masses: ten-year experience in 2598 patients. J Clin Endocrinol Metab 2011;96(6):1633–41.
24. Go JL, Rajamohan AG. Imaging of the sella and parasellar region. Radiol Clin North Am 2017;55(1):83–101.
25. Vasilev V, Rostomyan L, Daly AF, et al. Management of endocrine disease: pituitary 'incidentaloma': neuroradiological assessment and differential diagnosis. Eur J Endocrinol 2016;175(4):R171–84.
26. Hoang JK, Hoffman AR, González RG, et al. Management of incidental pituitary findings on CT, MRI, and (18)F-Fluorodeoxyglucose PET: a white paper of the ACR Incidental Findings Committee. J Am Coll Radiol 2018;15(7):966–72.
27. Chanson P, Daujat F, Young J, et al. Normal pituitary hypertrophy as a frequent cause of pituitary incidentaloma: a follow-up study. J Clin Endocrinol Metab 2001;86(7):3009–15.
28. Souteiro P, Maia R, Santos-Silva R, et al. Pituitary incidentalomas in paediatric age are different from those described in adulthood. Pituitary 2019;22(2):124–8.
29. Mete O, Lopes MB. Overview of the 2017 WHO classification of pituitary tumors. Endocr Pathol 2017;28(3):228–43.
30. Manojlovic-Gacic E, Engström BE, Casar-Borota O. Histopathological classification of non-functioning pituitary neuroendocrine tumors. Pituitary 2018;21(2):119–29.
31. Melmed S. Pituitary-tumor endocrinopathies. N Engl J Med 2020;382(10):937–50.
32. Daly AF, Beckers A. The epidemiology of pituitary adenomas. Endocrinol Metab Clin North Am 2020;49(3):347–55.
33. Anagnostis P, Adamidou F, Polyzos SA, et al. Pituitary incidentalomas: a single-centre experience. Int J Clin Pract 2011;65(2):172–7.
34. Esteves C, Neves C, Augusto L, et al. Pituitary incidentalomas: analysis of a neuroradiological cohort. Pituitary 2015;18(6):777–81.
35. Langlois F, Woltjer R, Cetas JS, et al. Silent somatotroph pituitary adenomas: an update. Pituitary 2018;21(2):194–202.
36. Ben-Shlomo A, Cooper O. Silent corticotroph adenomas. Pituitary 2018;21(2):183–93.
37. Culver SA, Grober Y, Ornan DA, et al. A case for conservative management: characterizing the natural history of radiographically diagnosed rathke cleft cysts. J Clin Endocrinol Metab 2015;100(10):3943–8.
38. Langlois F, Manea A, Lim DST, et al. High prevalence of adrenal insufficiency at diagnosis and headache recovery in surgically resected Rathke's cleft cysts-a large retrospective single center study. Endocrine 2019;63(3):463–9.

39. Müller HL, Merchant TE, Warmuth-Metz M, et al. Craniopharyngioma. Nat Rev Dis Primers 2019;5(1):75.

40. Chiloiro S, Giampietro A, Bianchi A, et al. Diagnosis of endocrine disease: primary empty sella: a comprehensive review. Eur J Endocrinol 2017;177(6): R275–85.

41. Donovan LE, Corenblum B. The natural history of the pituitary incidentaloma. Arch Intern Med 1995;155(2):181–3.

42. Karavitaki N, Collison K, Halliday J, et al. What is the natural history of nonoperated nonfunctioning pituitary adenomas? Clin Endocrinol (Oxf) 2007;67(6): 938–43.

43. Feldkamp J, Santen R, Harms E, et al. Incidentally discovered pituitary lesions: high frequency of macroadenomas and hormone-secreting adenomas - results of a prospective study. Clin Endocrinol (Oxf) 1999;51(1):109–13.

44. Reincke M, Allolio B, Saeger W, et al. The 'incidentaloma' of the pituitary gland. Is neurosurgery required? JAMA 1990;263(20):2772–6.

45. Fleseriu M, Hashim IA, Karavitaki N, et al. Hormonal replacement in hypopituitarism in adults: an endocrine society clinical practice guideline. J Clin Endocrinol Metab 2016;101(11):3888–921.

46. Langlois F, Varlamov EV, Fleseriu M. Hypopituitarism. In: Kellerman R, Rakel D, editors. Conn's current therapy. New York: Elsevier; 2021.

47. Katznelson L, Atkinson JL, Cook DM, et al. American association of clinical endocrinologists medical guidelines for clinical practice for the diagnosis and treatment of acromegaly-2011 update. Endocr Pract 2011;17:1–44.

48. Caron P, Brue T, Raverot G, et al. Signs and symptoms of acromegaly at diagnosis: the physician's and the patient's perspectives in the ACRO-POLIS study. Endocrine 2019;63(1):120–9.

49. Nieman LK, Biller BM, Findling JW, et al. The diagnosis of Cushing's syndrome: an Endocrine Society Clinical Practice Guideline. J Clin Endocrinol Metab 2008;93(5):1526–40.

50. Melmed S, Casanueva FF, Hoffman AR, et al. Diagnosis and treatment of hyperprolactinemia: an Endocrine Society clinical practice guideline. J Clin Endocrinol Metab 2011;96(2):273–88.

51. Milano W, Colletti C, Capasso A. Hyperprolactinemia induced by antipsychotics: from diagnosis to treatment approach. Endocr Metab Immune Disord Drug Targets 2017;17(1):38–55.

52. Vilar L, Vilar CF, Lyra R, et al. Pitfalls in the diagnostic evaluation of hyperprolactinemia. Neuroendocrinology 2019;109(1):7–19.

53. Richa V, Rahul G, Sarika A. Macroprolactin; a frequent cause of misdiagnosed hyperprolactinemia in clinical practice. J Reprod Infertil 2010;11(3):161–7.

54. Thakker RV, Newey PJ, Walls GV, et al. Clinical practice guidelines for multiple endocrine neoplasia type 1 (MEN1). J Clin Endocrinol Metab 2012;97(9): 2990–3011.

55. Suri H, Dougherty C. Clinical presentation and management of headache in pituitary tumors. Curr Pain Headache Rep 2018;22(8):55.

56. Levy MJ. The association of pituitary tumors and headache. Curr Neurol Neurosci Rep 2011;11(2):164–70.

57. Fleseriu M, Yedinak C, Campbell C, et al. Significant headache improvement after transsphenoidal surgery in patients with small sellar lesions. J Neurosurg 2009; 110(2):354–8.

58. Barkhoudarian G, Palejwala SK, Ansari S, et al. Rathke's cleft cysts: a 6-year experience of surgery vs. observation with comparative volumetric analysis. Pituitary 2019;22(4):362–71.

59. Nishioka H, Haraoka J, Izawa H, et al. Headaches associated with Rathke's cleft cyst. Headache 2006;46(10):1580–6.

60. Day PF, Guitelman M, Artese R, et al. Retrospective multicentric study of pituitary incidentalomas. Pituitary 2004;7(3):145–8.

61. Kerr NM, Chew SS, Eady EK, et al. Diagnostic accuracy of confrontation visual field tests. Neurology 2010;74(15):1184–90.

62. Lithgow K, Batra R, Matthews T, et al. Management of endocrine disease: visual morbidity in patients with pituitary adenoma. Eur J Endocrinol 2019;181(5):R185.

63. Heaney AP. Clinical review: pituitary carcinoma: difficult diagnosis and treatment. J Clin Endocrinol Metab 2011;96(12):3649–60.

64. Fernández-Balsells MM, Murad MH, Barwise A, et al. Natural history of nonfunctioning pituitary adenomas and incidentalomas: a systematic review and metaanalysis. J Clin Endocrinol Metab 2011;96(4):905–12.

65. Huang W, Molitch ME. Management of nonfunctioning pituitary adenomas (NFAs): observation. Pituitary 2018;21(2):162–7.

66. Arita K, Tominaga A, Sugiyama K, et al. Natural course of incidentally found nonfunctioning pituitary adenoma, with special reference to pituitary apoplexy during follow-up examination. J Neurosurg 2006;104(6):884–91.

67. Honegger J, Zimmermann S, Psaras T, et al. Growth modelling of non-functioning pituitary adenomas in patients referred for surgery. Eur J Endocrinol 2008;158(3): 287–94.

68. Wass JA, Reddy R, Karavitaki N. The postoperative monitoring of nonfunctioning pituitary adenomas. Nat Rev Endocrinol 2011;7(7):431–4.

69. Hinojosa-Amaya JM, Varlamov EV, McCartney S, et al. Pituitary magnetic resonance imaging use in teh posttreatment follow-up of secreting pituitary adenomas. In: Honegger J, Reincke M, Petersenn S, editors. Pituitary tumors: a comprehensive and interdisciplinary approach. New York: Elsevier; 2021.

70. Lombardi M, Lupi I, Cosottini M, et al. Lower prolactin levels during cabergoline treatment are associated to tumor shrinkage in prolactin secreting pituitary adenoma. Horm Metab Res 2014;46(13):939–42.

71. Varlamov EV, Hinojosa-Amaya JM, Fleseriu M. Magnetic resonance imaging in the management of prolactinomas; a review of the evidence. Pituitary 2020; 23(1):16–26.

72. Nachtigall LB, Karavitaki N, Kiseljak-Vassiliades K, et al. Physicians' awareness of gadolinium retention and MRI timing practices in the longitudinal management of pituitary tumors: a "Pituitary Society" survey. Pituitary 2019;22(1):37–45.

73. Fleseriu M, Bodach ME, Tumialan LM, et al. Congress of neurological surgeons systematic review and evidence-based guideline for pretreatment endocrine evaluation of patients with nonfunctioning pituitary adenomas. Neurosurgery 2016;79(4):E527–9.

74. Esposito D, Olsson DS, Ragnarsson O, et al. Non-functioning pituitary adenomas: indications for pituitary surgery and post-surgical management. Pituitary 2019; 22(4):422–34.

75. Jane JJ, Catalino M, Laws EJ. Surgical treatment of pituitary adenomas. In: Feingold K, Anawalt B, Boyce A, et al, editors. South Dartmouth, MA: MDText.com; 2000. Available at: https://www.ncbi.nlm.nih.gov/books/NBK278983/.

76. Casanueva FF, Barkan AL, Buchfelder M, et al. Criteria for the definition of Pituitary Tumor Centers of Excellence (PTCOE): a pituitary society statement. Pituitary 2017;20(5):489–98.

77. Colao A, Di Sarno A, Landi ML, et al. Macroprolactinoma shrinkage during cabergoline treatment is greater in naive patients than in patients pretreated with other dopamine agonists: a prospective study in 110 patients. J Clin Endocrinol Metab 2000;85(6):2247–52.

78. Molitch ME, Elton RL, Blackwell RE, et al. Bromocriptine as primary therapy for prolactin-secreting macroadenomas: results of a prospective multicenter study. J Clin Endocrinol Metab 1985;60(4):698–705.

79. Molitch ME. Dopamine agonists and antipsychotics. Eur J Endocrinol 2020; 183(3):C11–3.

80. Tewksbury A, Olander A. Management of antipsychotic-induced hyperprolactinemia. Ment Health Clin 2016;6(4):185–90.

81. Ioachimescu AG, Fleseriu M, Hoffman AR, et al. Psychological effects of dopamine agonist treatment in patients with hyperprolactinemia and prolactin-secreting adenomas. Eur J Endocrinol 2019;180(1):31.

82. Cooper O, Greenman Y. Dopamine agonists for pituitary adenomas. Front Endocrinol (Lausanne) 2018;9:469.

83. Feelders RA, Hofland LJ, van Aken MO, et al. Medical therapy of acromegaly: efficacy and safety of somatostatin analogues. Drugs 2009;69(16):2207–26.

84. Langlois F, McCartney S, Fleseriu M. Recent progress in the medical therapy of pituitary tumors. Endocrinol Metab (Seoul) 2017;32(2):162–70.

85. Langlois F, Chu J, Fleseriu M. Pituitary-directed therapies for Cushing's disease. Front Endocrinol (Lausanne) 2018;9:164.

86. Fleseriu M, Castinetti F. Updates on the role of adrenal steroidogenesis inhibitors in Cushing's syndrome: a focus on novel therapies. Pituitary 2016;19(6):643–53.

87. Bolfi F, Neves AF, Boguszewski CL, et al. Mortality in acromegaly decreased in the last decade: a systematic review and meta-analysis. Eur J Endocrinol 2018;179(1):59–71.

88. Graversen D, Vestergaard P, Stochholm K, et al. Mortality in Cushing's syndrome: a systematic review and meta-analysis. Eur J Intern Med 2012;23(3):278–82.

89. Tampourlou M, Fountas A, Ntali G, et al. Mortality in patients with non-functioning pituitary adenoma. Pituitary 2018;21(2):203–7.

90. Bonicki W, Kasperlik-Załuska A, Koszewski W, et al. Pituitary apoplexy: endocrine, surgical and oncological emergency. Incidence, clinical course and treatment with reference to 799 cases of pituitary adenomas. Acta Neurochir (Wien) 1993;120(3–4):118–22.

91. Fraioli B, Esposito V, Palma L, et al. Hemorrhagic pituitary adenomas: clinicopathological features and surgical treatment. Neurosurgery 1990;27(5):741–7 [discussion: 747–8].

92. Rajasekaran S, Vanderpump M, Baldeweg S, et al. UK guidelines for the management of pituitary apoplexy. Clin Endocrinol (Oxf) 2011;74(1):9–20.

93. Keane F, Egan AM, Navin P, et al. Gonadotropin-releasing hormone agonist-induced pituitary apoplexy. Endocrinol Diabetes Metab Case Rep 2016;2016: 160021.

94. Sasagawa Y, Tachibana O, Nakagawa A, et al. Pituitary apoplexy following gonadotropin-releasing hormone agonist administration with gonadotropin-secreting pituitary adenoma. J Clin Neurosci 2015;22(3):601–3.

95. Molitch ME. Diagnosis and treatment of pituitary adenomas: a review. JAMA 2017;317(5):516–24.

Practical Approach to Hyperandrogenism in Women

Anu Sharma, MD, Corrine K. Welt, MD*

KEYWORDS

- Hyperandrogenism • Women's health • Hirsutism • Polycystic ovarian syndrome

KEY POINTS

- Age must be considered in the differential diagnosis of hyperandrogenism.
- Total testosterone using liquid chromatography/mass spectrometry is the most useful laboratory test.
- Do not test testosterone or perform imaging in a patient on any form of hormonal contraception as it will suppress results.
- If a tumorous cause of hyperandrogenism is not identified, proceed with medical treatment.
- Hormonal contraceptives and anti-androgen medications, along with local treatment, are the most effective therapies to reduce hirsutism.

INTRODUCTION

The word androgen is derived from the Greek words andros and genao, which translate to "a man" and "produce or create," respectively. Hyperandrogenism is therefore any state with excess production of "male" hormones, although these hormones are normally found in women at lower levels. The most clinically relevant hormone in hyperandrogenism is testosterone, which is converted peripherally to dihydrotestosterone (DHT), its biologically active form. The most common symptom of hyperandrogenism in women is hirsutism, and the most prevalent cause is polycystic ovarian syndrome (PCOS).[1] The approach to hyperandrogenism in women differs depending on the stage of the woman's life. This article will serve as a concise review of hyperandrogenism in women at various stages of adult life.

Division of Endocrinology, Metabolism and Diabetes, University of Utah, EIHG 2110A, 15 N 2030 E, Salt Lake City, UT 84112, USA
* Corresponding author. Division of Endocrinology, Metabolism and Diabetes, University of Utah, Eccles Institute of Human Genetics, 15 North 2030 East, Salt Lake City, UT 84112.
E-mail address: cwelt@genetics.utah.edu

Med Clin N Am 105 (2021) 1099–1116
https://doi.org/10.1016/j.mcna.2021.06.008
0025-7125/21/© 2021 Elsevier Inc. All rights reserved.

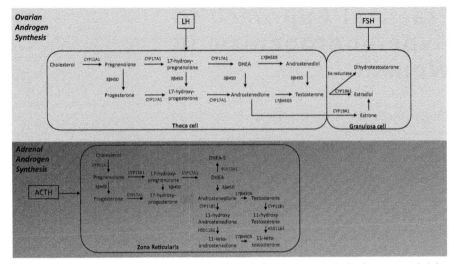

Fig. 1. Androgen synthesis in ovaries and adrenal glands. 3βHSD, 3β-hydroxysteroid dehydrogenase; CYP11A1, cytochrome P450 cholesterol side-chain cleavage; CYP11B1, cytochrome P450 11β-hydroxylase; CYP17A1, cytochrome P450 17α-hydroxylase/17,20-lyase; CYP19A1, cytochrome P450 aromatase demethylation/A-ring aromatization; FSH, follicle-stimulating hormone; HSD11B2, 11β-hydroxysteroid dehydrogenase type 2; LH, luteinizing hormone; SULT2A1, sulfotransferase 2A1.

Physiology of Androgens in Women

In women, the following are the two sources of androgens during the reproductive years: adrenal glands and ovaries (**Fig. 1**). It is estimated that 33% of circulating testosterone is produced by the theca cells of the ovaries.[2] The remaining testosterone is derived from androstenedione (A4), which is produced by both the ovaries and adrenal glands, and converted to testosterone in peripheral tissues. Testosterone is then converted by 5-α reductase to DHT both in the granulosa cell of the ovary and in peripheral tissues such as the skin.

A4 and dehydroepiandrosterone (DHEA) are secreted by the ovaries and the adrenal glands. Dehydroepiandrosterone sulfate (DHEA-S) is only produced in the zona reticularis of the adrenal gland.[3] DHEA is converted to A4. Adrenal androgen production is under adrenocorticotrophic hormone (ACTH) control, whereas ovarian androgen production is under control of luteinizing hormone (LH). The circulating concentration of all androgens, except DHEA-S, is therefore influenced by the phase of the menstrual cycle. Of note, androgens have a circadian rhythm, albeit mild, in women.[4]

DHEA, DHEA-S, and A4 are considered preandrogens as their action at the androgen receptor is far less potent than testosterone. In women, they can play a role in hyperandrogenic symptoms and signs because overall testosterone levels are relatively low.[5] The DHEA-S concentration in a woman increases from the age of 7 to 8 years (adrenarche), peaks in her 20s, and then decreases and plateaus in her 50s to 60s. Although the control of DHEA-S production is mainly by ACTH, it has a long half-life and is the best biomarker for adrenal hyperandrogenism in most situations. DHEA-S levels are increased by prolactin and insulin-like growth factor 1, which may explain the hyperandrogenism associated with other disorders.[5] Interestingly, circulating DHEA-S can be used as a precursor by ovarian follicles to produce DHEA, testosterone, and DHT.[6]

Androgens have direct effects on reproduction via the androgen receptor and indirect effects through conversion to estrogen. The androgen receptor is present on cells throughout the hypothalamic-pituitary-ovarian axis.[2] Therefore, high androgen levels can suppress hypothalamic and pituitary secretion of GnRH, LH, and follicle-stimulating hormone (FSH) directly and via aromatization to estradiol. Androgens also play a role in ovarian function, directly. Androgen receptor knockout mouse populations (complete,[7,8] granulosa cell specific,[9] and gonadotroph specific[10]) show decreased fertility, change in cycle length, poor follicle health, and decreased ovulation. Clinically and experimentally, excess androgens either from an endogenous[11] or exogenous source[12] result in increased follicle recruitment but then arrested follicle development. Androgen pretreatment during in vitro fertilization has resulted in improved ovarian response leading to increased pregnancy and live birth rates in some studies.[13,14] Optimal androgen concentrations are therefore required for ovarian follicle initiation, follicle growth, ovulation, and oocyte maturation.

Genetics

PCOS is by far the most common cause of hyperandrogenism in women, thus most of the genetic data on hyperandrogenism in women stem from PCOS studies. Genome-wide association studies (GWAS) of testosterone levels in women provide additional insight into testosterone production.[15] PCOS is a heritable, polygenic disorder with multiple risk loci contributing to disease.[16] The International PCOS Consortium performed a meta-analysis of more than 10,000 PCOS cases, with a control-to-case ratio of approximately 10:1, resulting in the identification of 19 loci that confer risk for PCOS in Han Chinese and European women.[17] Of those identified, 8 were associated with increased testosterone and/or hyperandrogenism phenotypes. Both *THADA* and *FSHβ* loci are associated with testosterone levels or regulation.[18,19] *DENND1A* is associated with hyperandrogenism (biochemical and clinical). However, the exact underlying mechanism by which it influences androgen concentrations and actions is unclear.[15] The *IRF1/RAD50* locus is associated with testosterone levels in the European GWAS;[17] however, its effect is likely indirect because of the lack of association in the GWAS of testosterone levels.[18] The other loci associated with hyperandrogenism are *SOD2*, *ERBB3/RAB5*, *TOX3*, and *C9orf3*.[17]

History/Physical

The three most important aspects when taking a history in the woman with hyperandrogenism are age, ethnicity, and duration of symptoms. The top differential diagnoses change depending on these features.

Age
Premenopausal women are more likely to have PCOS or nonclassic congenital adrenal hyperplasia (NCCAH). The top diagnoses would shift to ovarian hyperthecosis and androgen-producing tumors in postmenopausal women. If the woman is pregnant, gestational hyperandrogenism would be the likely culprit.

Ethnicity
Ethnicity influences the color, normal distribution, and quantity of body hair. Women of Mediterranean, Middle Eastern, South Asian, and Hispanic ethnicities have higher cut-offs for the modified Ferriman-Gallwey Score (mFG) (**Fig. 2**) compared with East Asians and Caucasians of Northern European ancestry.[20] Furthermore, self-perceived hirsutism scores are higher than clinician-perceived scores.[21] This should not negate the symptom of hirsutism, especially if it is of concern to the woman.[1]

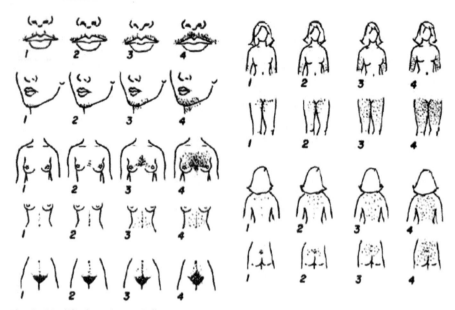

Fig. 2. Modified Ferriman-Gallwey score.

Duration of symptoms

Rapid onset (over months) of increased hair growth is concerning for an androgen-producing tumor compared with PCOS (12 months vs 42 months in one study).[22]

The most common symptoms of hyperandrogenism in women are as follows:

Hirsutism

Hirsutism is defined as male pattern terminal hair growth in a woman.[23] Both the location of hair growth that is bothersome to the woman and the type of hair growth influence the treatment plan. The distribution of terminal hair growth should be clearly documented. The mFG grades 9 androgen-sensitive areas on the quantity of hair growth and is useful for documentation (see **Fig. 2**). Scores range from 0 (absence of terminal hair) to 4 (fully covered). Abnormal total scores are as follows: ≥9 in Middle Eastern, Mediterranean, South Asian, and Hispanic women; ≥8 in Blacks and European Caucasians; ≥7 in Southern Chinese women; ≥6 in South American women; and ≥2 in Han Chinese women.[20,24] The mFG has significant interuser variability and is subjective to the scorer.[25,26] As noted earlier, self-reported scores are often higher than clinician scores and are limited by a patient's previous attempts at hair removal. In addition, the score limits the importance of local areas. For example, a woman with new-onset increased terminal hair growth on her face due to an androgen-producing tumor will receive a score of only 4.[27] It also fails to include the sideburns and lower buttocks.[1] Nevertheless, it remains the most common metric to score hirsutism.

Alopecia

The typical pattern of hair loss in women with hyperandrogenism follows a male pattern with vertex thinning/balding (male pattern hair loss or MPHL). MPHL or androgenic alopecia is commonly associated with elevated levels of circulating androgens. Female pattern hair loss (FPHL) usually occurs in the central scalp with preservation of the frontal hairline.[28] Elevated circulating androgens may or may not be associated, although the level of 5α reductase activity at the hair follicle cannot be easily assessed and may play a role in FPHL.[29,30] Interestingly, biochemical hyperandrogenism was found in 26% to 84% of women presenting with FPHL.[31–33]

Acne
Sebaceous glands are able to convert testosterone to DHT as they exhibit 5α reductase activity.[34] In addition, they express 3β-hydroxysteroid dehydrogenase, 17β hydroxysteroid dehydrogenase, and P450 side-chain cleavage activity,[35] all contributing to an increased androgenic environment, which promotes sebum formation in the presence of a proandrogenic environment.[36]

Oligomenorrhea/amenorrhea
Documentation of age at menarche, menstrual cycle history, and use of any hormonal contraception are important aspects in further elucidating an underlying etiology for hyperandrogenism. In the postmenopausal woman, hyperandrogenism can often lead to postmenopausal bleeding because of the increased conversion of testosterone to estrogen.

Of note, a thorough drug history should be performed to ensure there was no exposure to oral minoxidil, danazol, antiepileptics, anabolic steroids, and exogenous androgens. These exogenous androgens can include transfer from a family member's prescription,[37] DHEA supplements, bioidentical hormone creams/pills/pellets, hormone boosters, or antiaging cocktails supplied by wellness/antiaging clinics.[38]

Symptoms and signs of virilization are more likely to indicate an ovarian or adrenal tumor. These signs include deepening of the voice, clitoromegaly, and increased muscle mass. Clitoromegaly is defined as a clitoris length greater than 10 mm or a clitoral index (length × width) > 35 mm^2.[39]

Important clues to other underlying endocrine disorders include signs of Cushing syndrome (purple striae, supraclavicular fullness, facial plethora, and easy bruising) and acromegaly (enlarged jaw, macroglossia, and swollen hands/feet with an increase in shoe/ring size).

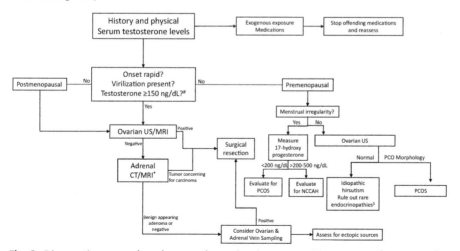

Fig. 3. Diagnostic approach to hyperandrogenism in women. CT – computed tomography; MRI – magnetic resonance imaging; NCCAH – non-classic congenital adrenal hyperplasia; PCOS – polycystic ovarian syndrome; US – ultrasound. *CT contraindicated in pregnancy, $See text for details, #Measured by LC-MS/MS.

Diagnostic Evaluation

Laboratory investigation

The most useful laboratory test is the total testosterone concentration (**Fig. 3**). The method of assay, however, influences the accuracy of this measurement. Liquid chromatography/mass spectrometry (LC-MS/MS) is the most reliable method in quantifying androgen excess in women.[40] Measurement of total testosterone by direct radioimmunoassay (RIA) is the most widely available method. RIA was designed to measure total testosterone concentrations in men. The interassay variation at low testosterone levels is high.[41] Therefore, although RIAs and other immunoassays are sufficient to identify moderate to severe androgen excess (as is seen in tumors), they often fail to detect mild elevations in PCOS.[41,42] Free testosterone correlates strongly with hyperandrogenism. However, its measurement is fraught with inaccuracies.[1] Free testosterone is most accurately measured by equilibrium dialysis, which is not readily available in most clinical laboratories.[41] Low levels of sex hormone-binding globulin (SHBG) can be used as an indirect marker of higher free testosterone levels.[43] The clinician should bear in mind that obesity, hypothyroidism, inflammation, SHBG polymorphisms, and mutations can cause low levels of SHBG and influence free testosterone.[44–47] Of note, laboratory testing should not be performed until at least 3 months after stopping hormonal contraception of any type and in the absence of progestin-coated IUDs. Hormones will suppress endogenous androgens and make measurements inaccurate for clinical diagnostic purposes.

In a premenopausal woman, a pregnancy test should be performed. If negative, measurement of prolactin, FSH, thyroid-stimulating hormone, and early morning 17-hydroxyprogesterone (7–9 AM) should be evaluated. Cushing's syndrome and acromegaly should be ruled out based on the presenting clinical symptoms and signs.

Measuring DHEA-S can be helpful to assess adrenal hyperandrogenism. DHEA-S can be elevated in both PCOS and adrenal tumors.[48] If the DHEA-S is >700 μg/dL, an adrenal tumor should be ruled out.[1] Concentrations of A4 and DHEA are not part of the routine evaluation for hyperandrogenism. The biochemical pattern of A4, DHEA, and DHT is variable and measurements add little value except in specific clinical cases.[49–51]

Imaging

If the physical examination reveals virilization or the laboratory measurements show severe biochemical androgen excess (total testosterone by LC/MS $\geq$150 ng/dL in a premenopausal woman or $\geq$64 ng/dL in a postmenopausal woman),[22] pelvic imaging should be the next step in evaluation. An ovarian source is the etiology in approximately 80% of cases.[22,52] Unless there is a concern for an ovarian tumor, imaging should also be delayed until at least 3 months after stopping hormonal contraception of any type and in the absence of progestin-coated IUDs. Hormones will cause the ovarian volume to decrease and make measurements inaccurate for PCOS clinical diagnostic purposes.

Owing to lower cost, transvaginal ultrasonography with color Doppler should be the first line of imaging.[53] However, ovarian tumors are generally small in size (Leydig cell tumors <3 cm) and isoechoic. They are easily missed by transabdominal ultrasonography. MRI would be the next best step if pelvic ultrasonography is negative. 18 Fluorodeoxyglucose ([18]FDG)-PET imaging is usually reserved for select cases.[54,55] Of note, ovarian hyperthecosis can be described on ultrasonography as a bilateral increase in ovarian size, a single ovarian nodule, or it can also appear normal.[56] The data comparing the different imaging techniques in the evaluation of severe hyperandrogenism are scant.[53,57] The absence of an ovarian tumor on imaging does not rule out the presence of an ovarian androgen-producing tumor. The presence of 12 or more antral follicles and/or ovarian volume greater than 10 cm³ would meet the Rotterdam criteria for PCOS.[58]

When pelvic imaging is negative or if androgen levels suggest an adrenal etiology (DHEA-S >700 μg/dL), adrenal computed tomography (CT) would be the next step. Adrenal CT should be performed with and without contrast so that the Hounsfield units, absolute and relative washout can be calculated. If CT is contraindicated, MRI with the measurement of chemical shift can be performed.[59] [18]FDG-PET/CT can also be considered second line in select cases.[60] Adrenal incidentalomas are common, especially in the postmenopausal age group.[61] Adrenal imaging should therefore only be pursued if clinically indicated. Adrenal imaging may reveal a solitary benign nodule, adrenal carcinoma, or bilateral hyperplasia. In the presence of an adrenal tumor, the woman should also be assessed for excess endogenous cortisol secretion. If cortisol excess is present, surgery for Cushing syndrome will decrease morbidity and mortality.[62] Bear in mind that the excess ACTH production in NCCAH would lead to bilateral adrenal cortical hyperplasia but there would not be excess cortisol present.[63]

Lastly, in the setting of severe hyperandrogenism, ovarian and adrenal vein sampling can be used when both pelvic and adrenal imaging are negative.[52] Right and left ovarian and adrenal veins are accessed and testosterone is measured to determine a left to right difference. This requires the skill set of a highly experienced interventional radiologist. Ovarian and adrenal vein sampling is useful in two scenarios: (1) in the premenopausal woman where preservation of fertility is desired and localization of one ovary for resection is required, and (2) in the postmenopausal woman with a small adrenal nodule but a suspected ovarian source.

Table 1
Differential diagnoses of hyperandrogenism

Stage of Life	Adrenal	Ovarian	Other
Premenopausal	Congenital adrenal hyperplasia (classic and nonclassic) Glucocorticoid resistance Cortisone reductase deficiency Adrenal adenoma Adrenal carcinoma Bilateral macronodular adrenal hyperplasia	PCOS Ovarian tumors: Sertoli-Leydig cell tumors Granulosa-theca cell tumors Hilus cell tumors	Idiopathic hirsutism Exogenous exposure Hyperprolactinemia Cushing's disease Acromegaly Insulin resistance syndromes Medications (danazol, valproic acid, oxcarbazepine)
Gestational	Adrenal adenoma Adrenal carcinoma	Luteoma Theca lutein cysts Sertoli-Leydig cell tumors	Exogenous exposure Placental aromatase deficiency
Postmenopausal	Adrenal adenoma Adrenal carcinoma Bilateral macronodular adrenal hyperplasia	Ovarian hyperthecosis Ovarian tumors: Sertoli-Leydig cell tumors Granulosa-theca cell tumors Teratomas Krukenberg tumors	Exogenous exposure Hyperprolactinemia Cushing's disease Acromegaly Medications (danazol, valproic acid, oxcarbazepine)

Differential Diagnoses

The top differential diagnoses differ based on the stage of the woman's life. We discuss the 3 most common diagnoses in premenopausal and postmenopausal women (**Table 1**). In addition, gestational hyperandrogenism is briefly explored.

Premenopausal hyperandrogenism

Polycystic ovarian syndrome. PCOS is the most common endocrine disorder in reproductive-age women, affecting approximately 10% of the population.[64] Two of 3 Rotterdam criteria are required to achieve the diagnosis: (1) oligomenorrhea/amenorrhea, (2) clinical or biochemical hyperandrogenism, and/or (3) polycystic ovaries on ultrasound, which is defined as 20 or more antral follicles and/or ovarian volume greater than 10 cm^3.[58] In women with hyperandrogenism, 57% to 82% meet the criteria for PCOS.[65,66] In women with PCOS, 65% to 75% have hyperandrogenism, with hirsutism being the most common symptom.[67] In one prospective study, only 2.3% of women with PCOS had another identifiable endocrine disorder to explain symptoms.[68]

Idiopathic hirsutism. When there are no abnormalities found on investigation, that is, elevated testosterone or DHEA-S and normal ovaries on ultrasound in a woman younger than 40 years and not on hormonal contraception, and there are no menstrual abnormalities, the diagnosis of idiopathic hirsutism is made.[69] Treatment is directed toward controlling hirsutism with shared decision-making to ensure the woman's perceived areas of concern are adequately addressed.

Non-classic congenital adrenal hyperplasia. Women with NCCAH present with menstrual irregularities and hyperandrogenism, often leading to a misdiagnosis of PCOS. NCCAH is due to 21-hydroxylase deficiency (P450c21) leading to increased 17-hydroxyprogesterone precursor available for the androgen pathway with increased production of androstenedione and testosterone.[70] The diagnosis can be made if the 7 to 9 AM 17-hydroxyprogesterone is >500 ng/dL. If the AM level is between 200 and 500 ng/dL, a stimulated 17-hydroxyprogesterone level 60 min after a 250 mcg injection of cosyntropin is needed, with a diagnostic 17-hydroxyprogesterone level ≥1500 ng/mL. Unlike the classic form, NCCAH rarely manifests with cortisol deficiency and thus glucocorticoid replacement and ACTH suppression is not needed unless fertility is desired. General hyperandrogenism treatments can be used (see section on Treatment: Glucocorticoids below).

Postmenopausal hyperandrogenism

Ovarian hyperthecosis. Ovarian hyperthecosis is a histologic diagnosis noted when there is the presence of nests of luteinized theca cells throughout the ovarian stroma. Postmenopausal women present with slow onset and progressive symptoms of hyperandrogenism. In severe cases, virilization can occur. Typical signs of insulin resistance are often present (acanthosis nigricans, skin tags, central obesity). The abundance of luteinized cells is thought to be due to increased gonadotrophin levels, which result in increased androgen production.[71] Postmenopausal bleeding, due to endometrial hyperplasia from testosterone aromatization to estrogen, can also be a presenting symptom. Women often have elevated testosterone and estradiol concentrations with inappropriately low LH and FSH for a menopausal woman.[72] Ultrasonography often reveals bilaterally enlarged, solid ovaries for the woman's stated age.[73] Therefore, it is important to evaluate ovarian size compared to age-based references as ovaries that are normal in size compared to a reproductive-aged woman are likely enlarged compared to normative data in postmenopausal women. In premenopausal women with hyperthecosis, ovaries may demonstrate an absence of small follicles on ultrasound in addition to enlarged ovaries.

Ovarian and adrenal neoplasms. Androgen-producing tumors are more common in postmenopausal women. Most ovarian sources are benign, whereas adrenal tumors can be either benign or malignant. Adrenocortical carcinoma often cosecretes other hormones (cortisol, aldosterone) in addition to excess androgens, thereby warranting further assessment. Women present with rapidly, progressive symptoms of hyperandrogenism, often with virilization.[56,74] Surgical resection results in rapid resolution of symptoms.

Iatrogenic hyperandrogenism. Androgens, including DHEA, are often prescribed to treat postmenopausal symptoms.[75] The currently available testosterone replacements were developed for male hypogonadism, but can be a cause of hyperandrogenism in women exposed to a partner's topical testosterone. If these products are used in women, they can lead to frank hyperandrogenism.[72] Antiepileptics (valproic acid and oxcarbazepine) have been associated with biochemical hyperandrogenism.[76,77]

Gestational hyperandrogenism

Hyperandrogenism in pregnancy is extremely rare.[78] During normal pregnancy, testosterone and A4 concentrations increase progressively in each trimester, returning to baseline concentrations postpartum.[79,80] The increase in androgens promotes cervical ripening[81] and contributes to the relaxation of the myometrium during pregnancy.[82] The increase in androgen concentrations is offset by an increase in SHBG, thereby limiting the biologically active fraction.[83] Rarely a pregnancy luteoma, the physiologic remnant of the corpus luteum from the menstrual cycle of conception, produces testosterone at high levels and results in hyperandrogenism. Placental aromatase cytochrome P450 converts androgens to estradiol, which is then metabolized to estriol by the fetal liver, protecting the fetus from maternal hyperandrogenism.[83] In rare cases of recessive placental aromatase deficiency, the placenta is unable to aromatize androgens and both the mother and fetus experience virilization.

In general, only hyperandrogenism internal to the fetus or placental aromatase deficiency cause fetal virilization.[84] Female fetal exposure to excess androgens between the 7th and 12th weeks of gestation can result in labial fusion and clitoromegaly. The hormonal milieu may also play a role in long-term fetal development with potential influence on fetal growth,[85] metabolism,[86] cardiovascular function,[87] reproductive function,[88] and behavior.[78,89] The most common fetal cause is fetal 21-hydroxylase CAH.[90] Treatment options are limited and dependent on fetal sex and fetal virilization risk.[83,91]

Treatment

The goals of management are 2-fold: (1) identify and surgically treat severe virilization and (2) decrease any perceived symptoms/signs of hyperandrogenism.[1]

Ovarian and adrenal tumors should undergo complete surgical resection if possible. Bilateral oophorectomy is the treatment of choice for ovarian hyperthecosis. If no tumor is identified in the postmenopausal woman, bilateral oophorectomy should be performed, given the high likelihood of an ovarian source.[22,56] In the premenopausal woman, fertility-sparing cytoreductive surgery should be considered.[92] For adrenal tumors, nonsurgical techniques can be used if surgery is contraindicated or not desired. Radiofrequency ablation and CT-guided cryoablation have been used in functional adrenal adenomas with similar outcomes compared to surgical resection.[93,94]

Medical management

Lifestyle. In obese women with PCOS, weight loss results in a small decrease in testosterone as measured by the free androgen index (mean difference −1.11, 95% confidence interval [CI] −1.96 to −0.26) and a concomitant mild improvement in hirsutism (mean difference −1.12 [95% CI (−2.16 to −0.08)].[95] Although lifestyle intervention is necessary for overall health, it has a limited impact in improving hyperandrogenism. It should not be the sole management strategy.[96]

Oral contraceptives. Oral contraceptives containing ethinyl estradiol (EE) suppress LH production and increase SHBG concentrations, resulting in decreased ovarian androgen production and decreased free testosterone concentrations, respectively.[97] The dose of EE, whether low dose (20 mcg) or average dose (30–35 mcg), both work to suppress androgens, and all progestins seem to work equally well regardless of the underlying androgenicity.[1] Hormonal contraception can also cause a small reduction in adrenal androgen secretion, inhibition of androgen binding to its receptor, and inhibition of 5α-reductase.[1] There is an increased risk of venous thromboembolism with oral contraceptives, with a greater risk in obese women over the age of 39 years who smoke.[98] Obesity itself is not a contraindication to using oral contraceptives.[99] In women with hirsutism or androgenic acne, oral contraceptives should be first-line medical management if fertility is not desired.[1,96] The effect on hyperandrogenic symptoms/signs should be reassessed in 6 months.[1]

Antiandrogens. After 6 months of oral contraceptive use, an antiandrogen can be added to improve symptoms of hyperandrogenism. The available antiandrogens in the United States are spironolactone (100–200 mg/d) and finasteride (2.5-5 mg/d). Use of any antiandrogen in women is considered off-label use.

Spironolactone. Spironolactone is an aldosterone receptor antagonist with a dose-dependent competitive inhibition of the androgen receptor. It is effective in reducing hirsutism scores.[100] It is contraindicated in pregnancy because of the blockade of androgen action critical for the formation of the external male genitalia. Therefore, it should be used with a reliable contraceptive method unless the woman is abstinent. It is a potassium-sparing diuretic and therefore can cause hypotension, dizziness, and hyperkalemia. Potassium levels should be monitored and caution should be taken in the setting of renal impairment.

Finasteride. Finasteride is a 5α reductase inhibitor, with specific activity against type 2 5α reductase. It decreases local DHT levels in hair follicles with comparable effects to other antiandrogens. The effect of finasteride is dose-dependent, with 2.5 mg and 5 mg having a similar reduction in hirsutism scores and 7.5 mg slightly more effective.[101] The most common side effects are low libido, depression/asthenia, and orthostatic hypotension.[102] Dutasteride is a 5α reductase inhibitor with activity against both type 1 and 2 5α reductase enzymes. There is limited data on the use of dutasteride in women.[103] Although there is no direct comparison of spironolactone to finasteride, pooled data suggest spironolactone to be more effective, although finasteride data are limited.[100]

Cyproterone acetate. Cyproterone acetate is a competitive inhibitor at the androgen receptor and commonly used outside of the United States.[69] It is available in combination with EE in the form of combined oral contraceptive pills. At a dose of 2 mg, its effect is equivalent to 50 mg of spironolactone.[104] However, the risk of venous thromboembolism is 50% to 100% higher than for oral contraceptives with levonorgestrel.[105] The use of an oral contraceptive containing cyproterone acetate results in a mildly better mFG on follow-up compared with the use of other oral contraceptives.[106] The Endocrine Society notes its effect on hirsutism is not clinically significant. Cyproterone acetate containing hormonal contraceptives are not recommended over other oral contraceptives.[1]

Local/topical treatment. If medical management is contraindicated or symptoms are not worrisome enough for the woman to warrant systemic therapy, local treatment options should be discussed. In addition, local treatment is an important adjunct to hormonal treatment as the improvement in hirsutism with hormonal treatment takes over 6 months, reflecting the cycle of the hair follicle. Direct hair removal via shaving, waxing, bleaching, chemical creams, photoepilation, or electrolysis can be used.[1] Topical antiandrogens have limited efficacy in hirsutism. Acne should be treated by a dermatologist. First-line therapy for alopecia is topical minoxidil, noting a synergistic effect when combined with systemic antiandrogens.[28] Other treatment options for alopecia are low-level laser light therapy,[107] hair transplantation,[108] and platelet-rich plasma.[109]

Glucocorticoids. In classic 21-hydroxylase congenital adrenal hyperplasia, glucocorticoids are effective in suppressing ACTH-stimulated adrenal androgen production.[70] In NCCAH, glucocorticoids should not be the first-line therapy to treat symptoms/signs of hyperandrogenism other than for ovulation induction. In fact, oral contraceptives are more effective in improving hirsutism compared with dexamethasone.[110]

GnRH agonists. GnRH agonists are equally effective as oral contraceptives in decreasing hirsutism.[111] These long-acting, modified GnRH peptides initially stimulate, but then suppress LH and FSH after approximately 1 week because of desensitization. GnRH agonists therefore induce hypoestrogenism, resulting in bone loss and hot flashes.[112] Its use should be reserved for the rare cases of virilization that are not amenable to other therapies.

Medications that reduce insulin levels or improve insulin action. In multiple meta-analyses, medications that reduce insulin levels or improve insulin action (metformin, troglitazone, and rosiglitazone) were no more effective than placebo in treating hyperandrogenism in PCOS.[1,96,100,113] Therefore, metformin should be reserved for the treatment of prediabetes or type 2 diabetes in women with PCOS, as it is not as effective as other medications for cosmetic concerns or for uterine protection in the case of irregular menses.

SUMMARY

The approach to hyperandrogenism in women varies depending on the woman's age and severity of symptoms. Once tumorous hyperandrogenism is excluded, the most common cause is PCOS. Hirsutism is the most common presenting symptom. The woman's concern about her symptoms plays an important role in the management of disease. Although measurement of testosterone is useful in identifying an underlying cause, care must be taken when interpreting the less accurate assays that are available commercially. Surgical resection is curative in tumorous etiologies, whereas medical management is the mainstay for nontumorous causes.

CLINICS CARE POINTS

- Age based diagnoses are important considerations

- Exclude androgen secreting tumors first
- Total testosterone is the best assay for hyperandrogenism
- Do not assess testosterone levels or ovarian morphology in a patient using any form of hormonal contraception
- Non-tumorous hyperandrogenism can be treated medically
- Total testosterone is the best assay for clinical hyperandrogenism

DISCLOSURE

The authors have nothing to disclose.

REFERENCES

1. Martin KA, Anderson RR, Chang RJ, et al. Evaluation and Treatment of Hirsutism in Premenopausal Women: An Endocrine Society Clinical Practice Guideline. J Clin Endocrinol Metab 2018;103(4):1233–57.
2. Walters KA, Handelsman DJ. Role of androgens in the ovary. Mol Cell Endocrinol 2018;465:36–47.
3. Schiffer L, Arlt W, Storbeck K-H. Intracrine androgen biosynthesis, metabolism and action revisited. Mol Cell Endocrinol 2018;465:4–26.
4. Davison SL, Bell R. Androgen Physiology. Semin Reprod Med 2006;24(02):071–7.
5. Burger HG. Androgen production in women. Fertil Steril 2002;77(Suppl 4):S3–5.
6. Haning RV Jr, Flood CA, Hackett RJ, et al. Metabolic Clearance Rate of Dehydroepiandrosterone Sulfate, Its Metabolism to Testosterone, and Its Intrafollicular Metabolism to Dehydroepiandrosterone, Androstenedione, Testosterone, and Dihydrotestosterone in Vivo*. J Clin Endocrinol Metab 1991;72(5):1088–95.
7. Shiina H, Matsumoto T, Sato T, et al. Premature ovarian failure in androgen receptor-deficient mice. Proc Natl Acad Sci U S A 2006;103(1):224–9.
8. Cheng XB, Jimenez M, Desai R, et al. Characterizing the neuroendocrine and ovarian defects of androgen receptor-knockout female mice. Am J Physiol Endocrinol Metab 2013;305(6):E717–26.
9. Walters KA, Middleton LJ, Joseph SR, et al. Targeted loss of androgen receptor signaling in murine granulosa cells of preantral and antral follicles causes female subfertility. Biol Reprod 2012;87(6):151.
10. Wu S, Chen Y, Fajobi T, et al. Conditional knockout of the androgen receptor in gonadotropes reveals crucial roles for androgen in gonadotropin synthesis and surge in female mice. Mol Endocrinol 2014;28(10):1670–81.
11. Hague WM, Adams J, Rodda C, et al. The prevalence of polycystic ovaries in patients with congenital adrenal hyperplasia and their close relatives. Clin Endocrinol 1990;33(4):501–10.
12. Becerra-Fernández A, Pérez-López G, Menacho Román M, et al. Prevalence of hyperandrogenism and polycystic ovary syndrome in female to male transsexuals. Endocrinología y Nutrición (English Edition) 2014;61(7):351–8.
13. Wiser A, Gonen O, Ghetler Y, et al. Addition of dehydroepiandrosterone (DHEA) for poor-responder patients before and during IVF treatment improves the pregnancy rate: A randomized prospective study. Humanit Rep 2010;25(10):2496–500.

14. Kim C-H, Howles CM, Lee H-A. The effect of transdermal testosterone gel pretreatment on controlled ovarian stimulation and IVF outcome in low responders. Fertil Steril 2011;95(2):679–83.
15. Welt CK. Genetics of polycystic ovary syndrome: What is new? Endocrinol Metab Clin North Am 2021;50(1):71–82.
16. Vink JM, Sadrzadeh S, Lambalk CB, et al. Heritability of polycystic ovary syndrome in a Dutch twin-family study. J Clin Endocrinol Metab 2006;91(6):2100–4.
17. Day F, Karaderi T, Jones MR, et al. Large-scale genome-wide meta-analysis of polycystic ovary syndrome suggests shared genetic architecture for different diagnosis criteria. Plos Genet 2018;14(12):e1007813.
18. Ruth KS, Day FR, Tyrrell J, et al. Using human genetics to understand the disease impacts of testosterone in men and women. Nat Med 2020;26(2):252–8.
19. Chen ZJ, Zhao H, He L, et al. Genome-wide association study identifies susceptibility loci for polycystic ovary syndrome on chromosome 2p16.3, 2p21 and 9q33.3. Nat Genet 2011;43(1):55–9.
20. Escobar-Morreale HF, Carmina E, Dewailly D, et al. Epidemiology, diagnosis and management of hirsutism: a consensus statement by the Androgen Excess and Polycystic Ovary Syndrome Society. Humanit Rep 2011;18(2):146–70.
21. Pasch L, He SY, Huddleston H, et al. Clinician vs Self-ratings of Hirsutism in Patients With Polycystic Ovarian Syndrome: Associations With Quality of Life and Depression. JAMA Dermatol 2016;152(7):783–8.
22. Sharma A, Kapoor E, Singh RJ, et al. Diagnostic Thresholds for Androgen-Producing Tumors or Pathologic Hyperandrogenism in Women by Use of Total Testosterone Concentrations Measured by Liquid Chromatography-Tandem Mass Spectrometry. Clin Chem 2018;64(11):1636–45.
23. Rosenfield RL. Clinical practice. Hirsutism N Engl J Med 2005;353(24):2578–88.
24. Afifi L, Saeed L, Pasch LA, et al. Association of ethnicity, Fitzpatrick skin type, and hirsutism: A retrospective cross-sectional study of women with polycystic ovarian syndrome. Int J Womens Dermatol 2017;3(1):37–43.
25. Wild RA, Vesely S, Beebe L, et al. Ferriman Gallwey self-scoring I: performance assessment in women with polycystic ovary syndrome. J Clin Endocrinol Metab 2005;90(7):4112–4.
26. Yildiz BO, Bolour S, Woods K, et al. Visually scoring hirsutism. Humanit Rep 2010;16(1):51–64.
27. Adefris M, Fekadu E. Postmenopausal mild hirsutism and hyperandrogenemia due to granulosa cell tumor of the ovary: a case report. J Med Case Rep 2017;11(1):242.
28. Carmina E, Azziz R, Bergfeld W, et al. Female Pattern Hair Loss and Androgen Excess: A Report From the Multidisciplinary Androgen Excess and PCOS Committee. J Clin Endocrinol Metab 2019;104(7):2875–91.
29. Montalto J, Whorwood CB, Funder JW, et al. Plasma C19 steroid sulphate levels and indices of androgen bioavailability in female pattern androgenic alopecia. Clin Endocrinol (Oxf) 1990;32(1):1–12.
30. Sánchez P, Serrano-Falcón C, Torres JM, et al. 5α-Reductase isozymes and aromatase mRNA levels in plucked hair from young women with female pattern hair loss. Arch Dermatol Res 2018;310(1):77–83.
31. Vexiau P, Chaspoux C, Boudou P, et al. Role of androgens in female-pattern androgenetic alopecia, either alone or associated with other symptoms of hyperandrogenism. Arch Dermatol Res 2000;292(12):598–604.

32. Karrer-Voegeli S, Rey F, Reymond MJ, et al. Androgen dependence of hirsutism, acne, and alopecia in women: retrospective analysis of 228 patients investigated for hyperandrogenism. Medicine (Baltimore) 2009;88(1):32–45.

33. Futterweit W, Dunaif A, Yeh HC, et al. The prevalence of hyperandrogenism in 109 consecutive female patients with diffuse alopecia. J Am Acad Dermatol 1988;19(5 Pt 1):831–6.

34. Makrantonaki E, Zouboulis CC. Testosterone metabolism to 5alpha-dihydrotestosterone and synthesis of sebaceous lipids is regulated by the peroxisome proliferator-activated receptor ligand linoleic acid in human sebocytes. Br J Dermatol 2007;156(3):428–32.

35. Thiboutot D, Jabara S, McAllister JM, et al. Human skin is a steroidogenic tissue: steroidogenic enzymes and cofactors are expressed in epidermis, normal sebocytes, and an immortalized sebocyte cell line (SEB-1). J Invest Dermatol 2003; 120(6):905–14.

36. Ju Q, Tao T, Hu T, et al. Sex hormones and acne. Clin Dermatol 2017;35(2): 130–7.

37. Merhi ZO, Santoro N. Postmenopausal virilization after spousal use of topical androgens. Fertil Steril 2007;87(4):976.e13-5.

38. Stuenkel CA, Manson JE. Compounded Bioidentical Hormone Therapy: Does the Regulatory Double Standard Harm Women? JAMA Intern Med 2017; 177(12):1719–20.

39. Tagatz GE, Kopher RA, Nagel TC, et al. The clitoral index: a bioassay of androgenic stimulation. Obstet Gynecol 1979;54(5):562–4.

40. Rosner W, Auchus RJ, Azziz R, et al. Utility, Limitations, and Pitfalls in Measuring Testosterone: An Endocrine Society Position Statement. J Clin Endocrinol Metab 2007;92(2):405–13.

41. Legro RS, Schlaff WD, Diamond MP, et al. Total testosterone assays in women with polycystic ovary syndrome: precision and correlation with hirsutism. J Clin Endocrinol Metab 2010;95(12):5305–13.

42. Chang WY, Knochenhauer ES, Bartolucci AA, et al. Phenotypic spectrum of polycystic ovary syndrome: clinical and biochemical characterization of the three major clinical subgroups. Fertil Steril 2005;83(6):1717–23.

43. Rosenfield RL. Plasma testosterone binding globulin and indexes of the concentration of unbound plasma androgens in normal and hirsute subjects. J Clin Endocrinol Metab 1971;32(6):717–28.

44. Goldman AL, Bhasin S, Wu FCW, et al. A Reappraisal of Testosterone's Binding in Circulation: Physiological and Clinical Implications. Endocr Rev 2017;38(4): 302–24.

45. Simó R, Barbosa-Desongles A, Lecube A, et al. Potential role of tumor necrosis factor-α in downregulating sex hormone-binding globulin. Diabetes 2012;61(2): 372–82.

46. Nestler JE, Powers LP, Matt DW, et al. A direct effect of hyperinsulinemia on serum sex hormone-binding globulin levels in obese women with the polycystic ovary syndrome. J Clin Endocrinol Metab 1991;72(1):83–9.

47. Hogeveen KN, Cousin P, Pugeat M, et al. Human sex hormone-binding globulin variants associated with hyperandrogenism and ovarian dysfunction. J Clin Invest 2002;109(7):973–81.

48. Elhassan YS, Idkowiak J, Smith K, et al. Causes, Patterns, and Severity of Androgen Excess in 1205 Consecutively Recruited Women. J Clin Endocrinol Metab 2018;103(3):1214–23.

49. Welt CK, Arason G, Gudmundsson JA, et al. Defining constant versus variable phenotypic features of women with polycystic ovary syndrome using different ethnic groups and populations. J Clin Endocrinol Metab 2006;91(11):4361–8.

50. O'Reilly MW, Taylor AE, Crabtree NJ, et al. Hyperandrogenemia predicts metabolic phenotype in polycystic ovary syndrome: the utility of serum androstenedione. J Clin Endocrinol Metab 2014;99(3):1027–36.

51. Livadas S, Pappas C, Karachalios A, et al. Prevalence and impact of hyperandrogenemia in 1,218 women with polycystic ovary syndrome. Endocrine 2014; 47(2):631–8.

52. Kaltsas GA, Mukherjee JJ, Kola B, et al. Is ovarian and adrenal venous catheterization and sampling helpful in the investigation of hyperandrogenic women? Clin Endocrinol (Oxf) 2003;59(1):34–43.

53. Outwater EK, Wagner BJ, Mannion C, et al. Sex cord-stromal and steroid cell tumors of the ovary. Radiographics 1998;18(6):1523–46.

54. McCarthy-Keith DM, Hill M, Norian JM, et al. Use of F 18-fluoro-D-glucose-positron emission tomography-computed tomography to localize a hilar cell tumor of the ovary. Fertil Steril 2010;94(2):753.e11-4.

55. Prassopoulos V, Laspas F, Vlachou F, et al. Leydig cell tumour of the ovary localised with positron emission tomography/computed tomography. Gynecol Endocrinol 2011;27(10):837–9.

56. Yance VRV, Marcondes JAM, Rocha MP, et al. Discriminating between virilizing ovary tumors and ovary hyperthecosis in postmenopausal women: clinical data, hormonal profiles and image studies. Eur J Endocrinol 2017;177(1):93.

57. Tanaka YO, Tsunoda H, Kitagawa Y, et al. Functioning ovarian tumors: direct and indirect findings at MR imaging. Radiographics 2004;24(Suppl 1):S147–66.

58. Teede HJ, Misso ML, Costello MF, et al. Recommendations from the international evidence-based guideline for the assessment and management of polycystic ovary syndrome. Fertil Steril 2018;110(3):364–79.

59. Nandra G, Duxbury O, Patel P, et al. Technical and Interpretive Pitfalls in Adrenal Imaging. Radiographics 2020;40(4):1041–60.

60. Delivanis DA, Bancos I, Atwell TD, et al. Diagnostic performance of unenhanced computed tomography and (18) F-fluorodeoxyglucose positron emission tomography in indeterminate adrenal tumours. Clin Endocrinol (Oxf) 2018; 88(1):30–6.

61. Fassnacht M, Arlt W, Bancos I, et al. Management of adrenal incidentalomas: European Society of Endocrinology Clinical Practice Guideline in collaboration with the European Network for the Study of Adrenal Tumors. Eur J Endocrinol 2016;175(2):G1.

62. Javanmard P, Duan D, Geer EB. Mortality in Patients with Endogenous Cushing's Syndrome. Endocrinol Metab Clin North Am 2018;47(2):313–33.

63. Kok HK, Sherlock M, Healy NA, et al. Imaging features of poorly controlled congenital adrenal hyperplasia in adults. Br J Radiol 2015;88(1053):20150352.

64. Bozdag G, Mumusoglu S, Zengin D, et al. The prevalence and phenotypic features of polycystic ovary syndrome: a systematic review and meta-analysis. Humanit Rep 2016;31(12):2841–55.

65. Azziz R, Sanchez LA, Knochenhauer ES, et al. Androgen excess in women: experience with over 1000 consecutive patients. J Clin Endocrinol Metab 2004;89(2):453–62.

66. Carmina E, Rosato F, Jannì A, et al. Extensive clinical experience: relative prevalence of different androgen excess disorders in 950 women referred because of clinical hyperandrogenism. J Clin Endocrinol Metab 2006;91(1):2–6.

67. Azziz R, Woods KS, Reyna R, et al. The prevalence and features of the polycystic ovary syndrome in an unselected population. J Clin Endocrinol Metab 2004; 89(6):2745–9.

68. O'Driscoll JB, Mamtora H, Higginson J, et al. A prospective study of the prevalence of clear-cut endocrine disorders and polycystic ovaries in 350 patients presenting with hirsutism or androgenic alopecia. Clin Endocrinol (Oxf) 1994; 41(2):231–6.

69. Azziz R, Carmina E, Sawaya ME. Idiopathic hirsutism. Endocr Rev 2000;21(4): 347–62.

70. Merke DP, Auchus RJ. Congenital Adrenal Hyperplasia Due to 21-Hydroxylase Deficiency. N Engl J Med 2020;383(13):1248–61.

71. Krug E, Berga SL. Postmenopausal hyperthecosis: functional dysregulation of androgenesis in climacteric ovary. Obstet Gynecol 2002;99(5 Pt 2):893–7.

72. Markopoulos MC, Kassi E, Alexandraki KI, et al. MANAGEMENT OF ENDOCRINE DISEASE: Hyperandrogenism after menopause. Eur J Endocrinol 2015;172(2):R79.

73. Rousset P, Gompel A, Christin-Maitre S, et al. Ovarian hyperthecosis on grayscale and color Doppler ultrasound. Ultrasound Obstet Gynecol 2008;32(5): 694–9.

74. Derksen J, Nagesser SK, Meinders AE, et al. Identification of virilizing adrenal tumors in hirsute women. N Engl J Med 1994;331(15):968–73.

75. Davis SR, Baber R, Panay N, et al. Global Consensus Position Statement on the Use of Testosterone Therapy for Women. J Clin Endocrinol Metab 2019;104(10): 4660–6.

76. Hu X, Wang J, Dong W, et al. A meta-analysis of polycystic ovary syndrome in women taking valproate for epilepsy. Epilepsy Res 2011;97(1–2):73–82.

77. Löfgren E, Tapanainen JS, Koivunen R, et al. Effects of carbamazepine and oxcarbazepine on the reproductive endocrine function in women with epilepsy. Epilepsia 2006;47(9):1441–6.

78. Hakim C, Padmanabhan V, Vyas AK. Gestational Hyperandrogenism in Developmental Programming. Endocrinology 2017;158(2):199-212.

79. Kuijper EA, Ket JC, Caanen MR, et al. Reproductive hormone concentrations in pregnancy and neonates: a systematic review. Reprod Biomed Online 2013; 27(1):33–63.

80. Sir-Petermann T, Maliqueo M, Angel B, et al. Maternal serum androgens in pregnant women with polycystic ovarian syndrome: possible implications in prenatal androgenization. Humanit Rep 2002;17(10):2573–9.

81. Ji H, Dailey TL, Long V, et al. Androgen-regulated cervical ripening: a structural, biomechanical, and molecular analysis. Am J Obstet Gynecol 2008;198(5): 543.e1-9.

82. Perusquía M, Navarrete E, Jasso-Kamel J, et al. Androgens induce relaxation of contractile activity in pregnant human myometrium at term: a nongenomic action on L-type calcium channels. Biol Reprod 2005;73(2):214–21.

83. Kaňová N, Bičíková M. Hyperandrogenic states in pregnancy. Physiol Res 2011; 60(2):243–52.

84. Wood RI, Foster DL. Sexual differentiation of reproductive neuroendocrine function in sheep. Rev Reprod 1998;3(2):130–40.

85. Carlsen SM, Jacobsen G, Romundstad P. Maternal testosterone levels during pregnancy are associated with offspring size at birth. Eur J Endocrinol 2006; 155(2):365–70.

86. Eisner JR, Dumesic DA, Kemnitz JW, et al. Timing of prenatal androgen excess determines differential impairment in insulin secretion and action in adult female rhesus monkeys. J Clin Endocrinol Metab 2000;85(3):1206–10.

87. Vyas AK, Hoang V, Padmanabhan V, et al. Prenatal programming: adverse cardiac programming by gestational testosterone excess. Sci Rep 2016;6:28335.

88. Abbott DH, Barnett DK, Bruns CM, et al. Androgen excess fetal programming of female reproduction: a developmental aetiology for polycystic ovary syndrome? Humanit Rep 2005;11(4):357–74.

89. Knickmeyer R, Baron-Cohen S, Fane BA, et al. Androgens and autistic traits: A study of individuals with congenital adrenal hyperplasia. Horm Behav 2006; 50(1):148–53.

90. Merke DP, Bornstein SR. Congenital adrenal hyperplasia. Lancet 2005; 365(9477):2125–36.

91. Masarie K, Katz V, Balderston K. Pregnancy luteomas: clinical presentations and management strategies. Obstet Gynecol Surv 2010;65(9):575–82.

92. Ertas IE, Taskin S, Goklu R, et al. Long-term oncological and reproductive outcomes of fertility-sparing cytoreductive surgery in females aged 25 years and younger with malignant ovarian germ cell tumors. J Obstet Gynaecol Res 2014;40(3):797–805.

93. Sarwar A, Brook OR, Vaidya A, et al. Clinical Outcomes following Percutaneous Radiofrequency Ablation of Unilateral Aldosterone-Producing Adenoma: Comparison with Adrenalectomy. J Vasc Interv Radiol 2016;27(7):961–7.

94. Fu YF, Cao C, Shi YB, et al. Computed tomography-guided cryoablation for functional adrenal aldosteronoma. Minim Invasive Ther Allied Technol 2019;1–5.

95. Lim SS, Hutchison SK, Van Ryswyk E, et al. Lifestyle changes in women with polycystic ovary syndrome. Cochrane Database Syst Rev 2019;3(3):Cd007506.

96. Legro RS, Arslanian SA, Ehrmann DA, et al. Diagnosis and Treatment of Polycystic Ovary Syndrome: An Endocrine Society Clinical Practice Guideline. J Clin Endocrinol Metab 2013;98(12):4565–92.

97. Fitzgerald C, Elstein M, Spona J. Effect of age on the response of the hypothalamo-pituitary-ovarian axis to a combined oral contraceptive. Fertil Steril 1999;71(6):1079–84.

98. Nightingale AL, Lawrenson RA, Simpson EL, et al. The effects of age, body mass index, smoking and general health on the risk of venous thromboembolism in users of combined oral contraceptives. Eur J Contracept Reprod Health Care 2000;5(4):265–74.

99. Curtis KM, Tepper NK, Jatlaoui TC, et al. U.S. Medical Eligibility Criteria for Contraceptive Use, 2016. MMWR Recomm Rep 2016;65(3):1–103.

100. Swiglo BA, Cosma M, Flynn DN, et al. Clinical review: Antiandrogens for the treatment of hirsutism: a systematic review and metaanalyses of randomized controlled trials. J Clin Endocrinol Metab 2008;93(4):1153–60.

101. Al-Khawajah MM. Finasteride for hirsutism: a dose finding study. Saudi Med J 1998;19(1):19–21.

102. Fertig RM, Gamret AC, Darwin E, et al. Sexual side effects of 5-α-reductase inhibitors finasteride and dutasteride: A comprehensive review. Dermatol Online J 2017;23(11).

103. Gupta AK, Mays RR, Dotzert MS, et al. Efficacy of non-surgical treatments for androgenetic alopecia: a systematic review and network meta-analysis. J Eur Acad Dermatol Venereol 2018;32(12):2112–25.

104. Muhn P, Fuhrmann U, Fritzemeier KH, et al. Drospirenone: a novel progestogen with antimineralocorticoid and antiandrogenic activity. Ann N Y Acad Sci 1995; 761:311–35.

105. Stegeman BH, de Bastos M, Rosendaal FR, et al. Different combined oral contraceptives and the risk of venous thrombosis: systematic review and network meta-analysis. Bmj 2013;347:f5298.

106. Van der Spuy ZM, le Roux PA. Cyproterone acetate for hirsutism. Cochrane Database Syst Rev 2003;4:Cd001125.

107. Afifi L, Maranda EL, Zarei M, et al. Low-level laser therapy as a treatment for androgenetic alopecia. Lasers Surg Med 2017;49(1):27–39.

108. Unger WP, Unger RH. Hair transplanting: an important but often forgotten treatment for female pattern hair loss. J Am Acad Dermatol 2003;49(5):853–60.

109. Giordano S, Romeo M, Lankinen P. Platelet-rich plasma for androgenetic alopecia: Does it work? Evidence from meta analysis. J Cosmet Dermatol 2017;16(3): 374–81.

110. Frank-Raue K, Junga G, Raue F, et al. [Therapy of hirsutism in females with adrenal enzyme defects of steroid hormone biosynthesis: comparison of dexamethasone with cyproterone acetate]. Klin Wochenschr 1990;68(12):597–601.

111. Heiner JS, Greendale GA, Kawakami AK, et al. Comparison of a gonadotropin-releasing hormone agonist and a low dose oral contraceptive given alone or together in the treatment of hirsutism. J Clin Endocrinol Metab 1995;80(12): 3412–8.

112. Dawood MY, Ramos J, Khan-Dawood FS. Depot leuprolide acetate versus danazol for treatment of pelvic endometriosis: changes in vertebral bone mass and serum estradiol and calcitonin. Fertil Steril 1995;63(6):1177–83.

113. van Zuuren EJ, Fedorowicz Z, Carter B, et al. Interventions for hirsutism (excluding laser and photoepilation therapy alone). Cochrane Database Syst Rev 2015;2015(4):Cd010334.

Update on Osteoporosis Screening and Management

Anika K. Anam, MD*, Karl Insogna, MD

KEYWORDS

- Bone loss • Dual-energy X-ray absorptiometry • Fracture • Menopause
- Osteoporosis

KEY POINTS

- All postmenopausal women and men aged 50 and older should be evaluated for risk of osteoporosis.
- Evaluation for osteoporosis should include a detailed history, physical exam, and laboratory tests to assess for secondary causes of bone loss and mineral metabolism.
- Osteoporosis treatment should be individualized to the patient and includes optimizing nutrition, weight-bearing exercise, fall prevention strategies, and use of anti-resorptive or anabolic pharmacologic therapies.

INTRODUCTION

Osteoporosis is a metabolic bone disease characterized by low bone mass and micro-architectural deterioration of the bone tissue, leading to reduced bone strength and increased risk of low-energy fractures or fragility fractures. Worldwide, osteoporosis is estimated to affect 200 million women, and 1 in 3 women over age 50 will experience osteoporosis-related fractures, as will 1 in 5 men aged over 50.[1–3] The most common osteoporotic-related fractures are those of the vertebrae (spine), proximal femur (hip), and distal forearm (wrist). Osteoporosis has many etiologies; the most common cause is estrogen deficiency-related bone loss, such as that occurring after menopause. This article mainly focuses on postmenopausal osteoporosis and newer pharmacologic therapies, although the therapeutic interventions discussed here are often but not always relevant to other pathophysiologic types of osteoporosis, including male osteoporosis. It provides guidance for health care providers on the proper screening, identification of secondary causes, and appropriate treatment of osteoporosis in postmenopausal women.

Department of Internal Medicine, Section of Endocrinology, Yale Bone Center, Yale University School of Medicine, 333 Cedar Street, FMP 107, PO Box 208020, New Haven, CT 06519, USA
* Corresponding author.
E-mail address: anika.anam@yale.edu

Med Clin N Am 105 (2021) 1117–1134
https://doi.org/10.1016/j.mcna.2021.05.016
0025-7125/21/© 2021 Elsevier Inc. All rights reserved.

PATHOPHYSIOLOGY OF OSTEOPOROSIS

The skeleton provides structural support for the body and storage for two essential minerals, calcium and phosphorus. Individual bone mass reaches a peak between 25 and 30 years of age and begins to decline around 40. The skeleton consists of a mineralized matrix with a highly active cellular fraction that includes osteocytes, osteoblasts, and osteoclasts. Osteoblasts are derived from marrow mesenchymal cells and form new bone and initiate bone resorption, which are the first steps in replacing old or damaged bone. Osteoclasts are involved in bone resorption and derived from hematopoietic progenitors. Both osteocytes and osteoblasts release receptor activator of nuclear factor kappa B ligand (RANKL), which is essential for osteoclastogenesis. In addition to RANKL, osteoblasts produce osteoprotegerin (OPG), an inhibitor of osteoclastogenesis. OPG is a soluble receptor for RANKL that binds this ligand and prevents interaction of RANKL with its cognate receptor, receptor activator of nuclear factor kappa B. RANKL is the primary stimulator of osteoclast formation. Osteoblasts and osteoclasts play critical roles in bone remodeling, a dynamic process during which old bone is removed and new bone is added to the skeleton. Osteocytes are thought to be the principal cell regulating remodeling, producing RANKL and a critical inhibitor of bone formation, sclerostin. Bone remodeling is affected by systemic hormones, including parathyroid hormone (PTH), 1,25-dihydroxyvitamin D, calcitonin, growth hormone, glucocorticoids, gonadal hormones, thyroid hormones, and cytokines. In addition, changes in mechanical force activate bone remodeling to improve skeletal strength and repair bone that has undergone microdamage. In the young adult skeleton, the amount of new bone formed by osteoblasts is equal to the amount resorbed by osteoclasts. However, bone loss occurs when this cycle is uncoupled, resulting in more removal than replacement of bone.[4]

The cycle of bone remodeling becomes uncoupled with menopause and advancing age, resulting in more bone resorption than bone formation. During the menopausal transition, serum estradiol levels decrease by 85% to 90%, and serum estrone decreases by 65% to 75%, relative to premenopausal values. With the decline in estrogen levels during menopause, the rate of bone remodeling increases by 2-fold to 4-fold. Increased bone resorption leads to a phase of accelerated bone loss and efflux of skeletal-derived calcium to the extracellular fluid. These changes lead to a negative balance of total body calcium, which further exacerbates skeletal losses.[5] At menopause, women undergo rapid trabecular bone loss that usually continues for 5 to 8 years after the cessation of menses. Initially, about 20% to 30% of the trabecular bone and 5% to 10% of the cortical bone are lost. During the second phase of bone loss, occurring 8 to 10 years after menopause, trabecular and cortical bone are lost at equal rates. Bone loss leads to deterioration in skeletal microarchitecture and increased fracture risk.

Later in menopause, age-related bone loss and accompanying changes in the material properties of bone further exacerbate estrogen deficiency-related bone loss.

Increased osteoclast number and activity disrupt trabecular connectivity and increase cortical porosity. Resorption pits caused by accelerated bone remodeling remain incompletely filled because new bone formation does not keep pace with bone resorption. Reduced bone density and quality cause increases in fracture risk.

Many other hormonal and systemic disorders can lead to accelerated bone loss regardless of age and estrogen status. These secondary causes of osteoporosis include vitamin D deficiency, hyperparathyroidism, hypercortisolism, hyperthyroidism, anorexia nervosa, inflammatory diseases (eg, rheumatoid arthritis), gastrointestinal disease (eg, chronic liver disease, celiac disease, and inflammatory bowel disease), plasma cell dyscrasias (eg, multiple myeloma and monoclonal gammopathy of undetermined significance), chronic renal disease, renal calcium leak, and drugs (eg, steroids, antiepileptics, depot medroxyprogesterone acetate, chronic heparin use, vitamin A, loop diuretics, and selective serotonin receptor uptake inhibitors). Excessive alcohol consumption and hypogonadism are secondary causes of bone loss in men.

DIAGNOSIS AND EVALUATION
Screening for Osteoporosis

The decision to perform bone density assessment should be based on the patient's fracture risk profile and skeletal health assessment. Regardless of clinical risk factors, women aged 65 and older and men aged 70 and older should undergo bone mineral density (BMD) testing. Bone density assessment should be considered in younger postmenopausal women, women in the menopausal transition, and men aged 50 to 69 with clinical risk factors for fracture. In addition, individuals who have a fracture at or over age 50 and those with conditions that predispose to low bone mass or bone loss (rheumatoid arthritis) or taking medications (chronic glucocorticoids) should be considered for bone density assessment. Individuals being considered for pharmacologic therapy for osteoporosis, anyone being treated for osteoporosis, anyone not receiving therapy and in whom evidence of bone loss would lead to treatment, and all postmenopausal women discontinuing estrogen should also be considered for bone density testing. BMD measurement is not routinely indicated in healthy young men or premenopausal women unless there is a significant fracture history or there are specific risk factors for bone loss.[6]

Measurement of Bone Mineral Density

Dual-energy x-ray absorptiometry (DXA) measurement of the hip (femoral neck and total hip) and spine is the preferred method of diagnosing osteoporosis, predicting future fracture risk, and monitoring patients. If the hip or spine cannot be measured, BMD measured by DXA at the one-third radius site can be used for diagnosis. DXA measures bone mineral content (BMC) in grams and bone area (BA) in square centimeters. The areal BMD in grams per square centimeter is calculated by dividing BMC by BA. The T-score, a value used for diagnosing osteoporosis, is calculated by subtracting the mean BMD of a young-adult reference population from the patient's BMD and dividing it by the standard deviation (SD) of the young-adult population. The Z-score, used to compare the patient's BMD with that of a population of peers, is calculated by subtracting the mean BMD of an age-matched, ethnicity-matched, and sex-matched reference population from the patient's BMD and dividing by the SD of the reference population.[7] BMD diagnoses of normal bone mass, osteopenia, and osteoporosis are

Table 1	
The World Health Organization definition of osteoporosis based on bone mineral density (BMD) measurement of the spine, hip, or forearm by dual-energy x-ray absorptiometry devices	
Normal	BMD within 1 SD of a young normal adult (T-score ≥ -1)
Low bone mass (osteopenia)	BMD between 1 and 2.4 SD less than that of a young normal adult (T-score between -1 and -2.4)
Osteoporosis	BMD 2.5 SD or more less than that of a young normal adult (T-score ≤ -2.5)
Severe osteoporosis	T-score ≤ -2.5 with one or more fractures

based on the World Health Organization (WHO) diagnostic classification (**Table 1**).[6] This classification should be used for postmenopausal women and should not be applied to premenopausal women. Of note, even if the BMD is in the normal range, osteoporosis can be diagnosed based on the presence of a previous fragility fracture. A fragility fracture is defined as a fracture in adult life occurring spontaneously or a fracture arising from trauma that, in a healthy individual, would not have resulted in a fracture. In premenopausal women, a diagnosis of osteoporosis should not be made from densitometric criteria alone. The International Society for Clinical Densitometry (ISCD) recommends that instead of T-scores, ethnic or race-adjusted Z-scores should be used in premenopausal women. Z-scores of −2.0 or lower are defined as either low BMD for chronologic age or less than the expected range for age; those more than −2.0 are defined as within the expected range for age.[7] When using DXA to monitor change in BMD with time and therapy, the absolute BMD value (grams per square centimeter) should be used. Statistically significant change in BMD is calculated as 2.77 multiplied by precision at the site of measurement to provide the least significant change. In an individual patient, an adequate time interval (usually 18–24 months) is required between measurements to show significant change unless larger changes in BMD are anticipated (eg, glucocorticoid treatment).[7] When using DXA to monitor change in BMD, it is important to use the same scanner and software because different manufacturers use different edge-detection algorithms and different x-ray beam technologies. Although not universally adopted, ISCD has recommended that T-scores for both men and women, regardless of race, should be calculated using a Caucasian female database. Z-scores are generated using sex and race reference databases.[7]

Additional Technologies to Measure Bone Mass

Peripheral dual-energy x-ray absorptiometry, computed tomography–based absorptiometry, quantitative computed tomography (QCT), peripheral QCT, and quantitative ultrasonography densitometry can predict both site-specific and overall fracture risk. When performed according to accepted standards, these techniques are accurate and highly reproducible. However, T-scores from these technologies are not equivalent to T-scores derived from DXA, and they cannot be used to diagnose osteoporosis based on the WHO classification.[6] Notably, DXA is the only method that has been used in all osteoporosis treatment trials.

Assessment of Fracture Risk

All postmenopausal women, and men aged 50 and older, should be evaluated for osteoporosis risk to determine the need for BMD testing. Generally, the greater the number of risk factors present, the higher the risk of fracture. Validated risk factors independent of BMD include advanced age, previous fracture, long-term glucocorticoid therapy, low body weight, family history of hip fracture, cigarette smoking, and excess alcohol intake.[8] Several of these risk factors are included in the University of Sheffield-launched Fracture Risk Assessment Tool—FRAX—available at (https://www.sheffield.ac.uk/FRAX/), which provides the 10-year probability of hip and major osteoporotic fracture and has developed from studying population-based cohorts from Europe, North America, Asia, and Australia. This set of risk factors increases fracture risk independently of BMD and is integrated with BMD measurements to assess an individual patient's risk of future fracture. Limitations of FRAX include underestimation of fracture risk when a patient is taking high-dose glucocorticoid therapy or has had multiple recent fragility fractures. Furthermore, FRAX is validated only in untreated patients and may overestimate fracture risk if an individual is already being treated.

Initial Evaluation

Initial evaluation for osteoporosis includes a detailed history to assess for clinical risk factors for fracture and secondary causes of bone loss, a thorough physical examination, and laboratory tests to assess general health, and specifically, mineral metabolism. The medical history should focus on risk factors for fracture (eg, prior fractures, family history of osteoporosis or hip fracture, recent falls), height loss, medications associated with bone loss, smoking, alcohol intake, and kidney stones. Patients should be clinically assessed for underlying medical conditions that may contribute to bone loss, including rheumatoid arthritis, hyperthyroidism, Cushing syndrome, hyperparathyroidism, multiple myeloma, celiac disease, and inflammatory bowel disease. Physical examination may reveal skeletal deformities due to unrecognized fractures (eg, kyphosis or diminished rib–pelvis space), identify possible secondary causes of skeletal fragility (eg, blue sclera with osteogenesis imperfecta or bone tenderness with osteomalacia). Height should be measured yearly, preferably with a stadiometer. Evaluating a patient's risk for falling should include inquiring about recent falls, assessing visual acuity, Romberg test, proximal muscle strength, and gait assessment.

Initial laboratory evaluation includes serum creatinine, calcium, phosphorus, magnesium, 25-hydroxyvitamin D, and liver function tests. If clinically indicated, a complete blood count, PTH, thyroid-stimulating hormone, serum protein electrophoresis, and 24-hour urine calcium and cortisol should be measured. If kyphosis is identified or a height loss of 2.5 cm (1 inch) or more is confirmed, radiographs of the thoracolumbar spine should be obtained to exclude vertebral compression fractures. The vertebral fracture assessment algorithm, an analysis that can be performed on certain DXA machines, is another way to determine whether a patient has a prevalent vertebral fracture.[9] Increasingly used in the management of osteoporosis, bone turnover markers can offer prognostic information on fracture risk and supplement bone density measurements. Bone turnover marker assays measure protein or protein derivative biomarkers released during bone remodeling by osteoblasts or osteoclasts. Bone-specific alkaline phosphatase, osteocalcin (OC), and N-terminal propeptide of type I procollagen (PINP) are markers specific to bone formation. N-terminal telopeptide of type I collagen (NTX) and C-terminal telopeptide of type I collagen (CTX) are available to assess bone resorption.[10] Although bone turnover markers are helpful in determining patient response to pharmacologic therapies for osteoporosis, testing must consider coexisting medical conditions and factors that can affect results. For example, CTX, NTX, monomeric PINP, and OC are renally cleared and generally increase with renal insufficiency.[11] Most bone turnover markers display circadian variation; serum CTX, NTX, and OC concentrations peak in the early morning between midnight and 8 AM with a nadir in the afternoon and early evening.[12] Thus, bone turnover markers should be measured on a fasting morning serum sample or a first or second voided urine to minimize variability.

TREATMENT
Nutrition

Optimal bone health requires a combination of mechanical load and adequate intake of macronutrients and micronutrients. The most important nutrients are calcium, vitamin D, and protein. Calcium is important for the bone formation phase of bone remodeling. Inadequate calcium intake can result in decreased calcium absorption and secondary hyperparathyroidism, which can cause increased bone resorption. With aging, the efficacy of intestinal calcium declines; thus, adequate calcium intake is crucial in maintaining bone health. Vitamin D generated from sunlight, food, or supplements is converted in the liver to 25-hydroxy vitamin D that serves as the substrate for 1,25-dihydroxyvitamin D, a key regulator of active intestinal calcium absorption. Recent systematic reviews and meta-analyses showed that supplementation with calcium and vitamin D results in a reduced risk of fractures and a modest increase in BMD.[13–15] The optimal amounts of calcium and vitamin D intake remain controversial, but generally, 1200 mg of calcium and 800 IU of vitamin D daily are recommended for most postmenopausal women and for men above age 70.[6] Calcium supplements have been associated with an increased risk of kidney stones in randomized clinical trials.[16] The preponderance of evidence indicates that neither calcium (up to 1000 mg daily) nor vitamin D supplements have been shown to increase cardiovascular or all-cause mortality.[17–19] Calcium supplements should be limited to patients who cannot achieve adequate dietary calcium intake. Although many studies have demonstrated a positive association between serum 25-hydroxyvitamin D levels and BMD, and low serum levels of 25-OH D have been associated with higher fracture risk, the optimal serum level of 25-OH D for fracture prevention remains unestablished.[20–23]

Nonetheless, a serum 25-hydroxyvitamin D level of 20 ng/mL seems to be adequate in protecting most of the population from adverse skeletal outcomes.[13] Data on the effect of protein intake on bone density are conflicting. Some studies suggest that higher protein intake is associated with a lower risk of hip fractures and bone loss, while others indicate increased bone resorption and calcium excretion with high protein intake.[24–26] Overall, available data suggest that an intake of 1.2 g/kg/d allows for normal calcium homeostasis.

Exercise

Although the beneficial effect of physical activity on bone density is small, it is associated with decreased risk of hip fractures in older women and decreased risk of falls by improving muscle strength, balance, and mobility. Individuals with osteoporosis (or seeking to prevent it) should exercise for at least 30 minutes 3 times per week. A meta-analysis of 43 randomized trials showed that multiple weight-bearing exercises, including resistance training, jogging, tennis, and walking, were effective. The most effective type of exercise for BMD of the femoral neck was non-weight-bearing, high-force exercise (eg, progressive resistance strength training), while a mixture of more than one exercise type was most effective for lumbar spine BMD.[27]

Fall Prevention

Given that the majority of osteoporosis-related fractures result from falls, risk factors for falling should be addressed. Risk factors for falls include a personal history of falling, muscle weakness, gait instability, medications (eg, narcotic analgesics, anticonvulsants, benzodiazepines, and antidepressants), home hazards, and visual deficits.[28] Falls can be reduced by several interventions, such as initiation of an exercise regimen that improves balance and strength, avoidance of polypharmacy, vision assessment and correction, and the use of assistive devices. Exercise programs tailored to reduce falls have consistently been shown to reduce fractures,[29,30] whereas hip protectors have not consistently been shown to decrease the risk of fractures.

PHARMACOLOGIC TREATMENT
Indications for Treatment

Currently, there are over 50 national guidelines in more than 30 countries regarding osteoporosis treatment. In the United States, pharmacologic therapy is recommended for postmenopausal women and men age 50 and older with hip or vertebral fractures; those with T-scores of −2.5 or less at the femoral neck, total hip, or lumbar spine; and those with T-scores of −1 to −2.5 and a 10-year probability of ≥20% for major osteoporotic fractures or ≥3% for hip fractures based on the US-adapted FRAX tool (NOF guidelines). An area of uncertainty is the efficacy of pharmacologic agents in otherwise healthy osteopenic patients with all central DXA T-scores better than −2.5, no prevalent vertebral fracture or recent fragility fracture, and FRAX scores in the treatment range. Because drug therapy trials only enroll patients based on BMD values and not FRAX scores, direct evidence to support treatment of such individuals based on FRAX scores is lacking. One recent study suggested a benefit to treatment in osteopenic older women, but the study included some women with osteoporosis.[31]

Treatment should be started without delay in patients with recent fractures to prevent more fractures, based on their fracture risk. Little data are available on the optimal timing of initiating therapy after a fracture. However, it is reasonable to start therapy 2 or more weeks after a hip fracture.[32] A suggested algorithm for diagnosis and management of postmenopausal osteoporosis is outlined in **Fig. 1**.

Approved Therapies

The pharmacologic arsenal for osteoporosis treatment includes drugs that inhibit bone resorption—bisphosphonates, estrogens, selective estrogen receptor modulators (SERMs), denosumab, and calcitonin; and anabolic agents that stimulate new bone formation—teriparatide, abaloparatide, and romosozumab (**Table 2**). Antiresorptive agents increase BMD in part by decreasing the rate of bone remodeling and altering the extracellular matrix. Teriparatide and abaloparatide are PTH and PTH-related protein analogs that stimulate new bone formation by directly activating PTH type 1 receptor to induce more bone formation than resorption, thus leading to an increase

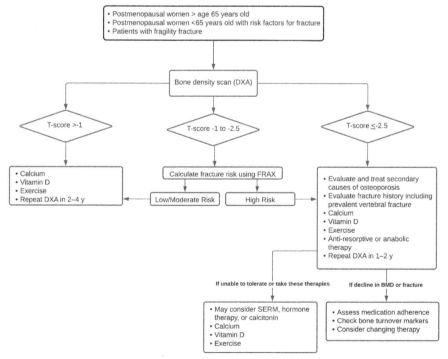

Fig. 1. Suggested algorithm for diagnosis and management of postmenopausal osteoporosis. Of note, a high FRAX score should not be the sole determinant for drug treatment.

Table 2
Summary of fracture risk reduction of pharmacologic therapies approved for postmenopausal osteoporosis

Drug	Vertebral Fracture	Hip Fracture	Nonvertebral Fracture
Alendronate	✔	✔	✔
Risedronate	✔	✔	✔
Ibandronate	✔	-	✔[a]
Zoledronic acid	✔	✔	✔
Denosumab	✔	✔	✔
Teriparatide	✔	-	✔
Abaloparatide	✔	-	✔
Romosozumab	✔	✔	✔
Estrogen	✔	✔	✔
Raloxifene	✔	-	-
Bazedoxifene	✔	-	-
Bazedoxifene and conjugated estrogen	-	-	-
Calcitonin	✔	-	-

[a] Effect shown in a post hoc analysis.

in BMD. Romosozumab is another anabolic agent and works by blocking the actions of sclerostin, an inhibitor of bone formation. These medications have been shown to decrease fracture risk in patients who have had fragility fractures or osteoporosis by DXA. These drugs may also reduce fractures in patients with low bone mass (osteopenia) without fractures, but that evidence is not as strong.

THE ANTIRESORPTIVE DRUGS
Bisphosphonates

Bisphosphonates are a cornerstone of osteoporosis treatment and are chemically stable derivatives of inorganic pyrophosphate. With their high affinity for calcium crystals, bisphosphonates concentrate selectively in the bone, decreasing bone resorption. Bisphosphonates are preferentially incorporated into sites of active bone remodeling and inhibit bone resorption by rapidly inhibiting the activity of osteoclasts. This abrupt reduction in bone resorption eventually results in the concomitant slowing of bone formation. A steady state is reached 3 to 6 months after exposure to these medications. Bisphosphonates also maintain or improve trabecular and cortical architecture and increase bone mineralization and BMD, with the net effect of decreasing fracture risk.[33,34] Bisphosphonates have low bioavailability with poor intestinal absorption (1%–5%) and rapid clearance from the circulation. About half of the absorbed dose concentrates in the bone, whereas the other half is excreted unmetabolized in the urine. Skeletal uptake primarily depends on renal function, bone turnover, binding site availability in bone, and bisphosphonate affinity for bone matrix. First-generation non–nitrogen-containing bisphosphonates (etidronate, clodronate, and tiludronate) are now rarely used because of low potency and increased risk of osteomalacia. Second-generation and third-generation bisphosphonates (alendronate, risedronate, ibandronate, pamidronate, and zoledronic acid) contain nitrogen and act primarily by inhibiting the enzyme farnesyl pyrophosphate (FPP) synthase in the mevalonate pathway (cholesterol biosynthetic pathway). Inhibition of FPP synthase disrupts protein prenylation, which creates cytoskeletal abnormalities in the osteo-clast and ultimately leads to osteoclast apoptosis.[35,36] Alendronate, risedronate, ibandronate, and zoledronic acid have been shown to improve BMD in postmeno-pausal women with underlying low bone density and to significantly decrease the risk of vertebral fractures. Alendronate, risedronate, and zoledronic acid have been proven to reduce the risk of hip and other nonvertebral fractures.[37–41] The most com-mon adverse effects of bisphosphonates include gastrointestinal problems such as esophagitis and esophageal ulcers with the oral preparations and myalgia and arthralgia with both oral and intravenous (IV) bisphosphonates. Flu-like symptoms (arthralgia, myalgia, fever, headache) occur in about 30% of patients after the first dose of IV zoledronic acid.[42] Because IV bisphosphonates have been associated with hypocalcemia, serum calcium and 25-hydroxyvitamin D levels should be checked before initiating treatment, and adequate supplementation should be provided. Kidney function should be checked before initiating treatment and then periodically because bisphosphonates are generally not recommended for patients with creatinine clear-ance of less than 30 to 35 mL/min. Ocular inflammation has rarely been reported. Other potential associations with bisphosphonate use include atrial fibrillation and esophageal cancer; however, a clear causal relationship has not been established.

Many articles have been published on the association of bisphosphonate therapy and the occurrence of osteonecrosis of the jaw (ONJ).[43] The incidence of ONJ is extremely low, and it occurs primarily in patients with cancer treated with high-dose IV bisphosphonates. Beginning in 2005, unusual fragility fractures in the subtrochan-teric region and along the femoral diaphysis in bisphosphonate-treated patients, now known as atypical femur fractures (AFFs), were first reported.[44,45] One possible under-lying mechanism of AFF is severely suppressed bone turnover. Because of concerns about atypical fractures, bisphosphonate use has declined considerably, and the magnitude of the association between these drugs and AFF remains controversial. Several studies have shown that the absolute risk of AFF is very low compared with the much greater number of fractures effectively prevented by bisphosphonates. In a large prospective cohort of women, risk factors for developing AFF include duration of bisphosphonate treatment (particularly with 8 or more years of use), Asian ancestry, shorter height, higher weight, and glucocorticoid use for 1 year or more.[46] Patients on long-term bisphosphonates (for example, greater than 3 years) reporting femoral shaft or hip pain should undergo a bone scan or MRI to exclude the presence of an insuf-ficiency fracture, which could be a harbinger for AFF. Because of the risk of ONJ and AFFs, there has been an increased focus on the optimal duration of bisphospho-nate therapy. The American Society for Bone and Mineral Research Task Force on Long-Term Bisphosphonates has proposed that AFF risk might be reduced by taking a temporary holiday from oral bisphosphonates after 5 years and IV bisphosphonates after 3 years in patients who are not at high risk of fracture.[47] The suggested approach for long-term bisphosphonate use does not replace the need for clinical judgment, and continuation of therapy may be warranted in patients remaining at high fracture risk, such as those continuing to have osteoporosis of the femoral neck (T-score ≤ -2.5) after 3 to 5 years of treatment or those with an existing vertebral fracture and a femoral neck T-score less than -2.[48] However, it has to be acknowledged that if a femoral neck T-score remains ≤ -2.5 after a complete course of bisphosphonate therapy, it is less likely that continued therapy will further improve the BMD at that site. Several studies support the notion that fracture efficacy is maintained during a bisphospho-nate holiday. Long-term randomized trials with alendronate and zoledronic acid indi-cate that after stopping treatment, BMD gains remain but are slowly lost over the next

3 to 5 years. Bone turnover marker levels initially remain low but slowly increase, though the risk of nonvertebral fractures is not increased more than 5 years after discontinuation.[48,49] After starting a drug holiday, fracture risk and BMD should be reevaluated every 2 to 4 years after discontinuation. A significant decrease in BMD or increase in bone turnover markers should lead to restarting osteoporosis therapy, depending on the patient's fracture risk before the 5-year maximum holiday is completed.

Menopausal Hormone Therapy—Estrogen

Estrogen therapy is suggested for use in women under 60 years of age or less than 10 years past menopause, who have vasomotor or climacteric symptoms associated with menopause, and those in whom bisphosphonates or denosumab are not appropriate. However, given potential risks (eg, myocardial infarction, stroke, invasive breast cancer, pulmonary emboli, and deep vein thrombophlebitis) associated with hormonal therapy, especially when combined with a progestin, non-estrogen treatments should first be considered for treatment and prevention of osteoporosis. In the Women's Health Initiative, 5 years of combined estrogen and progestin therapy (Prempro) reduced the risk of clinical vertebral fractures and hip fractures by 34% and other osteoporotic fractures by 23%.[50]

Selective Estrogen Receptor Modulators—Raloxifene (Brand Name Evista), Bazedoxifene (Duavee)

SERMs bind with high affinity to the estrogen receptor and have estrogen agonist and antagonist properties depending on the target organ. Raloxifene (60 mg once daily) has estrogenic activity in bone, thus preventing bone loss, improving BMD, and reducing fracture risk. In a 3-year trial, raloxifene reduced the risk of vertebral fractures by about 30% in patients with a prior vertebral fracture and by about 55% in patients without a prior vertebral fracture. Raloxifene does not reduce the risk of hip or nonvertebral fractures.[51,52] Several side effects limit use, including venous thromboembolism, stroke, hot flashes, and leg cramps.[53] The effect of raloxifene on BMD is less than that of menopausal hormone therapy, but there are no comparative fracture data.[54] Bazedoxifene is only approved in the United States and Canada in combination with conjugated estrogens for the treatment of hot flashes or prevention of osteoporosis in patients for whom other treatments are not suitable. The combination of conjugated estrogens and bazedoxifene results in less increase in spinal BMD at 1 year compared with conjugated estrogens and progestin, but less breast tenderness and more amenorrhea.[55] Conjugated estrogens/bazedoxifene have not been shown to reduce the risk of fracture.

Denosumab (Brand Name Prolia)

Denosumab is a fully human monoclonal antibody to RANKL. It reduces osteoclastogenesis, induces osteoclast apoptosis, decreases bone resorption, increases BMD, and reduces fracture risk. Denosumab can be offered as an alternative initial treatment to postmenopausal women with osteoporosis at high risk for fractures. A meta-analysis that compared denosumab with placebo found that fracture risk was reduced by 68% for vertebral fractures, 39% for hip fractures, and 19% for nonvertebral fractures.[52] Denosumab increases lumbar spine BMD by 9% and total hip BMD by 4%.[56] In the 7-year extension of the denosumab registration trial, the FREEDOM Extension study, continued low rates of new radiographic vertebral, nonvertebral, and hip fractures supported a stable level of fracture reduction for up to 10 years.[57] The recommended dosage of denosumab is 60 mg subcutaneously every 6 months. Decreased bone remodeling by denosumab is reflected in bone turnover markers, but these changes reverse after 6 months if the drug is not taken on schedule. In addition, several studies have shown that stopping denosumab treatment is associated with a risk of multiple or severe vertebral fractures.[58] To decrease the risk of rebound rapid BMD loss and to prevent fractures, denosumab administration should not be delayed or stopped without subsequent antiresorptive (e.g., bisphosphonate, hormone therapy, or SERM) therapy. Unlike bisphosphonates, denosumab is not cleared by the kidney. It may be used in patients with CKD and those with eGFRs of ≤35 mL/min. However, patients should be monitored for hypocalcemia because the drug rapidly and significantly lowers bone turnover, blocking calcium mobilization from bone. Adverse effects of denosumab include ONJ, AFFs, and hypocalcemia. Adequate calcium and vitamin D levels should be ensured before initiating denosumab. In the FREEDOM trial, denosumab was also associated with increased infections (cellulitis, cystitis), but it was not statistically significant.[59] A recent meta-analysis evaluating the risk of infection with denosumab reached essentially the same conclusion.[60] There are no published data on the use of denosumab beyond 10 years of treatment.

Calcitonin (Brand Names Miacalcin or Fortical)

Salmon calcitonin (intranasal or injectable) is approved to treat osteoporosis in women who are at least 5 years postmenopausal. The intranasal preparation at a dose of 200 IU daily is almost exclusively used in clinical practice. Studies show that calcitonin reduces the risk of vertebral but not nonvertebral fractures.[61,62] There is some evidence for an analgesic effect in patients with acute painful vertebral fractures.[63] Nasal calcitonin has been withdrawn from the market in Europe and Canada because of concerns about a possible association with certain malignancies, prompting the FDA to request that prescribing information note this possible association. A recent meta-analysis has concluded that there is no plausible mechanism for this association.[64]

THE ANABOLIC DRUGS
Parathyroid Hormone and Related Protein Analogs—Teriparatide (Brand Name Forteo), Abaloparatide (Brand Name Tymlos)

Anabolic agents increase BMD by increasing bone formation when administered intermittently. There are now two approved peptides that are anabolic for bone: PTH (1–34) (teriparatide) and a PTH-related protein analog (abaloparatide). Switching to an anabolic agent may be considered when a patient on bisphosphonates continues to lose bone mass or sustains a fracture. A meta-analysis comparing teriparatide with placebo showed a 74% reduction in the risk of vertebral fractures and 39% reduction in the risk of nonvertebral fractures. Comparison of abaloparatide with placebo showed an 87% reduction in the risk of vertebral fractures and a 46% reduction in the risk of nonvertebral fractures.[52] Since benefits of anabolic therapy are quickly lost after discontinuation, most clinical guidelines recommend a course of teriparatide or abaloparatide followed by a bisphosphonate, raloxifene, denosumab, or menopausal hormone therapy. There is some controversy about the efficacy of anabolic agents following bisphosphonate therapy. Several studies have suggested that while teriparatide retains its anabolic effect, the magnitude of the effect is blunted, and the timing of onset may be delayed.[65] Both teriparatide and abaloparatide are limited to a maximum of 24 months of therapy based on increased osteosarcoma in rats given lifelong treatment with these agents. However, since the introduction of teriparatide in 2002, with more than 1 million human users, the rate of osteosarcoma has not been greater than expected, and no cases have been reported in the Forteo Patient Registry established since 2009.[66,67] Adverse effects of teriparatide include dizziness and leg cramps, and side effects of abaloparatide include nausea, postural hypotension, headache, and palpitations.[68] Both agents can cause hypercalciuria and increase serum calcium, but persistent hypercalcemia is uncommon. These agents should be used cautiously in patients with calcium oxalate nephrolithiasis. Serum calcium should be assessed before treatment, and neither agent should be used in patients with hypercalcemia. It may be preferable to administer these drugs in the evening to avoid complications from occasional hypotension.

Romosozumab (Brand Name Evenity)

Romosozumab is the newest anabolic agent approved for the treatment of osteoporosis, and it increases bone formation as it reduces bone resorption. Romosozumab blocks the actions of sclerostin, an inhibitor of bone formation that binds to the low-density lipoprotein receptor-related protein (LRP)5/6 component of the LRP5/6-frizzled coreceptor complex that transduces Wnt signaling.[69] The drug is administered as a 210 mg monthly subcutaneous injection for 12 months. There have been 2 large phase 3 trials of romosozumab. In the Fracture Study in Postmenopausal Women with Osteoporosis (FRAME) trial, romosozumab led to a 73% reduction in the risk of vertebral fractures but with no significant effect on the risk of hip or nonvertebral fractures compared with placebo. At 24 months, those treated with romosozumab (initial 12 months) followed by denosumab demonstrated a 75% lower risk for new vertebral fractures.[70] The Active-Controlled Fracture Study in Postmenopausal Women with Osteoporosis at High Risk (ARCH) trial compared 1 year of treatment with romosozumab followed by 1 year of alendronate to 2 years of treatment with alendronate only in postmenopausal women at high risk of fracture.[59] The ARCH trial suggests that romosozumab/alendronate versus alendronate/alendronate resulted in a 48% reduction in the risk of vertebral fractures, a 38% reduction in the risk of hip fractures, and a 19% reduction in the risk of nonvertebral fractures at 24 months. Romosozumab should be considered a first-line therapy in patients with severe osteoporosis and multiple vertebral fractures or hip fracture (eg, T-score < −2.5 and fractures) and can also be used in individuals who have failed antiresorptive treatments. In the ARCH trial, a composite endpoint of cardiovascular death, nonfatal myocardial infarction, and nonfatal stroke was more common in the romosozumab group. Thus, individuals at high risk of cardiovascular disease or stroke or those with prior myocardial infarction or stroke within the past year should not be offered romosozumab.[71,72] Additional adverse effects observed with romosozumab included small numbers of ONJ, AFFs, and injection-site reactions. Romosozumab treatment resulted in large increases in BMD compared with controls in both FRAME and ARCH trials. In FRAME at 12 months, the difference in BMD between romosozumab and placebo was 13% (spine), 7% (total hip), and 5% (femoral neck). In ARCH at 12 months, BMD had significantly increased with romosozumab, by 14% (spine), 6% (total hip), and 5% (femoral neck), compared with increased BMD with alendronate of 5% (spine), 3% (total hip), and 1.7% (femoral neck).[71] At 12 months, romosozumab appears to be more potent than teriparatide in its effect on BMD. A head-to-head comparison of teriparatide and romosozumab showed that BMD had significantly increased with romosozumab, by 11% (spine), 4% (total hip), and 4% (femoral neck), compared with increased BMD with teriparatide of 7% (spine), 1.3% (total hip), and 1.1% (femoral neck).

Romosozumab should be followed by an antiresorptive agent to maintain BMD gains and prevent accelerated bone loss after completing the treatment course.

CHOOSING ANTIOSTEOPOROTIC THERAPY

In addition to recommending adequate calcium and vitamin D intake, resistance and weight-bearing exercises, smoking cessation, limited alcohol consumption, pharmacologic therapy should be selected based on cost, safety profile, and efficacy. For patients with osteoporosis of the hip, drugs proven to be effective at this site should be used, and thus, ibandronate, raloxifene, and calcitonin should not be considered in this scenario. Owing to their lower costs and lengthier clinical experience, bisphosphonates are often used as first-line treatment for osteoporosis. However, drug choice should be individualized to the patient, and there may be specific patient factors that help determine the optimal drug. For example, IV bisphosphonates or denosumab could be alternatives for patients who cannot tolerate oral bisphosphonates because of gastrointestinal side effects. As noted, adherence to oral antiresorptive therapy is often poor. Despite their greater cost, this has led to increased use of parenterally administered drugs in this class.

Combination Therapy

Combination therapy, usually a bisphosphonate with a nonbisphosphonate, is not recommended. It can provide additional, small increases in BMD compared with monotherapy; however, the effect on fracture rates is unknown. The added cost and potential side effects, such as oversuppression of bone turnover, should be weighed against potential benefits. From a practical standpoint, insurers can be reluctant to provide coverage for combined therapy.

Monitoring Response to Treatment

Several studies have shown poor adherence with osteoporosis medications. One year after initiating treatment of osteoporosis, about 45% of patients do not refill the prescriptions. Thus, it is important to confirm whether patients are taking their medications and to encourage adherence.

Sharing the bone density results with patients modestly increases adherence to therapy. Various approaches have also been suggested to improve adherence, such as counseling programs and health care system interventions.[73,74] Central DXA measurement of the spine and hip is the preferred method for serial assessment of BMD. There is no consensus on the optimal frequency of monitoring and the preferred site to monitor. The NOF recommends repeating the BMD assessment every 2 years but recognizes that testing more frequently may be warranted in certain clinical situations.[6] A stable or increasing BMD is an acceptable response to therapy. Generally, a loss of BMD greater than the least significant change (typically 5% in the lumbar spine, 4% in the total hip, and 5% in the femoral neck) over 2 years and a less than expected reduction in bone turnover markers on antiresorptive drugs is considered "failure" of therapy. In addition, poor adherence, malabsorption, secondary diseases affecting skeletal health should be investigated if there is a decrease in BMD during ongoing antiosteoporotic therapy. Bone turnover markers can be followed to evaluate the efficacy of therapy. A significant decrease in bone turnover markers with antiresorptive therapy or an increase in bone turnover with anabolic therapy provides evidence of compliance and drug efficacy.

SUMMARY

Osteoporosis is a global public health concern that is underdiagnosed and undertreated. Fragility fractures of the spine and hip can result in chronic pain, depression, disability, and death. Central DXA measurements are the gold standard for the assessment of BMD. Secondary causes and risk factors for bone loss should be identified and treated. Pharmacologic agents in conjunction with a well-balanced diet, exercise, smoking cessation, and fall prevention should be recommended in all patients at high risk for fracture.

CLINICS CARE POINTS

- Pharmacologic therapies should be recommended in postmenopausal women at high risk for fracture.
- Bisphosphonates or denosumab can be offered as initial treatments.
- Anabolic therapy with teriparatide, abaloparatide, or romosozumab is recommended in postmenopausal women with osteoporosis and at very high risk for fracture, especially those with severe fragility fractures or multiple vertebral fractures.

DISCLOSURE

The authors have nothing to disclose.

REFERENCES

1. Kanis JA. Diagnosis of osteoporosis and assessment of fracture risk. Lancet 2002;359:1929–36.
2. Melton LJ, Atkinson EJ, O'Connor MK, et al. Bone density and fracture risk in men. J Bone Miner Res 1998;13:1915–23.
3. Curtis EM, van der Velde R, Moon RJ, et al. Epidemiology of fractures in the United Kingdom 1988-2012: Variation with age, sex, geography, ethnicity and socioeconomic status. Bone 2016;87:19–26.
4. Bartl R, Frisch B. Osteoporosis: diagnosis, prevention, therapy. Springer Science & Business Media; 2009.
5. Khosla S, Atkinson EJ, Melton LJ, et al. Effects of Age and Estrogen Status on Serum Parathyroid Hormone Levels and Biochemical Markers of Bone Turnover in Women: A Population-Based Study. J Clin Endocrinol Metab 1997;82:1522–7.
6. Cosman F, de Beur SJ, LeBoff MS, et al. Clinician's Guide to Prevention and Treatment of Osteoporosis. Osteoporos Int 2014;25:2359–81.
7. ISCD. 2019 Official Positions Adult.pdf | Powered by Box. Available at: https://iscd.app.box.com/s/5r713cfzvf4gr28q7zdccg2i7169fv86. Accessed March 11, 2021.
8. Kanis JA, Borgstrom F, De Laet C, et al. Assessment of fracture risk. Osteoporos Int 2005;16:581–9.
9. Rosen HN, Vokes TJ, Malabanan AO, et al. The Official Positions of the International Society for Clinical Densitometry: vertebral fracture assessment. J Clin Densitom 2013;16:482–8.
10. Greenblatt MB, Tsai JN, Wein MN. Bone Turnover Markers in the Diagnosis and Monitoring of Metabolic Bone Disease. Clin Chem 2017;63:464–74.
11. Woitge HW, Pecherstorfer M, Li Y, et al. Novel serum markers of bone resorption: clinical assessment and comparison with established urinary indices. J Bone Miner Res 1999;14:792–801.
12. Qvist P, Christgau S, Pedersen BJ, et al. Circadian variation in the serum concentration of C-terminal telopeptide of type I collagen (serum CTx): effects of gender, age, menopausal status, posture, daylight, serum cortisol, and fasting. Bone 2002;31:57–61.

13. Ross AC, Manson JE, Abrams SA, et al. The 2011 Report on Dietary Reference Intakes for Calcium and Vitamin D from the Institute of Medicine: What Clinicians Need to Know. J Clin Endocrinol Metab 2011;96:53–8.
14. Lips P, Bouillon R, van Schoor NM, et al. Reducing fracture risk with calcium and vitamin D. Clin Endocrinol 2010;73:277–85.
15. Yao P, Bennett D, Mafham M, et al. Vitamin D and Calcium for the Prevention of Fracture: A Systematic Review and Meta-analysis. JAMA Netw Open 2019;2: e1917789.
16. Heller HJ, Greer LG, Haynes SD, et al. Pharmacokinetic and pharmacodynamic comparison of two calcium supplements in postmenopausal women. J Clin Pharmacol 2000;40:1237–44.
17. Langsetmo L, Berger C, Kreiger N, et al. Calcium and vitamin D intake and mortality: results from the Canadian Multicentre Osteoporosis Study (CaMos). J Clin Endocrinol Metab 2013;98:3010–8.
18. Chung M, Tang AM, Fu Z, et al. Calcium Intake and Cardiovascular Disease Risk: An Updated Systematic Review and Meta-analysis. Ann Intern Med 2016;165: 856–66.
19. Wallace TC, Weaver CM. Calcium Supplementation and Coronary Artery Disease: A Methodological Confound? J Am Coll Nutr 2020;39:383–7.
20. Kuchuk NO, van Schoor NM, Pluijm SM, et al. Vitamin D status, parathyroid function, bone turnover, and BMD in postmenopausal women with osteoporosis: global perspective. J Bone Miner Res 2009;24:693–701.
21. Bischoff-Ferrari HA, Dietrich T, Orav EJ, et al. Positive association between 25-hydroxy vitamin D levels and bone mineral density: a population-based study of younger and older adults. Am J Med 2004;116:634–9.
22. Looker AC. Serum 25-hydroxyvitamin D and risk of major osteoporotic fractures in older U.S. adults. J Bone Miner Res 2013;28:997–1006.
23. Cauley JA, Lacroix AZ, Wu LL, et al. Serum 25-hydroxyvitamin D concentrations and risk for hip fractures. Ann Intern Med 2008;149:242–50.
24. Wengreen HJ, Munger RG, West NA, et al. Dietary protein intake and risk of osteoporotic hip fracture in elderly residents of Utah. J Bone Miner Res 2004;19: 537–45.
25. Hannan MT, Tucker KL, Dawson-Hughes B, et al. Effect of dietary protein on bone loss in elderly men and women: the Framingham Osteoporosis Study. J Bone Miner Res 2000;15:2504–12.
26. Kerstetter JE, Mitnick ME, Gundberg CM, et al. Changes in bone turnover in young women consuming different levels of dietary protein. J Clin Endocrinol Metab 1999;84:1052–5.
27. Howe TE, Shea B, Dawson LJ, et al. Exercise for preventing and treating osteoporosis in postmenopausal women. Cochrane Database Syst Rev 2011;CD000333. https://doi.org/10.1002/14651858.CD000333.pub2.
28. Guideline for the prevention of falls in older persons. American Geriatrics Society, British Geriatrics Society, and American Academy of Orthopaedic Surgeons Panel on Falls Prevention. J Am Geriatr Soc 2001;49:664–72.
29. El-Khoury F, Cassou B, Charles M-A, et al. The effect of fall prevention exercise programmes on fall induced injuries in community dwelling older adults: systematic review and meta-analysis of randomised controlled trials. BMJ 2013;347: f6234.
30. Gillespie LD, Roberston CM, Gillespie WJ, et al. Interventions for preventing falls in older people living in the community. Cochrane Database Syst Rev 2012. https://doi.org/10.1002/14651858.CD007146.pub3.

31. Reid IR, Horne AM, Mihov B, et al. Fracture Prevention with Zoledronate in Older Women with Osteopenia. N Engl J Med 2018;379:2407–16.
32. Lyles KW, Colon-Emeric CS, Magaziner JS, et al. Zoledronic acid and clinical fractures and mortality after hip fracture. N Engl J Med 2007;357:1799–809.
33. Rodan GA, Fleisch HA. Bisphosphonates: mechanisms of action. J Clin Invest 1996;97:2692–6.
34. Hughes DE, Wright KR, Uy HL, et al. Bisphosphonates promote apoptosis in murine osteoclasts in vitro and in vivo. J Bone Miner Res 1995;10:1478–87.
35. Drake MT, Clarke BL, Khosla S. Bisphosphonates: Mechanism of Action and Role in Clinical Practice. Mayo Clin Proc 2008;83:1032–45.
36. Russell RGG. Bisphosphonates: Mode of Action and Pharmacology. Pediatrics 2007;119:S150–62.
37. Cummings SR, Black DM, Thompson DE, et al. Effect of alendronate on risk of fracture in women with low bone density but without vertebral fractures: results from the Fracture Intervention Trial. JAMA 1998;280:2077–82.
38. Chesnut CH, Skag A, Christiansen C, et al. Effects of oral ibandronate administered daily or intermittently on fracture risk in postmenopausal osteoporosis. J Bone Miner Res 2004;19:1241–9.
39. McClung MR, Geusens P, Miller PD, et al. Effect of Risedronate on the Risk of Hip Fracture in Elderly Women. N Engl J Med 2001;344:333–40.
40. Black DM, Cummings SR, Karpf DB, et al. Randomised trial of effect of alendronate on risk of fracture in women with existing vertebral fractures. Lancet 1996; 348:1535–41.
41. Black DM, Delmas PD, Eastell R, et al. Once-Yearly Zoledronic Acid for Treatment of Postmenopausal Osteoporosis. N Engl J Med 2007;356:1809–22.
42. Reid IR, Gamble GD, Mesenbrink P, et al. Characterization of and risk factors for the acute-phase response after zoledronic acid. J Clin Endocrinol Metab 2010; 95:4380–7.
43. Khosla S, Burr D, Cauley J, et al. Bisphosphonate-Associated Osteonecrosis of the Jaw: Report of a Task Force of the American Society for Bone and Mineral Research. J Bone Miner Res 2007;22:1479–91.
44. Odvina CV, Zerwekh JE, Rao DS, et al. Severely suppressed bone turnover: a potential complication of alendronate therapy. J Clin Endocrinol Metab 2005;90: 1294–301.
45. Goh S-K, Yang KY, Koh JSB, et al. Subtrochanteric insufficiency fractures in patients on alendronate therapy: a caution. J Bone Joint Surg Br 2007;89:349–53.
46. Black DM, Geiger EJ, Eastell R, et al. Atypical Femur Fracture Risk versus Fragility Fracture Prevention with Bisphosphonates. N Engl J Med 2020;383: 743–53.
47. Adler RA, El-Hajj Fuleihan G, Bauer D, et al. Managing Osteoporosis in Patients on Long-Term Bisphosphonate Treatment: Report of a Task Force of the American Society for Bone and Mineral Research. J Bone Miner Res 2016;31:16–35.
48. Black DM, Bauer DC, Schwartz AV, et al. Continuing Bisphosphonate Treatment for Osteoporosis — For Whom and for How Long? N Engl J Med 2012;366: 2051–3.
49. Black DM, Schwartz AV, Ensrud KE, et al. Effects of continuing or stopping alendronate after 5 years of treatment: the Fracture Intervention Trial Long-term Extension (FLEX): a randomized trial. JAMA 2006;296:2927–38.
50. Rossouw JE, Anderson GL, Prentice RL, et al. Risks and benefits of estrogen plus progestin in healthy postmenopausal women: principal results From the Women's Health Initiative randomized controlled trial. JAMA 2002;288:321–33.

51. Ettinger B, Black DM, Mitlak BH, et al. Reduction of vertebral fracture risk in post-menopausal women with osteoporosis treated with raloxifene: results from a 3-year randomized clinical trial. Multiple Outcomes of Raloxifene Evaluation (MORE) Investigators. JAMA 1999;282:637–45.

52. Barrionuevo P, Kapoor E, Asi N, et al. Efficacy of Pharmacological Therapies for the Prevention of Fractures in Postmenopausal Women: A Network Meta-Analysis. J Clin Endocrinol Metab 2019;104:1623–30.

53. Crandall CJ, Newberry SJ, Diamant A, et al. Comparative effectiveness of pharmacologic treatments to prevent fractures: an updated systematic review. Ann Intern Med 2014;161:711–23.

54. Reid IR, Eastell R, Fogelman I, et al. A comparison of the effects of raloxifene and conjugated equine estrogen on bone and lipids in healthy postmenopausal women. Arch Intern Med 2004;164:871–9.

55. Pinkerton JV, Harvey JA, Lindsay R, et al. Effects of bazedoxifene/conjugated estrogens on the endometrium and bone: a randomized trial. J Clin Endocrinol Metab 2014;99:E189–98.

56. Cummings SR, Martin JS, McClung MR, et al. Denosumab for Prevention of Fractures in Postmenopausal Women with Osteoporosis. N Engl J Med 2009;361:756–65.

57. Bone HG, Wagman RB, Brandi ML, et al. 10 years of denosumab treatment in postmenopausal women with osteoporosis: results from the phase 3 randomised FREEDOM trial and open-label extension. Lancet Diabetes Endocrinol 2017;5:513–23.

58. Tsourdi E, Langdahl B, Cohen-Solal M, et al. Discontinuation of Denosumab therapy for osteoporosis: A systematic review and position statement by ECTS. Bone 2017;105:11–7.

59. Watts NB, Roux C, Modlin JF, et al. Infections in postmenopausal women with osteoporosis treated with denosumab or placebo: coincidence or causal association? Osteoporos Int 2012;23:327–37.

60. Diker-Cohen T, Rosenberg D, Avni T, et al. Risk for Infections During Treatment With Denosumab for Osteoporosis: A Systematic Review and Meta-analysis. J Clin Endocrinol Metab 2020;105:1641–58.

61. Chesnut CH, Silverman S, Andriano K, et al. A randomized trial of nasal spray salmon calcitonin in postmenopausal women with established osteoporosis: the prevent recurrence of osteoporotic fractures study. Am J Med 2000;109:267–76.

62. Overgaard K, Hansen MA, Jensen SB, et al. Effect of salcatonin given intranasally on bone mass and fracture rates in established osteoporosis: a dose-response study. Br Med J 1992;305:556–61.

63. Lyritis GP, Paspati I, Karachalios T, et al. Pain relief from nasal salmon calcitonin in osteoporotic vertebral crush fractures. A double blind, placebo-controlled clinical study. Acta Orthop Scand Suppl 1997;275:112–4.

64. Wells G, Chernoff J, Gilligan JP, et al. Does salmon calcitonin cause cancer? A review and meta-analysis. Osteoporos Int 2016;27:13–9.

65. Geusens P, Marin F, Kendler DL, et al. Effects of Teriparatide Compared with Risedronate on the Risk of Fractures in Subgroups of Postmenopausal Women with Severe Osteoporosis: The VERO Trial. J Bone Miner Res 2018;33:783–94.

66. Black DM, Rosen CJ. Clinical Practice. Postmenopausal Osteoporosis. N Engl J Med 2016;374:254–62.

67. Gilsenan A, Harding A, Kellier-Steele N, et al. The Forteo Patient Registry linkage to multiple state cancer registries: study design and results from the first 8 years. Osteoporos Int 2018;29:2335–43.

68. Miller PD, Hattersley G, Riis BJ, et al. Effect of Abaloparatide vs Placebo on New Vertebral Fractures in Postmenopausal Women With Osteoporosis: A Randomized Clinical Trial. JAMA 2016;316:722–33.
69. Holdsworth G, Roberts SJ, Ke HZ. Novel actions of sclerostin on bone. J Mol Endocrinol 2019;62:R167–85.
70. Lewiecki EM, Dinavahi RJ, Lazaretti-Castro M, et al. One Year of Romosozumab Followed by Two Years of Denosumab Maintains Fracture Risk Reductions: Results of the FRAME Extension Study. J Bone Miner Res 2019;34:419–28.
71. Saag KG, Petersen J, Brandi ML, et al. Romosozumab or Alendronate for Fracture Prevention in Women with Osteoporosis. N Engl J Med 2017;377:1417–27.
72. McClung MR, Grauer A, Boonen S, et al. Romosozumab in postmenopausal women with low bone mineral density. N Engl J Med 2014;370:412–20.
73. Jaleel A, Saag KG, Danila MI. Improving drug adherence in osteoporosis: an update on more recent studies. Ther Adv Musculoskelet Dis 2018;10:141–9.
74. Diez-Perez A, Adachi JD, Agnusdei D, et al. Treatment failure in osteoporosis. Osteoporos Int 2012;23:2769–74.

Evaluation and Management of Elevated Parathyroid Hormone Levels in Normocalcemic Patients

Natalie E. Cusano, MD, MS

KEYWORDS

- Normocalcemic primary hyperparathyroidism • Normocalcemic
- Primary hyperparathyroidism • Hyperparathyroidism

KEY POINTS

- Patients can be diagnosed with normocalcemic primary hyperparathyroidism in the setting of elevated PTH concentrations on at least 3 occasions over a period of 3 to 6 months with consistently normal serum calcium.
- It is important to measure ionized calcium, monitor biochemical parameters over time, and exclude secondary causes of hyperparathyroidism in order to make a diagnosis of normocalcemic disease.
- Most patients with normocalcemic primary hyperparathyroidism are diagnosed in the setting of kidney stones or bone disease.
- There are limited data regarding optimal medical and surgical management.

INTRODUCTION

Primary hyperparathyroidism is a common endocrine disorder. It used to present as a highly symptomatic disease with severe hypercalcemia before the advent of the multichannel blood autoanalyzer. In the developed world, primary hyperparathyroidism now usually presents as mild asymptomatic hypercalcemia incidentally noted on routine blood tests. A newer presentation of primary hyperparathyroidism has been increasingly identified in the past 2 decades, in which patients present with elevated parathyroid hormone concentrations and consistently normal serum calcium. Patients with this phenotype, normocalcemic primary hyperparathyroidism, are usually symptomatic at the time of diagnosis, with parathyroid hormone levels measured in the setting of evaluation for kidney stones or osteoporosis. It is important to exclude causes of secondary hyperparathyroidism, including vitamin D deficiency, chronic

Division of Endocrinology, Department of Medicine, Lenox Hill Hospital, 110 East 59th Street, Suite 8B, New York, NY, USA
E-mail address: ncusano@northwell.edu

Med Clin N Am 105 (2021) 1135–1150
https://doi.org/10.1016/j.mcna.2021.05.017
0025-7125/21/© 2021 Elsevier Inc. All rights reserved.

medical.theclinics.com

renal failure, and use of certain medications, which can cause an appropriate elevation in parathyroid hormone levels. This review focuses on the evaluation and management of elevated parathyroid hormone levels in patients who are normocalcemic.

DEFINITION AND EVALUATION

Although normocalcemic primary hyperparathyroidism was formally recognized at the time of the Third International Workshop on the Management of Asymptomatic Primary Hyperparathyroidism in 2008, recommendations for diagnosis and management were not proposed until the Fourth International Workshop in 2013.[1] A review of the literature is confounded by the lack of consistency in diagnostic criteria, and these guidelines provided an important step forward for future research to better understand the disease. The guidelines recommend an elevated serum parathyroid hormone (PTH) on at least 3 occasions over a period of 3 to 6 months in order to make a diagnosis of normocalcemic primary hyperparathyroidism. The importance of repeated measurements has been demonstrated by multiple studies showing a lack of persistence of hyperparathyroidism in some patients diagnosed with the disease, with concern for misclassification of individuals with secondary hyperparathyroidism. In general, individuals with secondary hyperparathyroidism have serum calcium concentrations toward the lower end of the normal range, whereas for those with normocalcemic primary hyperparathyroidism, calcium levels tend to be in the upper end of the normal range. There is unfortunately some overlap. In one population-based study of disease prevalence, 108 of 3450 men and women were noted to have normal serum calcium and elevated PTH using a single measurement after exclusion of secondary causes of hyperparathyroidism. Of the 64 of 108 individuals with follow-up data 8 years later, 1 individual had developed hypercalcemia and only 13 (20%) demonstrated a persistently elevated PTH concentration.[2]

Although patients with traditional hypercalcemic primary hyperparathyroidism can occasionally have normal serum calcium as a part of their clinical course, serum total (albumin-corrected) and ionized calcium levels must be consistently normal to make a diagnosis of normocalcemic primary hyperparathyroidism. Reliable measurement of ionized calcium is not universally available because it requires particular sample handling techniques and is more labor intensive and expensive than total calcium. Studies have shown the importance of ionized calcium, however, with reports that 4%–64% of patients with an initial diagnosis of normocalcemic primary hyperparathyroidism would be subsequently reclassified as having traditional hypercalcemic disease with measurement of ionized calcium.[3–5]

There must also be a rigorous evaluation for secondary causes of hyperparathyroidism in order to make the diagnosis, which are discussed in the following section.

Vitamin D Deficiency

Low 25-hydroxyvitamin D is a major stimulus for PTH secretion, and PTH levels can remain elevated for several months after improvement in vitamin D levels. A minimum goal level of at least 20 ng/mL (50 nmol/L) is needed to exclude secondary hyperparathyroidism; however, levels of at least 30 ng/mL (>75 nmol/L) are favored by many experts.[1,6] As part of a larger investigation, Rosário and Calsolari studied 25 patients initially diagnosed with normocalcemic primary hyperparathyroidism using a 25-hydroxyvitamin D level greater than 20 ng/mL followed every 8 weeks with vitamin D supplementation to increase levels to greater than 30 ng/mL. The 20 individuals (or 80%) who achieved a 25-hydroxyvitamin D level greater than 30 ng/mL at 6 months had subsequent normalization of hyperparathyroidism. They also evaluated individuals with elevated PTH levels undergoing planned thyroid surgery and investigated the parathyroid glands at the time of surgery, noting whether the glands were normal or "altered" (not further defined). They noted that among those with a 25-hydroxyvitamin D level greater than 30 ng/mL and estimated glomerular filtration rate (eGFR) greater than 60 mL/min, 80% had altered parathyroid glands and thus more likely a diagnosis of normocalcemic primary hyperparathyroidism compared with only 8.7% of patients with biochemical cut-offs of 25-hydroxyvitamin D greater than 20 ng/mL and eGFR greater than 40 mL/min, most of whom were presumed to have had secondary hyperparathyroidism.[7] The Institute of Medicine acknowledged that there is no widespread agreement in the literature regarding a 25-hydroxyvitamin D level by which there is a plateau in PTH concentrations,[8] suggesting that a range of values may be needed.[9] In addition, some patients with traditional primary hyperparathyroidism can become hypercalcemic when vitamin D deficiency is treated.[10] Of note, 1,25-dihydroxyvitamin D is not a marker for vitamin D stores and can be normal or even elevated in patients with vitamin D deficiency due to stimulation of renal 1α-hydroxylase by PTH.[1]

Renal Failure

Population studies have demonstrated that PTH levels increase as eGFR declines.[11,12] The guidelines state that eGFR must be at least 60 mL/min in order to make a diagnosis of normocalcemic primary hyperparathyroidism.

Medications Associated with Elevated Parathyroid Levels

Lithium alters feedback mechanisms within the parathyroid gland, increasing the set point at which calcium suppresses PTH secretion, and can also induce increased calcium reabsorption within the loop of Henle.[13] Thiazide diuretics increase renal calcium reabsorption and have been reported to increase PTH concentrations, although this has not been a consistent finding.[14,15] The guidelines recommend exclusion of lithium and thiazide diuretic therapy in order to make a diagnosis of normocalcemic primary hyperparathyroidism if these medications can be discontinued safely. Antiresorptive medications including bisphosphonates[16,17] and denosumab[18] can cause physiologic elevations in PTH concentrations in order to prevent hypocalcemia. With antiresorptive therapy, PTH levels may increase to a level higher than the normal range within the first 24 hours to 3 months of treatment initiation but usually normalize by 24 months for bisphosphonate therapy and 6 months for denosumab.

Hypercalciuria

It is recommended to exclude hypercalciuria, defined as a 24-hour urine calcium excretion greater than 250 mg for women and greater than 300 mg for men, or a weight-based limit of 4 mg/kg/d for lean individuals; this is based on an early understanding that renal calcium wasting could precipitate secondary hyperparathyroidism[19] However, more recent work has demonstrated that many individuals with idiopathic hypercalciuria may not develop secondary hyperparathyroidism despite net renal calcium losses.[20] Some experts advocate for a trial of a thiazide diuretic in those found to be hypercalciuric in order to determine if a decrease in renal calcium excretion leads to normalization of PTH values.[21]

Insufficient Calcium Intake or Calcium Malabsorption

Low calcium intake is a stimulus for PTH secretion. Celiac disease and other gastrointestinal disorders causing calcium malabsorption should also be excluded, especially in the setting of vitamin D deficiency or hypocalciuria.[22] Patients should be recommended to have sufficient calcium intake through diet and/or supplements to meet the Institute of Medicine recommendations.[8] Low calcium intake and malabsorption will be marked by hypocalciuria—another reason to assess urinary calcium excretion in these evaluations.

There are 2 studies evaluating the use of the calcium/phosphate ratio to improve the diagnosis of primary hyperparathyroidism, with the aim of replacing the need for PTH testing.[23,24] Although the studies show a relatively robust sensitivity and specificity for hypercalcemic disease, the sensitivity for normocalcemic disease was lower. Another study evaluated use of a parathyroid function index incorporating calcium, PTH, and phosphorus to differentiate between normocalcemic primary hyperparathyroidism and secondary hyperparathyroidism.[25] Prospective studies are needed to further investigate the utility of these measurements.

PATHOPHYSIOLOGY

There are several hypotheses regarding the pathophysiology of normocalcemic primary hyperparathyroidism. One is that normocalcemic primary hyperparathyroidism is an early or mild form of traditional hypercalcemic disease. With this theory, one would expect that many or most patients would manifest with hypercalcemia over time; however, the natural history data detailed later do not support this. Some investigators have proposed that PTH secretion is lower in normocalcemic than hypercalcemic individuals, although there is considerable overlap in PTH levels between these groups.[26] Another perspective relates to the fact that although the population range for normal serum calcium is quite broad (generally 8.5–10.5 mg/dL), the range for a given individual is much more narrow.[27] An increase in serum calcium from the 8.8 to 9.0 mg/dL range to the 10.1 to 10.3 mg/dL range, while technically remaining within normal for the assay, would represent relative hypercalcemia for this individual. Maruani and colleagues[28] proposed a partial tissue resistance to PTH in normocalcemic patients. Polymorphisms in the calcium sensing receptor gene (CASR) may also play a role, leading to PTH resistance.[29] The fact that PTH levels increase with age has led some experts to propose age-specific PTH values.[30] A recent review by Zavatta and Clarke provides further detail regarding possible pathogenic mechanisms.[31] The lack of a clear unifying mechanism underscores the need for more research in this area.

EPIDEMIOLOGY

Although there are good data regarding the epidemiology of traditional hypercalcemic primary hyperparathyroidism around the world, the incidence and prevalence of normocalcemic primary hyperparathyroidism remain unclear, due to several causes. Normocalcemic primary hyperparathyroidism is often diagnosed when PTH levels are measured in the setting of symptoms of nephrolithiasis or fracture, with a clear bias from referral centers. There are few population-based studies investigating the prevalence in healthy patients because ionized calcium or PTH levels are not often ordered in the absence of hypercalcemia or symptoms. In addition, there are significant differences in the exclusion of secondary causes of hyperparathyroidism across different studies, especially in cut-offs for 25-hydroxyvitamin D and eGFR. Of note, few of the studies monitored biochemical parameters over time or evaluated ionized calcium levels, which can overestimate the disease prevalence. The disease seems to be relatively rare, with most studies using established criteria demonstrating a prevalence of 0.1% to 0.7% (**Table 1**).[2,7,30,32–38]

Table 1
Epidemiology of normocalcemic primary hyperparathyroidism

Study	Population	Prevalence	Diagnostic Criteria
Palermo et al,[32] 2015	2677 community-dwelling women investigated for a bone imaging study (The Osteoporosis and Ultrasound Study [OPUS], United Kingdom, France, Germany)	0.1% (baseline) 0.0% (follow-up)	Elevated PTH concentration and normal albumin-adjusted total serum calcium on at least 2 occasions; exclusion of renal failure (GFR <60 mL/min), vitamin D deficiency (25-hydroxyvitamin D <20 ng/mL); medication effect not excluded
Schini et al,[30] 2020	6280 men and women referred for bone density testing (United Kingdom)	0.2%	Elevated PTH concentration and normal albumin-adjusted total serum calcium on at least 2 occasions; exclusion of renal failure (GFR <60 mL/min), vitamin D deficiency (25-hydroxyvitamin D <20 ng/mL)
Cusano et al,[2] 2013	2364 unselected community-dwelling men, age 65 y or older, investigated for fracture risk factors (The Osteoporotic Fractures in Men Study [MrOS] cohort, United States)	0.4%	Elevated PTH concentration and normal albumin-adjusted total serum calcium; exclusion of renal failure (GFR <60 mL/min), vitamin D deficiency (25-hydroxyvitamin D <20 ng/mL), medication effect
Vignali et al,[33] 2015	685 adult men and women living in a village in Southern Italy (Italy)	0.4%	Elevated PTH concentration and normal albumin-adjusted total serum calcium; exclusion of renal failure (GFR <60 mL/min), vitamin D deficiency (25-hydroxyvitamin D <30 ng/mL), medication effect, overt gastrointestinal or metabolic bone diseases

(continued on next page)

Table 1
(continued)

Study	Population	Prevalence	Diagnostic Criteria
Lundgren et al,[34] 1997	5202 postmenopausal women age 55–75 y attending a population-based mammography screening (Sweden)	0.5%	Elevated PTH concentration with normal albumin-adjusted total serum calcium and normal ionized calcium on repeat measure; none had history of malabsorption
Rosário & Calsolari,[7] 2019	676 adults without history of nephrolithiasis or fracture with planned thyroidectomy for thyroid disease (Brazil)	0.7% (eGFR >60 mL/min, 25-hydroxyvitamin D >30 ng/mL), 1.8% (eGFR >40 mL/min, 25-hydroxyvitamin D >30 ng/mL), 4.4% (eGFR >60 mL/min, 25-hydroxyvitamin D >20 ng/mL), 6.8% (eGFR >40 mL/min, 25-hydroxyvitamin D >40 ng/mL)	Elevated PTH concentration and normal albumin-adjusted total serum calcium; exclusion of renal failure (GFR <40 mL/min), vitamin D deficiency (25-hydroxyvitamin D <20 ng/mL), medication effect, malabsorption (by history and measurement of tissue transglutaminase IgA)
Kontogeorgos et al,[35] 2015	608 men and women, age 25–64 y, investigated for cardiovascular disease (World Health Organization MONitoring of trends and determinants for CArdiovascular disease project [WHO MONICA])	2.0% (baseline) 0.2% (follow-up)	Elevated PTH concentration and normal total serum calcium; exclusion of renal failure (eGFR <60 mL/min), vitamin D deficiency (25-hydroxyvitamin D <20 ng/mL); medication effect not excluded
Cusano et al,[2] 2013	3450 community-dwelling men and women, age 18–65 y, investigated for cardiovascular disease (Dallas Heart Study cohort, United States)	3.1% (baseline) 0.6% (follow-up)	Elevated PTH concentration and normal albumin-adjusted total serum calcium; exclusion of renal failure (eGFR < 60 mL/min), vitamin D deficiency (25-hydroxyvitamin D < 20 ng/mL), medication effect

Berger et al,[36] 2015	1872 community-dwelling men and women, age 35 y and older investigated for fracture risk factors (Canadian Multicentre Osteoporosis Study, Canada)	3.3%	Elevated PTH concentration and normal albumin-adjusted total serum calcium; exclusion of renal failure (eGFR <60 mL/min), vitamin D deficiency (25-hydroxyvitamin D <20 ng/mL); medication effect not excluded and most of the patients on diuretic and/or antiresorptive therapy
Garcia-Martin et al,[37] 2012	100 healthy, unselected postmenopausal women (Spain)	6% (baseline) 6% (follow-up)	Elevated PTH concentration and normal albumin-adjusted total serum calcium; exclusion of renal failure (creatinine clearance <70 mL/min), vitamin D deficiency (25-hydroxyvitamin D <30 ng/mL)
Marques et al,[38] 2011	156 women referred for osteoporosis screening (Brazil)	8.9%	Elevated PTH concentration and normal albumin-adjusted total serum calcium; exclusion of renal failure (eGFR <40 mL/min), vitamin D deficiency (25-hydroxyvitamin D <30 ng/mL), history of metabolic bone disease, liver disease, malabsorption syndromes, medication effect

Abbreviation: IgA, immunoglobulin A.

Table 2
Clinical summary of skeletal and renal complications in cohorts of patients with normocalcemic primary hyperparathyroidism

Study	Cohort Size	Age (years)	Female (%)	Osteoporosis	Nephrolithiasis	Comments
Symptomatic cohorts						
Lowe et al,[39] 2007	37	58 ± 2	95	57% 11% with fragility fracture	14%	Ionized calcium not available for all
Maruani et al,[28] 2003	34	53 ± 14	68	Radiographic bone demineralization in 18% (bone density not performed)	35%	-
Marques et al,[38] 2011	14	61 ± 15	100[c]	36% 21% with fragility fracture	21%	-
Tordjman et al,[40] 2004	32	61 ± 11	84	36%	9%	-
Amaral et al.[41] 2012	33	64 ± 14	79	15%[a]	18%	Ionized calcium not measured
Cakir et al.[42] 2012	18	50 ± 2	47	47%	11%	Ionized calcium not measured
Wade et al,[43] 2012	8	60	63	25% 13% with fragility fracture	25%	Surgical cohort
Šiprová et al,[44] 2016	137	61	81	42% described as having "reduced bone density"	4%	-
Palermo et al,[45] 2020	47	64 ± 9	91	28%[b]	13%	-
Asymptomatic cohort						
Garcia-Martin et al,[37] 2012	6	56 ± 3	100[c]	0%	0%	Ionized calcium not measured Population-based cohort
Rosário & Calsolari,[7] 2019	5	53	80%	0%	0%	Patients undergoing planned thyroid surgery 80% of patients had confirmed parathyroid pathology

Mean ± SD.
[a] Only fracture history available.
[b] Only vertebral fracture history available.
[c] Study design.

CLINICAL FEATURES
Classic Manifestations

In the published literature, cohorts with normocalcemic primary hyperparathyroidism have high rates of nephrolithiasis, osteoporosis, and fracture; this is not surprising because many patients with normal serum calcium undergoing PTH testing are doing so during evaluation of these conditions, with selection bias accounting for the highly symptomatic form of the disease that has so far been described. Although traditional hypercalcemic primary hyperparathyroidism is now usually diagnosed incidentally on routine blood tests, normocalcemic primary hyperparathyroidism is primarily diagnosed in the setting of a target organ abnormality, and the prevalence of symptomatic disease in the reported cohorts is in some cases higher than for hypercalcemic disease. A summary of the reported clinical features is provided in **Table 2**.[7,28,37–45] Few population-based, unselected cohorts have been described; in these patients identified through biochemical testing, clinical indices, bone turnover markers, and bone mass do not seem to be different to euparathyroid patients or patients with secondary hyperparathyroidism.[2,7,37]

Nonclassical Manifestations

Although patients with severe hypercalcemic primary hyperparathyroidism have been described to have cardiovascular manifestations, studies have shown only the possibility of more subtle indices of cardiovascular risk in patients with mild, asymptomatic hypercalcemic primary hyperparathyroidism.[46] A few studies of glucose metabolism have demonstrated a small but statistically significant increase in mean fasting glucose levels, although no differences have been observed in either hemoglobin A1c or insulin sensitivity between men and women with normocalcemic primary hyperparathyroidism and controls.[47–51] A study of various noninvasive measures of arterial compliance (as a surrogate for vascular risk) noted no differences in individuals with normocalcemic primary hyperparathyroidism and controls.[52] One study demonstrated an increase in coronary artery calcium score in patients with normocalcemic primary hyperparathyroidism,[53] whereas another showed no difference.[54] The effect of mild, asymptomatic hypercalcemic primary hyperparathyroidism on quality of life also remains unclear[46]; one study has demonstrated a reduction in quality of life in patients with normocalcemic primary hyperparathyroidism.[55]

NATURAL HISTORY

There are few studies investigating the natural history of the normocalcemic phenotype of the disease, with most studies involving relatively small cohorts of patients showing that a small number, if any, develop hypercalcemia.[35,37,39,40,44,56] In a longitudinal cohort study of symptomatic patients referred to an endocrine clinic published by Tordjman and colleagues,[40] none of the 20 patients followed-up for a median of 4 years without surgery developed hypercalcemia or hypercalciuria. Twelve patients with positive localization studies underwent parathyroidectomy, with 9 patients having a single adenoma and 2 having hyperplasia (pathology not available for the remaining patient). In a longitudinal cohort study of symptomatic patients referred to a metabolic bone diseases unit published by Lowe and colleagues, 7 of 37 patients (19%) developed hypercalcemia over a median of 3 years. During the follow-up period, 41% in total developed evidence of progressive disease, including hypercalcemia, new hypercalciuria, nephrolithiasis, and/or fracture.[39] In the cohort, 7 patients underwent parathyroid surgery, 3 of whom had developed hypercalcemia and the other 4 with persistently normal serum calcium, with findings of adenoma or hyperplasia. In a symptomatic cohort of 187 patients with normocalcemic primary hyperparathyroidism followed-up for 6 years by Šiprová and colleagues,[44] 36 patients (19%) became hypercalcemic, with the majority (67%) transitioning to hypercalcemia within the first 2 years of follow-up but a small cohort (6%) becoming hypercalcemic after 4 years. Nine of thirty-six patients who became hypercalcemic underwent parathyroid surgery, and in 7 patients an adenoma was removed. One patient underwent a successful reoperation, whereas the remaining patient declined subsequent surgery. One year postoperatively, 8 patients had normal serum calcium and 5 patients had normalization of PTH concentrations. In the population-based study of Garcia-Martin and colleagues,[37] all 6 of 100 women identified with normocalcemic primary hyperparathyroidism had persistently elevated PTH levels at 1 year. None of the women had evidence of hypercalcemia, nephrolithiasis, or fracture after 1-year follow-up.

MEDICAL MANAGEMENT

Parathyroidectomy is the only definitive therapy for patients with primary hyperparathyroidism. There are no data regarding when to recommend surgery and limited data regarding medical management of patients with normocalcemic primary hyperparathyroidism. Guidelines from the Fourth International Workshop on the Management of Asymptomatic Primary Hyperparathyroidism, based on expert opinion, recommend monitoring of patients with normocalcemic primary hyperparathyroidism with biochemical parameters annually and bone density testing every 1 to 2 years.[57] Surgery is recommended for normocalcemic patients with progression of disease, including kidney stone, fracture, or worsening bone density. If the patient becomes hypercalcemic, the usual guidelines for hypercalcemic primary hyperparathyroidism can be followed.

Alendronate has been demonstrated to increase bone density in patients with hypercalcemic primary hyperparathyroidism,[58,59] and a small study has shown benefit for patients with normocalcemic disease as well.[60] Thirty postmenopausal women with normocalcemic primary hyperparathyroidism and osteoporosis were randomized to alendronate 70 mg weekly with cholecalciferol, or cholecalciferol alone for 12 months. There were significant improvements in bone density in the alendronate arm, with +4.7% increase at the lumbar spine and +4.0% at the total hip, in the same general range as in euparathyroid individuals, whereas patients in the cholecalciferol-alone arm experienced declines. Alendronate therapy did not result in any change in biochemical safety parameters.

Cinacalcet is an approved therapy to reduce serum calcium for patients with hypercalcemic primary hyperparathyroidism for whom parathyroidectomy is indicated but not able to be performed. A small unblinded pilot study of cinacalcet was performed with the aim of reducing number and size of kidney stones in 10 patients with primary hyperparathyroidism followed-up over 10 months, including six with normocalcemic disease.[61] The investigators found that cinacalcet, at a dose sufficient to decrease PTH levels, was able to decrease the number and diameter of kidney stones. Because these reductions occurred in the absence of changes to urinary calcium, there is a suggestion that PTH affects other aspects of urine chemistry; however, this remains inconclusive due to the small sample size.

SURGICAL MANAGEMENT

Limited data demonstrate that patients with normocalcemic disease who undergo surgical resection may have improvement in bone density,[62] nephrolithiasis,[63] cardiovascular parameters,[64] and quality of life[65]; these biochemical and surgical outcomes following surgery were recently reviewed by Dawood and colleagues.[66] However, parathyroidectomy in patients with normocalcemic disease is associated with lower long-term cure rates than for hypercalcemic disease,[67] likely due to smaller adenomas,[62,68] increased risk of multiglandular disease, and decreased sensitivity of preoperative localization studies as discussed later.

The presence of multiglandular disease or hyperplasia is an important factor in surgical management, because a minimally invasive parathyroidectomy (which targets a single culprit gland) would not be an appropriate surgical approach. Four-gland exploration is a more challenging operation with increased surgical risk. Pandian and colleagues[69] reported that patients with normocalcemic disease were more likely to have hyperplasia (43.1% vs 21.9%) and less likely to have a single adenoma (47.5% vs 73.3%) compared with patients with hypercalcemic primary hyperparathyroidism. There was also an increased risk of needing remedial surgery in the normocalcemic cohort (6.4% vs 4.5%). Lim and colleagues[70] also found that patients with normocalcemic primary hyperparathyroidism were more likely to have hyperplasia (45% vs 9%). Using logistic regression analysis, normocalcemic disease and family history were the only factors associated with multiglandular disease. Patients with normocalcemic primary hyperparathyroidism had a greater than 8-fold risk of multiglandular disease (odds ratio 8.17, 95% confidence interval 4.49–14.83). Trinh and colleagues[71] noted an increased risk of conversion from a targeted surgery to bilateral neck exploration in patients with normocalcemic versus hypercalcemic disease (13% vs 4%).

Preoperative localization studies are critical for surgical management in primary hyperparathyroidism, and less likely to be positive in patients with normocalcemic disease, likely due to decreased adenoma size and risk of hyperplasia. Šiprová and colleagues[44] noted that sestamibi localization was successful in only 14% of normocalcemic patients, increasing to 73% success in patients who subsequently became hypercalcemic. Cunha-Bezerra and colleagues[72] evaluated different imaging modalities in a cohort of patients with normocalcemic primary hyperparathyroidism and found that the sensitivity of all imaging procedures was lower for patients with normocalcemic compared with hypercalcemic disease. Four-dimensional computed tomography performed the best for normocalcemic patients (56% vs 75% in normocalcemic vs hypercalcemic individuals) followed by ultrasound (22% vs 58%) and scintigraphy (11% vs 75%).

SUMMARY

Despite the increasing diagnosis of individuals with normocalcemic primary hyperparathyroidism, much remains unknown regarding the disorder. It is important to measure ionized calcium, monitor biochemical parameters over time, and exclude secondary causes of hyperparathyroidism in order to make a diagnosis of normocalcemic disease. Most of the patients are diagnosed in the setting of kidney stones or bone disease. Because most publications are from referral populations with selection bias, there is limited information regarding a mild, asymptomatic form of the disease. There are limited data for medical management, and surgical management is complicated due to decreased sensitivity of localization procedures and increased risk of multiglandular disease. Further prospective studies are needed to determine optimal diagnostic criteria as well as improve medical and surgical therapeutic options.

CLINICS CARE POINTS

- Patients can be diagnosed with normocalcemic primary hyperparathyroidism in the setting of elevated PTH concentrations on at least 3 occasions over a period of 3 to 6 months with consistently normal serum calcium.

- It is important to measure ionized calcium, monitor biochemical parameters over time, and exclude secondary causes of hyperparathyroidism in order to make a diagnosis of normocalcemic disease.

- Most patients with normocalcemic primary hyperparathyroidism are diagnosed in the setting of kidney stones or bone disease.

- There are limited data regarding optimal medical and surgical management.

DISCLOSURES

Dr Cusano is a consultant for Shire/Takeda and Radius Pharmaceuticals and received research support from Shire/Takeda.

REFERENCES

1. Eastell R, Brandi ML, Costa AG, et al. Diagnosis of asymptomatic primary hyperparathyroidism: proceedings of the fourth international workshop. J Clin Endocrinol Metab 2014;99(10):3570–9.
2. Cusano NE, Maalouf NM, Wang PY, et al. Normocalcemic hyperparathyroidism and hypoparathyroidism in two community-based nonreferral populations. J Clin Endocrinol Metab 2013;98(7):2734–41.
3. Nordenström E, Katzman P, Bergenfelz A. Biochemical diagnosis of primary hyperparathyroidism: analysis of the sensitivity of total and ionized calcium in combination with PTH. Clin Biochem 2011;44(10–11):849–52.
4. Ong GS, Walsh JP, Stuckey BG, et al. The importance of measuring ionized calcium in characterizing calcium status and diagnosing primary hyperparathyroidism. J Clin Endocrinol Metab 2012;97(9):3138–45.
5. Gómez-Ramírez J, Gómez-Valdazo A, Luengo P, et al. Comparative prospective study on the presentation of normocalcemic primary hyperparathyroidism. Is it more aggressive than the hypercalcemic form? Am J Surg 2020;219(1):150–3.
6. Cusano NE, Silverberg SJ, Bilezikian JP. Normocalcemic Primary Hyperparathyroidism. J Clin Densitom 2013;16(1):33–9.
7. Rosário PW, Calsolari MR. Normocalcemic primary hyperparathyroidism in adults without a history of nephrolithiasis or fractures: a prospective study. Horm Metab Res 2019;51(4):243–7.
8. IOM (Institute of Medicine). Dietary reference intakes for calcium and vitamin D. Washington, DC: The National Academies Press; 2011.
9. Fuleihan Gel -H, Bouillon R, Clarke B, et al. Serum 25-Hydroxyvitamin D levels: variability, knowledge gaps, and the concept of a desirable range. J Bone Miner Res 2015;30(7):1119–33.
10. Eller-Vainicher C, Cairoli E, Zhukouskaya VV, et al. Prevalence of subclinical contributors to low bone mineral density and/or fragility fracture. Eur J Endocrinol 2013;169(2):225–37.
11. Martinez I, Saracho R, Montenegro J, et al. The importance of dietary calcium and phosphorous in the secondary hyperparathyroidism of patients with early renal failure. Am J Kidney Dis 1997;29:496–502.

12. KDIGO clinical practice guideline for the diagnosis, evaluation, prevention, and treatment of Chronic Kidney Disease-Mineral and Bone Disorder (CKD-MBD). Kidney Int Supplements 2009;S1–130.
13. Haden ST, Stoll AL, McCormick S, et al. Alterations in parathyroid dynamics in lithium-treated subjects. J Clin Endocrinol Metab 1997;82(9):2844–8.
14. Rejnmark L, Vestergaard P, Heickendorff L, et al. Effects of thiazide-and loop-diuretics, alone or in combination, on calcitropic hormones and biochemical bone markers: a randomized controlled study. J Intern Med 2001;250(2):144–53.
15. Yacobi-Bach M, Serebro M, Greenman Y, et al. Letter to the Editor: thiazides are not inducers of PTH secretion: a comment on normocalcemic hyperparathyroidism. J Clin Endocrinol Metab 2015;100(2):L27.
16. Chesnut CH, McClung MR, Ensrud KE, et al. Alendronate treatment of the postmenopausal osteoporotic woman: effect of multiple dosages on bone mass and bone remodeling. Am J Med 1995;99(2):144–52.
17. Cipriani C, Pepe J, Clementelli C, et al. Effect of a single intravenous zoledronic acid administration on biomarkers of acute kidney injury (AKI) in patients with osteoporosis: a pilot study. Br J Clin Pharmacol 2017;83(10):2266–73.
18. McClung MR, Lewiecki EM, Cohen SB, et al. Denosumab in postmenopausal women with low bone mineral density. N Engl J Med 2006;354(8):821–31.
19. Coe FL, Canterbury JM, Firpo JJ, et al. Evidence for secondary hyperparathyroidism in idiopathic hypercalciuria. J Clin Invest 1973;52(1):134.
20. Worcester EM, Coe FL. New insights into the pathogenesis of idiopathic hypercalciuria. Semin Nephrol 2008;28(2):120–32.
21. Souberbielle JC, Cavalier E, Cormier C. How to manage an isolated elevated PTH? Ann Endocrinol (Paris) 2015;76(2):134–41.
22. Collin P, Kaukinen K, Valimaki M, et al. Endocrinological disorders and celiac disease. Endocr Rev 2002;23(4):464–83.
23. Madeo B, Kara E, Cioni K, et al. Serum calcium to phosphorous (Ca/P) ratio is a simple, inexpensive, and accurate tool in the diagnosis of primary hyperparathyroidism. JBMR Plus 2018;2(2):109–17.
24. Madeo B, De Vincentis S, Repaci A, et al. The calcium-to-phosphorous (Ca/P) ratio in the diagnosis of primary hyperparathyroidism and hypoparathyroidism: aa multicentric study. Endocrine 2020;68(3):679–87.
25. Guo Y, Wang Q, Lu C, et al. New parathyroid function index for the differentiation of primary and secondary hyperparathyroidism: a case-control study. BMC Endocr Disord 2020;20(1):5.
26. Farquharson RF, Tibbetts DM. Studies of calcium and phosphorus metabolism: XVIII. On temporary fluctuations in the level of calcium and inorganic phosphorus in blood serum of normal individuals. J Clin Invest 1931;10(2):271–86.
27. Cusano NE, Cipriani C, Bilezikian JP. Management of normocalcemic primary hyperparathyroidism. Best Pract Res Clin Endocrinol Metab 2018;32(6):837–45.
28. Maruani G, Hertig A, Paillard M, et al. Normocalcemic primary hyperparathyroidism: evidence for a generalized target-tissue resistance to parathyroid hormone. J Clin Endocrinol Metab 2003;88(10):4641–8.
29. Díaz-Soto G, Romero E, Castrillón JLP, et al. Clinical expression of calcium sensing receptor polymorphism (A986S) in normocalcemic and asymptomatic hyperparathyroidism. Horm Metab Res 2016;48(3):163–8.
30. Schini M, Jacques RM, Oakes E, et al. Normocalcemic hyperparathyroidism: study of its prevalence and natural history. J Clin Endocrinol Metab 2020; 105(4):e1171–86.

31. Zavatta G, Clarke BL. Normocalcemic hyperparathyroidism: a heterogeneous disorder often misdiagnosed? JBMR Plus 2020;4(8):e10391.
32. Palermo A, Jacques R, Gossiel F, et al. Normocalcaemic hypoparathyroidism: prevalence and effect on bone status in older women. The OPUS study. Clin Endocrinol (Oxf) 2015;82(6):816–23.
33. Vignali E, Cetani F, Chiavistelli S, et al. Normocalcemic primary hyperparathyroidism: a survey in a small village of Southern Italy. Endocr Connect 2015;4(3): 172–8.
34. Lundgren E, Rastad J, Thurfjell E, et al. Population-based screening for primary hyperparathyroidism with serum calcium and parathyroid hormone values in menopausal women. Surgery 1997;121(3):287–94.
35. Kontogeorgos G, Trimpou P, Laine CM, et al. Normocalcaemic, vitamin D-sufficient hyperparathyroidism – high prevalence and low morbidity in the general population: A long-term follow-up study, the WHO MONICA project, Gothenburg, Sweden. Clin Endocrinol (Oxf) 2015;83(2):277–84.
36. Berger C, Almohareb O, Langsetmo L, et al. Characteristics of hyperparathyroid states in the Canadian multicentre osteoporosis study (CaMos) and relationship to skeletal markers. Clin Endocrinol (Oxf) 2015;82(3):359–68.
37. García-Martín A, Reyes-García R, Muñoz-Torres M. Normocalcemic primary hyperparathyroidism: one-year follow-up in one hundred postmenopausal women. Endocrine 2012;1–3.
38. Marques TF, Vasconcelos R, Diniz E, et al. Normocalcemic primary hyperparathyroidism in clinical practice: an indolent condition or a silent threat? Arq Bras Endocrinol Metabol 2011;55(5):314–7.
39. Lowe H, McMahon D, Rubin M, et al. Normocalcemic primary hyperparathyroidism: further characterization of a new clinical phenotype. J Clin Endocrinol Metab 2007;92(8):3001–5.
40. Tordjman KM, Greenman Y, Osher E, et al. Characterization of normocalcemic primary hyperparathyroidism. Am J Med 2004;117(11):861–3.
41. Amaral L, Queiroz D, Marques T, et al. Normocalcemic versus hypercalcemic primary hyperparathyroidism: more stone than bone? J Osteoporos 2012;2012: 128352.
42. Cakir I, Unluhizarci K, Tanriverdi F, et al. Investigation of insulin resistance in patients with normocalcemic primary hyperparathyroidism. Endocrine 2012;42(2): 419–22.
43. Wade TJ, Yen TW, Amin AL, et al. Surgical management of normocalcemic primary hyperparathyroidism. World J Surg 2012;36(4):761–6.
44. Šiprová H, Fryšák Z, Souček M. Primary hyperparathyroidism, with a focus on management of the normocalcemic form: to treat or not to treat? Endocr Pract 2016;22(3):294–301.
45. Palermo A, Naciu AM, Tabacco G, et al. Clinical, biochemical, and radiological profile of normocalcemic primary hyperparathyroidism. J Clin Endocrinol Metab 2020;105(7):dgaa174.
46. Silverberg SJ, Clarke BL, Peacock M, et al. Current issues in the presentation of asymptomatic primary hyperparathyroidism: proceedings of the Fourth International Workshop. J Clin Endocrinol Metab 2014;99(10):3580–94.
47. Hagström E, Lundgren E, Rastad J, et al. Metabolic abnormalities in patients with normocalcemic hyperparathyroidism detected at a population-based screening. Eur J Endocrinol 2006;155(1):33–9.
48. Temizkan S, Kocak O, Aydin K, et al. Normocalcemic hyperparathyroidism and insulin resistance. Endocr Pract 2014;21(1):23–9.

49. Yener Ozturk F, Erol S, Canat MM, et al. Patients with normocalcemic primary hyperparathyroidism may have similar metabolic profile as hypercalcemic patients. Endocr J 2016;63(2):111–8.
50. Chen G, Xue Y, Zhang Q, et al. Is normocalcemic primary hyperparathyroidism harmful or harmless? J Clin Endocrinol Metab 2015;100(6):2420–4.
51. Karras SN, Koufakis T, Tsekmekidou X, et al. Increased parathyroid hormone is associated with higher fasting glucose in individuals with normocalcemic primary hyperparathyroidism and prediabetes: a pilot study. Diabetes Res Clin Pract 2020;160:107985.
52. Tordjman KM, Yaron M, Izkhakov E, et al. Cardiovascular risk factors and arterial rigidity are similar in asymptomatic normocalcemic and hypercalcemic primary hyperparathyroidism. Eur J Endocrinol 2010;162(5):925–33.
53. Mesquita PN, Dornelas Leão Leite AP, Chagas Crisóstomo SD, et al. Evaluation of coronary calcium score in patients with normocalcemic primary hyperparathyroidism. Vasc Health Risk Management 2017;13:225–9.
54. Koubaity O, Mandry D, Nguyen-Thi PL, et al. Coronary artery disease is more severe in patients with primaryhyperparathyroidism. Surgery 2020;167(1):149–54.
55. Voss L, Nóbrega M, Bandeira L, et al. Impaired physical function and evaluation of quality of life in normocalcemic and hypercalcemic primary hyperparathyroidism. Bone 2020;141:115583.
56. Diri H, Unluhizarci K, Kelestimur F. Investigation of glucose intolerance in patients with normocalcemic primary hyperparathyroidism: 4-year follow-up. Endocrine 2014;47(3):971–2.
57. Bilezikian JP, Brandi ML, Eastell R, et al. Guidelines for the management of asymptomatic primary hyperparathyroidism: summary statement from the Fourth International Workshop. J Clin Endocrinol Metab 2014;99(10):3561–9.
58. Khan AA, Bilezikian JP, Kung AW, et al. Alendronate in primary hyperparathyroidism: a double-blind, randomized, placebo-controlled trial. J Clin Endocrinol Metab 2004;89(7):3319–25.
59. Khan AA, Bilezikian JP, Kung A, et al. Alendronate therapy in men with primary hyperparathyroidism. Endocr Pract 2009;15(7):705–13.
60. Cesareo R, Di Stasio E, Vescini F, et al. Effects of alendronate and vitamin D in patients with normocalcemic primary hyperparathyroidism. Osteoporos Int 2014;26(4):1295–302.
61. Brardi S, Cevenini G, Verdacchi T, et al. Use of cinacalcet in nephrolithiasis associated with normocalcemic or hypercalcemic primary hyperparathyroidism: results of a prospective randomized pilot study. Arch Ital Urol Androl 2015;87(1):66–71.
62. Koumakis E, Souberbielle J-C, Sarfati E, et al. Bone mineral density evolution after successful parathyroidectomy in patients with normocalcemic primary hyperparathyroidism. J Clin Endocrinol Metab 2013;98(8):3213–20.
63. Sho S, Kuo EJ, Chen AC, et al. Biochemical and skeletal outcomes of parathyroidectomy for normocalcemic (Incipient) primary hyperparathyroidism. Ann Surg Oncol 2019;26(2):539–46.
64. Beysel S, Caliskan M, Kizilgul M, et al. Parathyroidectomy improves cardiovascular risk factors in normocalcemic and hypercalcemic primary hyperparathyroidism. BMC Cardiovasc Disord 2019;19(1):106.
65. Bannani S, Christou N, Guérin C, et al. Effect of parathyroidectomy on quality of life and non-specific symptoms in normocalcaemic primary hyperparathyroidism. Br J Surg 2018;105(3):223–9.

66. Dawood NB, Yan KL, Shieh A, et al. Normocalcaemic primary hyperparathyroidism: an update on diagnostic and management challenges. Clin Endocrinol (Oxf) 2020;93(5):519–27.

67. Singh Ospina NM, Rodriguez-Gutierrez R, Maraka S, et al. Outcomes of parathyroidectomy in patients with primary hyperparathyroidism: a systematic review and meta-analysis. World J Surg 2016;40(10):2359–77.

68. Traini E, Bellantone R, Tempera SE, et al. Is parathyroidectomy safe and effective in patients with normocalcemic primary hyperparathyroidism? Langenbecks Arch Surg 2018;403(3):317–23.

69. Pandian TK, Lubitz CC, Bird SH, et al. Normocalcemic hyperparathyroidism: a collaborative endocrine surgery quality improvement program analysis. Surgery 2020;167(1):168–72.

70. Lim JY, Herman MC, Bubis L, et al. Differences in single gland and multigland disease are seen in low biochemical profile primary hyperparathyroidism. Surgery 2017;161(1):70–7.

71. Trinh G, Rettig E, Noureldine SI, et al. Surgical management of normocalcemic primary hyperparathyroidism and the impact of intraoperative parathyroid hormone testing on outcome. Otolaryngol Head Neck Surg 2018;159(4):630–7.

72. Cunha-Bezerra P, Vieira R, Amaral F, et al. Better performance of four-dimension computed tomography as a localization procedure in normocalcemic primary hyperparathyroidism. J Med Imaging Radiat Oncol 2018;62(4):493–8.

UNITED STATES POSTAL SERVICE®

Statement of Ownership, Management, and Circulation
(All Periodicals Publications Except Requester Publications)

1. Publication Title	2. Publication Number	3. Filing Date
MEDICAL CLINICS IN NORTH AMERICA	337 – 340	9/18/2021

4. Issue Frequency	5. Number of Issues Published Annually	6. Annual Subscription Price
JAN, MAR, MAY, JUL, SEP, NOV	6	$304.00

7. Complete Mailing Address of Known Office of Publication (Not printer) (Street, city, county, state, and ZIP+4®)

ELSEVIER INC.
230 Park Avenue, Suite 800
New York, NY 10169

Contact Person
STEPHEN R. BUSHING

Telephone (Include area code)
215-239-3688

8. Complete Mailing Address of Headquarters or General Business Office of Publisher (Not printer)

ELSEVIER INC.
230 Park Avenue, Suite 800
New York, NY 10169

9. Full Names and Complete Mailing Addresses of Publisher, Editor, and Managing Editor (Do not leave blank)

Publisher (Name and complete mailing address)

DOLORES MELONI, ELSEVIER INC.
1600 JOHN F KENNEDY BLVD, SUITE 1800
PHILADELPHIA, PA 19103-2899

Editor (Name and complete mailing address)

KATERINA HEIDHAUSEN, ELSEVIER INC.
1600 JOHN F KENNEDY BLVD, SUITE 1800
PHILADELPHIA, PA 19103-2899

Managing Editor (Name and complete mailing address)

PATRICK MANLEY, ELSEVIER INC.
1600 JOHN F KENNEDY BLVD, SUITE 1800
PHILADELPHIA, PA 19103-2899

10. Owner (Do not leave blank. If the publication is owned by a corporation, give the name and address of the corporation immediately followed by the names and addresses of all stockholders owning or holding 1 percent or more of the total amount of stock. If not owned by a corporation, give the names and addresses of the individual owners. If owned by a partnership or other unincorporated firm, give its name and address as well as those of each individual owner. If the publication is published by a nonprofit organization, give its name and address.)

Full Name	Complete Mailing Address
WHOLLY OWNED SUBSIDIARY OF REED/ELSEVIER, US HOLDINGS	1600 JOHN F KENNEDY BLVD, SUITE 1800 PHILADELPHIA, PA 19103-2899

11. Known Bondholders, Mortgagees, and Other Security Holders Owning or Holding 1 Percent or More of Total Amount of Bonds, Mortgages, or Other Securities. If none, check box ☐ None

Full Name	Complete Mailing Address
N/A	

12. Tax Status (For completion by nonprofit organizations authorized to mail at nonprofit rates) (Check one)
The purpose, function, and nonprofit status of this organization and the exempt status for federal income tax purposes:
☒ Has Not Changed During Preceding 12 Months
☐ Has Changed During Preceding 12 Months (Publisher must submit explanation of change with this statement)

PS Form 3526, July 2014 [Page 1 of 4 (see instructions page 4)] PSN: 7530-01-000-9931   PRIVACY NOTICE: See our privacy policy on www.usps.com

13. Publication Title	14. Issue Date for Circulation Data Below
MEDICAL CLINICS IN NORTH AMERICA	JULY 2021

15. Extent and Nature of Circulation

		Average No. Copies Each Issue During Preceding 12 Months	No. Copies of Single Issue Published Nearest to Filing Date
a. Total Number of Copies (Net press run)		452	392
b. Paid Circulation (By Mail and Outside the Mail)	(1) Mailed Outside-County Paid Subscriptions Stated on PS Form 3541 (include paid distribution above nominal rate, advertiser's proof copies, and exchange copies)	265	234
	(2) Mailed In-County Paid Subscriptions Stated on PS Form 3541 (include paid distribution above nominal rate, advertiser's proof copies, and exchange copies)	0	0
	(3) Paid Distribution Outside the Mails Including Sales Through Dealers and Carriers, Street Vendors, Counter Sales, and Other Paid Distribution Outside USPS®	129	116
	(4) Paid Distribution by Other Classes of Mail Through the USPS (e.g., First-Class Mail®)	0	0
c. Total Paid Distribution (Sum of 15b (1), (2), (3), and (4))		394	350
d. Free or Nominal Rate Distribution (By Mail and Outside the Mail)	(1) Free or Nominal Rate Outside-County Copies included on PS Form 3541	39	27
	(2) Free or Nominal Rate In-County Copies Included on PS Form 3541	0	0
	(3) Free or Nominal Rate Copies Mailed at Other Classes Through the USPS (e.g., First-Class Mail)	0	0
	(4) Free or Nominal Rate Distribution Outside the Mail (Carriers or other means)	0	0
e. Total Free or Nominal Rate Distribution (Sum of 15d (1), (2), (3) and (4))		39	27
f. Total Distribution (Sum of 15c and 15e)		433	377
g. Copies not Distributed (See Instructions to Publishers #4 (page #3))		19	15
h. Total (Sum of 15f and g)		452	392
i. Percent Paid (15c divided by 15f times 100)		90.99%	92.83%

* If you are claiming electronic copies, go to line 16 on page 3. If you are not claiming electronic copies, skip to line 17 on page 3.

16. Electronic Copy Circulation

	Average No. Copies Each Issue During Preceding 12 Months	No. Copies of Single Issue Published Nearest to Filing Date
a. Paid Electronic Copies		
b. Total Paid Print Copies (Line 15c) + Paid Electronic Copies (Line 16a)		
c. Total Print Distribution (Line 15f) + Paid Electronic Copies (Line 16a)		
d. Percent Paid (Both Print & Electronic Copies) (16b divided by 16c × 100)		

☒ I certify that 50% of all my distributed copies (electronic and print) are paid above a nominal price.

17. Publication of Statement of Ownership
☒ If the publication is a general publication, publication of this statement is required. Will be printed ☐ Publication not required.
in the NOVEMBER 2021 issue of this publication.

18. Signature and Title of Editor, Publisher, Business Manager, or Owner		Date
Malathi Samayan - Distribution Controller *Malathi Samayan*		9/18/2021

I certify that all information furnished on this form is true and complete. I understand that anyone who furnishes false or misleading information on this form or who omits material or information requested on the form may be subject to criminal sanctions (including fines and imprisonment) and/or civil sanctions (including civil penalties).

PS Form 3526, July 2014 (Page 3 of 4)   PRIVACY NOTICE: See our privacy policy on www.usps.com

Moving?

Make sure your subscription moves with you!

To notify us of your new address, find your **Clinics Account Number** (located on your mailing label above your name), and contact customer service at:

Email: journalscustomerservice-usa@elsevier.com

800-654-2452 (subscribers in the U.S. & Canada)
314-447-8871 (subscribers outside of the U.S. & Canada)

Fax number: 314-447-8029

Elsevier Health Sciences Division
Subscription Customer Service
3251 Riverport Lane
Maryland Heights, MO 63043

*To ensure uninterrupted delivery of your subscription, please notify us at least 4 weeks in advance of move.

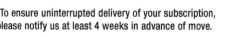

Printed and bound by CPI Group (UK) Ltd, Croydon, CR0 4YY

03/10/2024

01040481-0001